Challenges in Foot and Ankle Reconstructive Surgery

Harry John Visser

Challenges in Foot and Ankle Reconstructive Surgery

A Case-based Approach

Springer

Harry John Visser
SSM Health Care
St. Louis, MO, USA

ISBN 978-3-031-07892-7 ISBN 978-3-031-07893-4 (eBook)
https://doi.org/10.1007/978-3-031-07893-4

This Springer imprint is published by the registered company Springer Nature Switzerland AG
The registered company address is: Gewerbestrasse 11, 6330 Cham, Switzerland

Humbly, as a child growing up in a small rural town in Northeast Ohio called Huntsburg, I can say that a major source and force in my life was from my mother. Without her, I do not believe this book would have been created or my professional goals would have been met.

She was like a storm that gathers its coming fury

She was there as I made the stand

Crafting its nebula with a sharp cavalcade

She would not allow any situation to blight but would see there is constant progression

She reminded me always that I will become erumpent

I also owe great gratitude to my wife, Melody. Her constant assurance and love were a driving force for the completion of this book. She made my life easy and assured, as I sacrificed full weekends of time with her support. Such is my wife jocose

I am also fortunate that my son Jared has followed in my footsteps. He has been a source of great personal and professional joy. My son Tyler also has been a source of pride, serving as a Pedorthist in our practice.

I am also in great debt to my profession that allowed me to serve as a Residency Director for 35 years training over 100 residents.

Acknowledgments

The following is the list of contributors who were essentials for the composition and formation of the book. Without their praxis, knowledge, and parlance, the book would have never come to fruition. I would truly like to thank each and every one of them for their time and devotion.

Editors
Blake T. Savage, DPM
Rekha Kouri, DPM
Nicole M. Smith, DPM

Case Management
Raul Aviles, DPM

References
Robert K. Duddy, DPM
Carmina Quiroga, DPM
Jared J. Visser, DPM
Shirley C. Visser, DPM
Brittany R. Staples, DPM
Joshua Wolfe, DPM
Melinda Nicholes, DPM
Hannan Zahid, DPM
Kalen Farr, DPM
Kiera Benge-Shea, DPM

Contents

Part V Tendinopathies

Part VI The Cavus Foot and Ankle

Part VII Complex Foot Deformity Correction with Hexapod External Fixator

Part I

Forefoot Maladies

Case #1: Revision of a Scarf Osteotomy and Lapidus Procedure with Antibiotic Polymethylmethacrolate Spacer for an Infected Second Metatarsophalangeal Joint Implant

1

Case Presentation
This is a 60-year-old female patient who presents with a recurrent bunion deformity. The original procedure was SCARF osteotomy of the first metatarsal. Also there were three prior operations performed for a second toe hammertoe deformity that included an intramedullary implant and a silastic flexible hinge lesser toe implant.

Diagnosis and Assessment

The patient presents with the main problem of a recurrent hallux abductovalgus deformity after a failed (Scarf joint) shaft type osteotomy. The osteotomy did not excessively shorten the first metatarsal and produced proper plantarflexion. Thus, there was no need for an interpositional bone graft. Correction needed to reduce the intermetatarsal angle and provide triplane stability. Interestingly, despite the operation for a "floating toe" for a probable unrecognized plantar plate rupture, the toe remains well aligned noted on the weight bearing (WB) lateral view and is not excessively shortened (Fig. 1.1).

Management

The recurrent hallux valgus deformity was managed with a Lapidus type first metatarsal—medial cuneiform arthrodesis (Fig. 1.2) [1]. Preparation of the joint was by cartilage curettage and subchondral fragmentation of the joint surface. Positioning is critical with medial to lateral compression to reduce the intermetatarsal angle

H. J. Visser, *Challenges in Foot and Ankle Reconstructive Surgery*,
https://doi.org/10.1007/978-3-031-07893-4_1

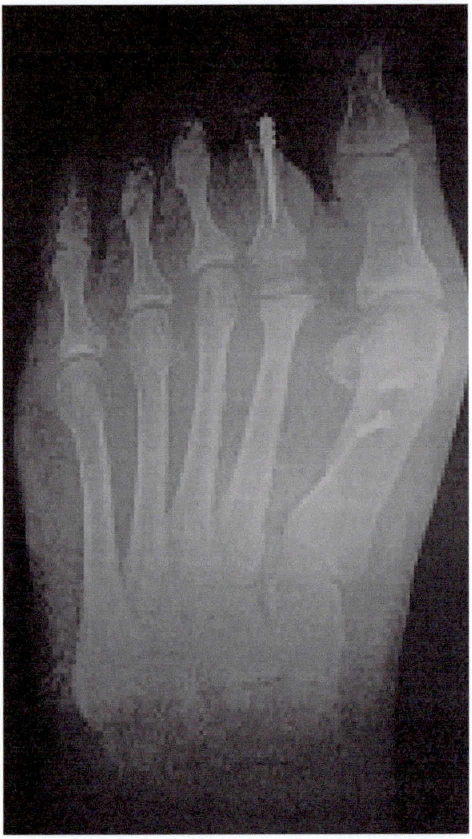

Fig. 1.1 Post recurrent hallux abducto valgus deformity post Scarf osteotomy, left foot

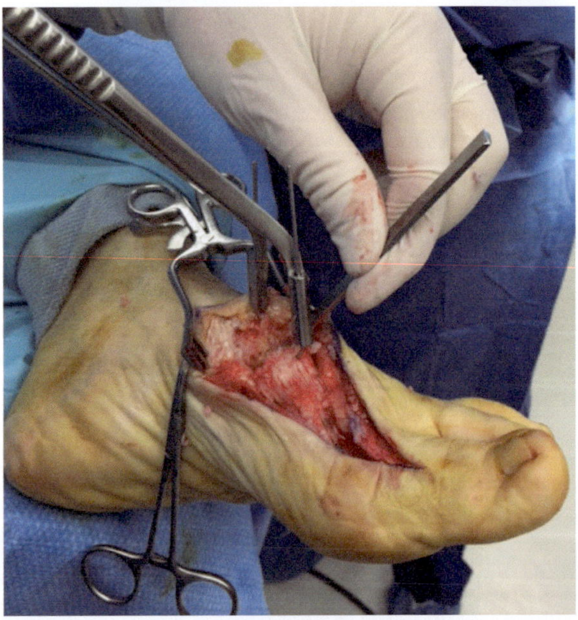

Fig. 1.2 Revision with Lapidus arthrodesis

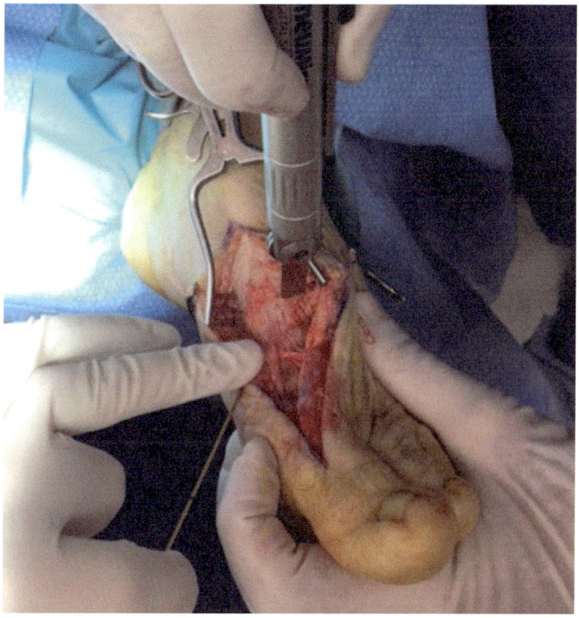

Fig. 1.3 Kerfing technique for further closure of intermetatarsal angle

(transverse plane). The hallux was dorsiflexed to produce retrograde plantarflexion of the first metatarsal (sagittal plane). Inversion (internal rotation) of the hallux corrected the frontal plane position. This creates a retrograde eversion of the first metatarsal. Further correction of the IM angle can be attained with a kerfing technique (Fig. 1.3). Fixation included a locking plate, placed dorsal medial and a 4.0 mm compression screw (Fig. 1.4a, b) [2]. Patient was kept non-weight bearing (NWB) for 2 weeks then followed by WB for further 4 weeks in a controlled ankle motion (CAM)boot [3].

Outcome

Postoperatively, the patient did well with the Lapidus arthrodesis but developed problems with the second metatarsophalangeal joint (MPJ) which was not involved in the revision operation. When physical therapy began, the patient did well initially for the first 4 weeks. However, at 10 weeks the patient presented with swelling, pain, and erythema about the second MPJ. No drainage or fistula was noted (Fig. 1.5). The patient was treated initially with prednisone for possible gouty arthropathy and doxycycline for possible infection. The patient returned in 1 week and demonstrated no positive response. Laboratory work up noted a normal white blood cell (WBC) (8.2, no left shift) count. The sedimentation rate (ESR) was 45 mm/h and C-reactive protein (CRP) was 3.0 mg/L, these were elevated.

Due to obvious concern for infection, radionuclear imaging involving a Ceretec scan (Tc99m HMPAO—Hexamethyl Propylene Amine Oxime) was performed (Fig. 1.6) [4]. As can be seen the scan uptake was positive for potential osteomyelitis of second metatarsal, proximal phalanx, and implant of the left foot.

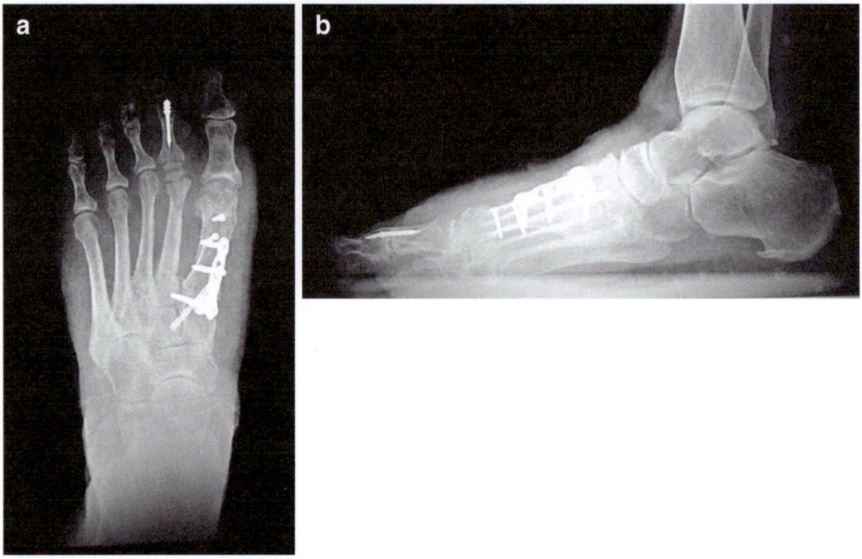

Fig. 1.4 (**a**, **b**) Post-operative revision Lapidus arthrodesis with triplane first metatarsal cuneiform correction

Fig. 1.5 Swelling, pain, erythema, second MPJ, left foot

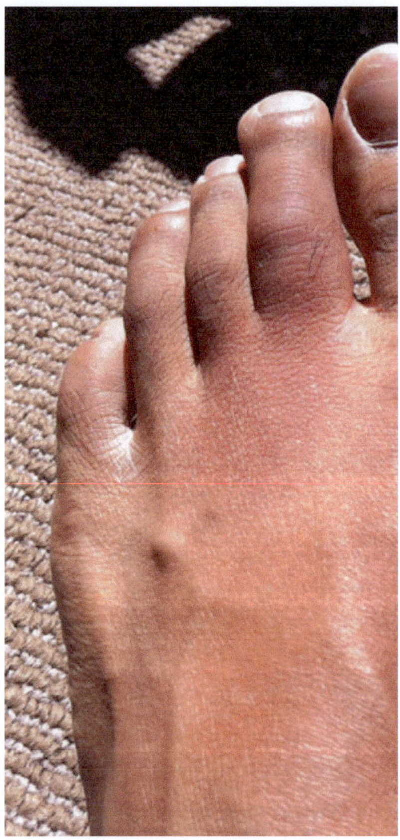

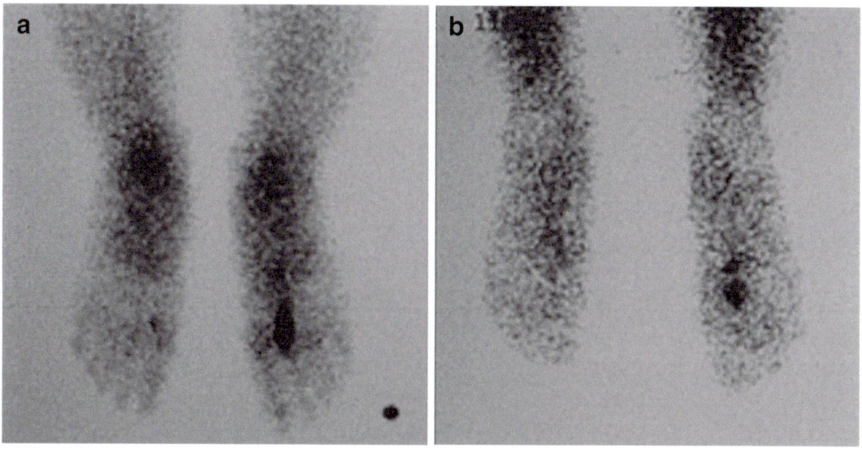

Fig. 1.6 (**a**) Technetium 99 MDP scan showing increased focal uptake of the second MPJ, during the stage 3 bone phase (**b**) Ceretec Tc 99 HMPAO scan showing symmetrical uptake of the second MPJ

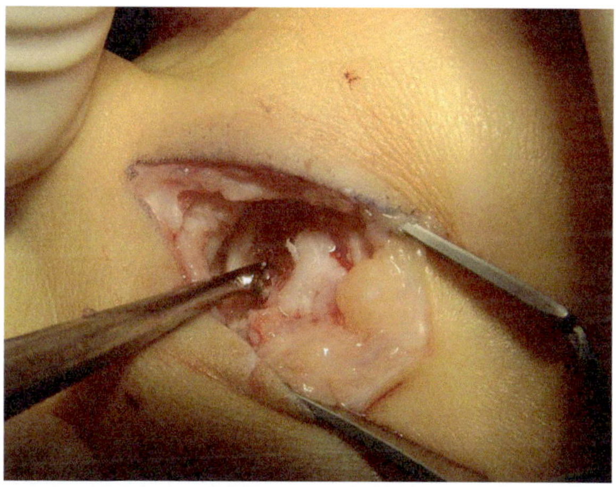

Fig. 1.7 Removal silastic implant, debridement of intramedullary canals in preparation for PMMA spacer

Percutaneous bone biopsy with a Jamshidi needle confirmed osteomyelitis. Cultures grew methicillin—resistant staphylococcus aureus (MRSA). The silastic implant was removed and the second metatarsal was debrided (Fig. 1.7). A polymethylmethacrylate (PMMA) spacer impregnated with vancomycin was inserted [5]. The size of the spacer was such to maintain digital length by ligamentotaxis. Oral antibiotics with doxycycline for 14 days led to complete healing. The patient has done extremely well and is currently 2 years now functioning with the spacer as a "form of "implant (Fig. 1.8a–c).

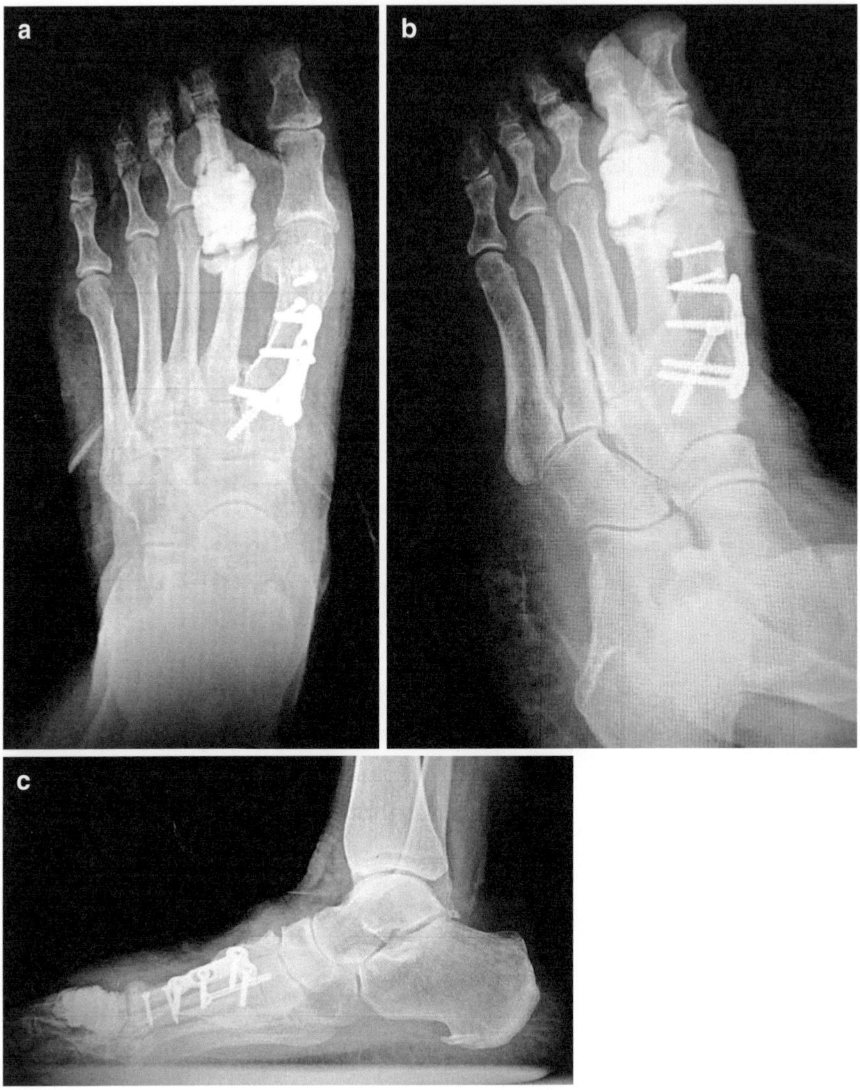

Fig. 1.8 (**a–c**) Post-operative revision of Lapidus arthrodesis and insertion of PMMA spacer to the second MPJ for a septic joint

Clinical Pearls and Pitfalls

Revision of a failed prior (SCARF) procedure usually is due to failure of the initial procedure [6]. The SCARF is described as a bone cut osteotomy originating from architecture and carpentry. It refers to fastening two pieces of bone by notching and grooving. While designed for higher IM (intermetatarsal) angles, often attributed positioning leads to "undercorrection." The Lapidus procedure allows excellent correction of hallux abductovalgus (HAV) deformity in all three planes. Once joint preparation occurs "dialing" in final correction is done by a "feathering" (Kerfing) technique (carpentry term for feathering edges so they may meet), laterally to reduce the intermetatarsal (IM) angle with a sagittal saw. With curettage of the joint surfaces, this leads to minimal shortening. Application of a locking plate on the dorsal medial side of the first metatarsal protects or neutralizes the lag screw by being halfway between the tension and compression sides. This allows early WB to occur.

Utilization of implants can lead to delayed forms of infection [7]. In this case, the implant (silastic) had been in place for 2 years without event. By active utilization of physical therapy (PT) in the postoperative period, the glycocalyx on biomembrane coating the implant/bone interface was damaged, showering bacteria into the surrounding soft tissue space. Management of pedal implant infection is similar to that of the hip and knee. Removal with bone debridement and use of an antibiotic spacer. This allows elution of high concentrations of antibiotic to the bone locally. This is supplemented with either oral or IV antibiotics dependent on the anatomic area.

Maintenance of proper anatomical length and position is important which the PMMA spacer provides by ligamentotaxis [8]. When the second stage procedure is considered, grafting with a "fresh" second metatarsal head allograft can be performed. Also consideration can be given to resecting the fifth metatarsal head and metaphyseal neck and use as an autograft. Purse stringing (quilting) the resected fifth metatarsal head capsule can reduce shortening of the fifth digit. In some cases, as in this case, maintenance of the spacer may allow the patient to function pain free though not with anatomic function.

References

1. Coetzee JC, Resig SJ, Kuskowski M, Khaled S. The Lapidus procedure as salvage after failed surgical treatment of hallux valgus. J Bone Joint Surg. 2003;85(1):60–5.
2. Klos K, Gueorguieve B, Mückley T, Fröber R, Hofmann GO, Schwieger K, Windolf M. Stability of medial locking plate and compression screw versus two crossed screws for lapidus arthrodesis. Foot Ankle Int. 2010;31(2):158–63.
3. Sorensen MD, Hyer CH, Berlet GC. Results of lapidus arthrodesis and locked plating with early weight bearing. Foot Ankle Spec. 2009;2(5):227–33.
4. Williams MT, Molloy AP, Simmonds DJ, Butcher CK. Infection rates in foot and ankle surgery. Orthopaed Proc. 2018;94(B):28.
5. Elmarsafi T, Oliver NG, Steinberg JS, Evans KK, Attinger CE, Kim PJ. Long-term outcomes of permanent cement spacers in the infected foot. J Foot Ankle Surg. 2017;56(2):287–90.
6. Weil LS. Scarf osteotomy for correction of hallux valgus. Historical perspective, surgical technique, and results. Foot Ankle Clin. 2000;5(3):559–80.
7. Shereff MJ, Jahss MH. Complications of silastic implant arthroplasty in the hallux. Foot Ankle. 2000;1(2):95–101.
8. Schade VL, Roukis TS. The role of polymethylmethacrylate antibiotic-loaded cement in addition to debridement for the treatment of soft tissue and osseous infections of the foot and ankle. J Foot Ankle Surg. 2018;49(1):55–62.

2 Case #2: Utilization of a Cancellous Titanium Wedge for a Revisional Reconstruction of a Lapidus Procedure

Case Presentation

This is a 50-year-old Caucasian female with a history of a failed Lapidus first metatarsal cuneiform arthrodesis for correction of a bunion deformity 3 years prior [1]. The patient due to continued pain had the hardware removed from that sight 1 year prior [2]. The patient continued to demonstrate pain despite hardware removal. She also noted further flattening of her foot and persistent pain at the surgical site.

Diagnosis and Assessment

On evaluation of the radiographs, there is recurrent deformity. Shortening of the first metatarsal with a persistent increase in the intermetatarsal (IM) angle is present. Also, a nonunion of the first metatarsal medial cuneiform joint is present on the DP (dorsal plantar) view. A significant increase in the TC (talo-calcaneal) angle (Harris Beath) is noted with a lateral peritalar subluxation. A retained broken screw from prior fixation was noted in the medial cuneiform (MC) (Fig. 2.1a). The lateral view demonstrated significant loss of arch height with the medial cuneiform parallel to the fifth metatarsal base (Fig. 2.1b).

Management

Revision of the residual deformity included (1) interposition of a cancellous titanium wedge at the first metatarsal-MC joint [3], (2) gastrocnemius recession [4], (3) posterior displacement calcaneal osteotomy [5], and (4) talonavicular (TN) arthrodesis

H. J. Visser, *Challenges in Foot and Ankle Reconstructive Surgery*,
https://doi.org/10.1007/978-3-031-07893-4_2

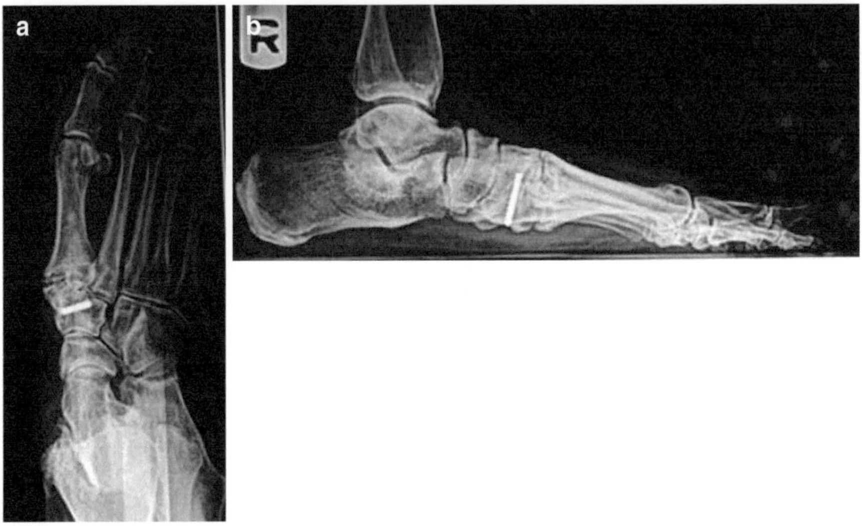

Fig. 2.1 (**a**) Post failed Lapidus arthrodesis with non-union; recurrent increased IM angle; Shortening of first metatarsal; peritalar subluxation. (**b**) Loss of arch height; broken hardware medial cuneiform; medical cuneiform parallel to fifth metatarsal, right foot

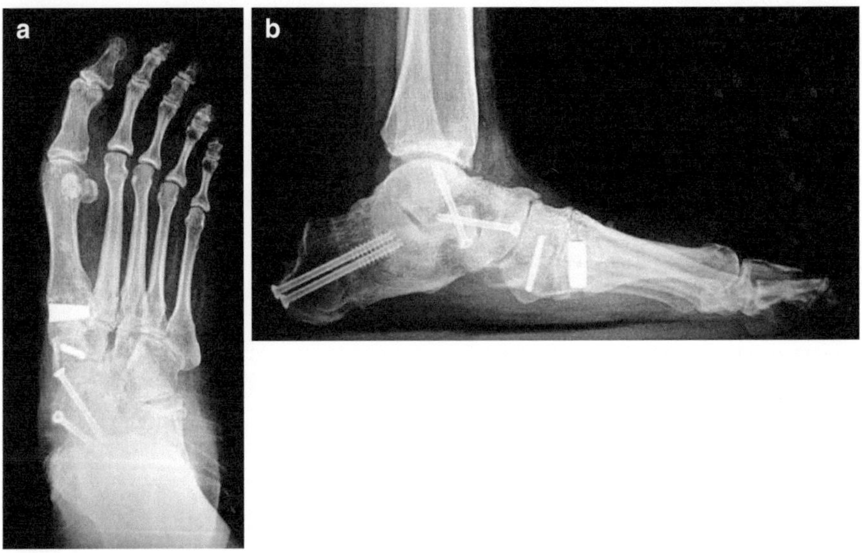

Fig. 2.2 (**a**) Utilization of cotton type cancellous titanium wedge to restore IM angle and first metatarsal length, right foot. (**b**) TN arthrodesis; posterior calcaneal osteotomy; gastrocnemius recession; restoration of medial longitudinal arch

[6]. The utilization of the biofoam intrapositioned "cotton wedge" of cancellous titanium was used in an "off label" manner to restore length, correct the IM angle, and attain proper position of plantarflexion to restore a tripod position (Fig. 2.2a).

The posterior calcaneal osteotomy and TN arthrodesis help reduce the lateral peritalar subluxation of the foot and restore arch height (Fig. 2.2b). The gastrocnemius recession (Strayer type) is also essential to reduce midfoot strain once heel valgus and recreation of arch height occur. Postoperatively, the patient was maintained 6 weeks NWB (non-weight bearing) then allowed WB (weight bearing) via CAM (controlled ankle motion) boot for a further 6 weeks. The patient began intensive strengthening exercises during the WB phase.

Outcome

The patient did very well postoperatively with no noted complications. It can be seen that the cancellous titanium wedge incorporated well. It has the consistency of cancellous bone. Also a solid TN arthrodesis was attained as well as a healed calcaneal osteotomy. Arch height and overall alignment were attained. As is typical with this type of procedure the patient was back to normal activity at approximately 6 months. However, residual discomfort and mild edema persisted for a full year. Orthotics were also utilized and began use at 14 weeks to support the re-established foot structure.

Clinical Pearls and Pitfalls

Utilization of an "off label" cotton titanium wedge can be considered in a Lapidus first metatarsal-MC nonunion. The rhomboid shaped wedge placed "dorsal-medial" can (1) add length (2) as well as correct the IM angle and (3) also plantarflex the first metatarsal and maintain plantar weight bearing integrity.

Incorporation is by osseointegration [7]. Repositioning of the first metatarsal occurs with a Hintermann retractor. The nonunion surfaces must be prepared in the same way as if utilizing an auto or allograft. Curettage of fibrous tissue and creation of cancellous bleeding by fenestration of the subchondral and cancellous bone must be performed at the first metatarsal MC joint site.

Fixation of the titanium wedge is dependent on intraoperative compression. When the distractor is released, detection of motion by stressing the implant is performed. If it remains tight and no clinical movement is noted, no further fixation is needed. If there is noted movement or gapping at the surface interface, a plate or staple may be used to add compression.

Despite calcaneocuboid arthrosis noted at the lateral edge of the joint, reduction of the lateral peritalar subluxation created by the posterior calcaneal osteotomy and talonavicular arthrodesis provides a distraction or an arthrodiastasis effect at the calcaneocuboid (CC) joint level. It is extremely important to maintain lateral column mobility. An associated cheilectomy and subchondral drilling is performed at the degenerative site. This allows increased mobility and can allow fibrocartilage repair.

References

1. Toolan B. Surgical strategies: the Lapidus procedure. Foot Ankle Int. 2007;28(10):1108–14.
2. Hamilton GA, Mullins S, Schuberth JM, Rush SM, Ford L. Revision Lapidus arthrodesis: rate of union in 17 cases. J Foot Ankle Surg. 2007;46(6):447–50.
3. Matthews M, Cook EA, Cook J, Johnson L, Karthas T, Collier B, Hansen D, Manning E, McKenna B, Basile P. Long-term outcomes of corrective osteotomies using porous titanium wedges for flexible flatfoot deformity correction. J Foot Ankle Surg. 2018;57(5):924–30.
4. Pinney SJ, Sangeorzan BJ, Hansen ST. Surgical anatomy of the gastrocnemius recession (Strayer procedure). Foot Ankle Int. 2004;24(4):247–50.
5. Lombardi CM, Dennis LN, Connolly FG, Silhanek AD. Talonavicular joint arthrodesis and Evans calcaneal osteotomy for treatment of posterior tibial tendon dysfunction. J Foot Ankle Surg. 1999;38(2):116–22.
6. Rammelt S, Marti RK, Zwipp H. Arthrodesis of the talonavicular joint. Der Orthopade. 2006;35(4):428–34.
7. Libicher M, Hillmeier J, Liegibel U, Sommer U, Pyerin W, Vetter M, Meinzer HP, Grafe I, Meeder P, Nöldge G, Nawroth P, Kasperk C. Osseous integration of calcium phosphate in osteoporotic vertebral fractures after kyphoplasty: initial results from a clinical and experimental pilot study. Osteoporos Int. 2006;17(1):1208–15.

3 Case #3: Revision of Displaced Capital First Metatarsal Head Osteotomy with Intramedullary K-wire & Dual Locking Plates

Case Presentation

This is a 64-year-old Caucasian female who underwent a double osteotomy Austin-Akin type procedure at the first MPJ (metatarsal phalangeal joint) for hallux valgus deformity. The patient was doing well with the wound healed and sutures removed at 2 weeks. However, at 3 weeks postoperatively the patient fell while missing a step. She sustained a hyperextension injury to the first MPJ [1]. She presented with increased significant pain and considerable edema. She was unable to bear weight and presented in a wheelchair.

Diagnosis and Assessment

Radiographs were taken and noted loosening of the (2) 2.0 mm screws with medial, dorsal displacement of the first metatarsal head. Considerable gapping was noted at the dorsal wing (Fig. 3.1a, b). Clinically, there was crepitus noted on manual manipulation of the first metatarsal osteotomy site thus noting instability. The proximal phalanx remained intact [2]. The patient presents with an obvious displaced first metatarsal head osteotomy noted on the medial oblique (MO) and lateral views (Fig. 3.1b, c). The presence of the two loose screws indicates loss of osteotomy compression. Also, it serves to provide a distraction force and thus will not allow any form of secondary bone healing with protected weight bearing (WB). A post-traumatic medial displacement deformity and elevation of the first metatarsal are noted on the dorsal plantar (DP) and lateral views. There is also concern for the potential development of avascular necrosis (AVN) [3]. This can be due to the tenuous nature of the blood supply to the first metatarsal head [4].

H. J. Visser, *Challenges in Foot and Ankle Reconstructive Surgery*,
https://doi.org/10.1007/978-3-031-07893-4_3

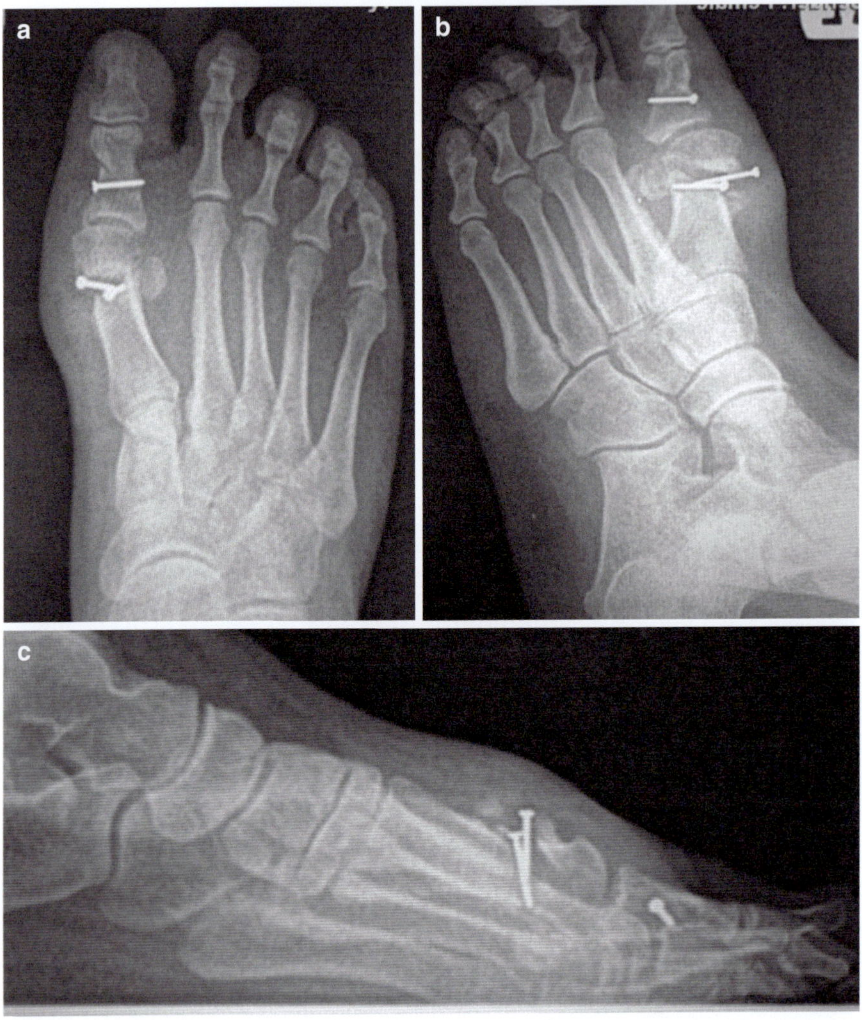

Fig. 3.1 (**a**) Medial displacement of the capital fragment with hardware loosening (**b**) Dorsal displacement of the capital fragment with loosening of 2.0 mm screws (**c**) Gapping of dorsal wing with dorsal displacement of capital fragment

Management

The operational approach was to realign the displaced first metatarsal head in the sagittal, transverse, and frontal planes. A 0.045″ Kirschner (K)-wire was utilized to stabilize the first metatarsal head to the proximal shaft [5]. Dual locking plates were applied medial and dorsal to support the repositioned first metatarsal head. Bone grafting was performed to support the dorsal wing. Proper position by correcting the intermetatarsal (IM) angle and re-establishing plantarflexion in the sagittal plane

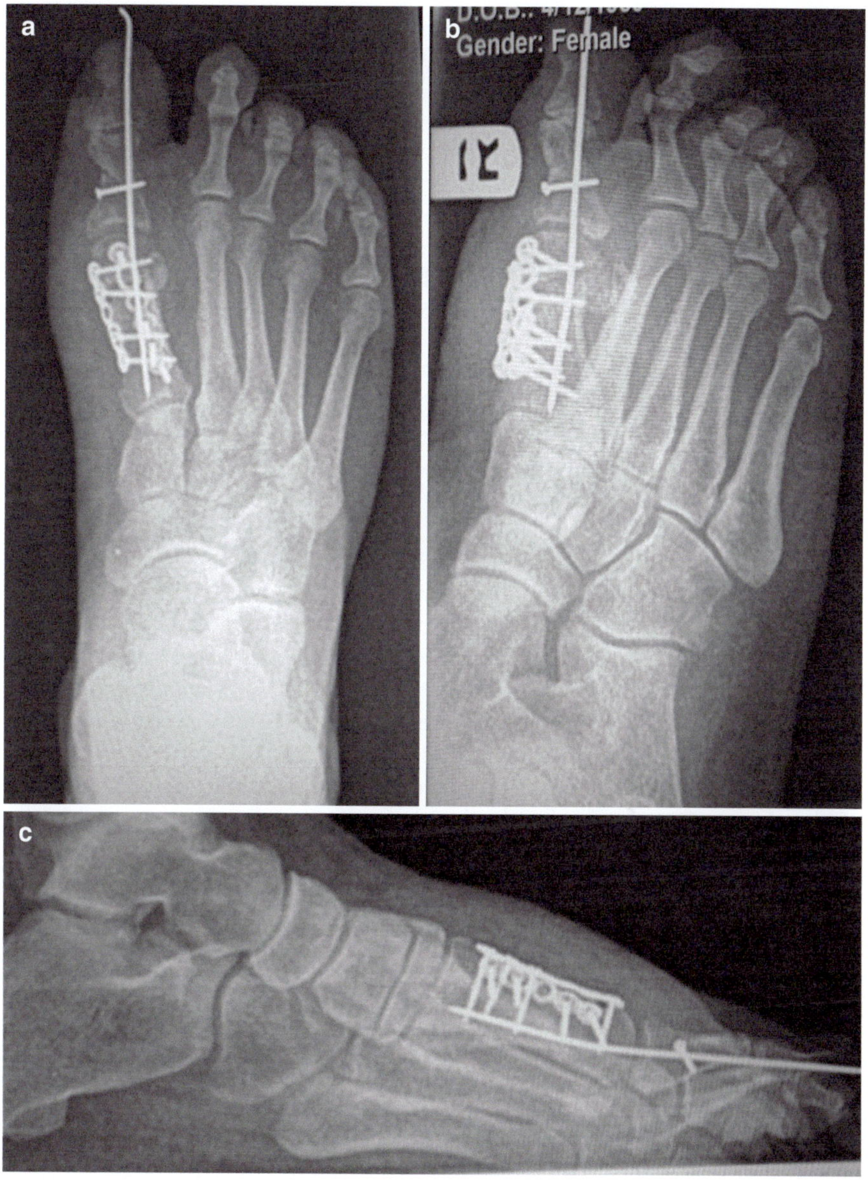

Fig. 3.2 (**a**, **b**) Anatomic alignment of the first metatarsal head with intramedullary K-wire and dual locking plates (**c**) dual locking plate to resist tension, shear, and bending force

occurred, frontal rotation of the first metatarsal head was also attained (Fig. 3.2a–c). The patient was kept non-weight bearing (NWB) for 4 weeks. The K-wire was removed at that time. Range of motion (ROM) of first MPJ occurred and guarded

WB in controlled ankle motion (CAM) boot for a further 4 weeks was performed until radiographic healing occurred. Physical therapy was instilled for 4 further weeks.

Outcome

She returned to shoe wear at 9 weeks and began home physical therapy (PT). The patient was monitored carefully by radiographs for 6 months to assure osteotomy healing and lack of presence of AVN. She was back to full activity at 6 months. She maintained good ROM and first MPJ function. As being an older patient, there was no need for increased functional demand and the patient was very happy with the outcome.

Clinical Pearls and Pitfalls

Displaced first metatarsal head osteotomies can present a significant challenge. Reoperation with the presence of edema increases the risk of hematoma formation and infection. Also, there is the major concern for the development of AVN [6].

The key to positioning is realignment of the dorsal wing which is comminuted. There is very little "real estate" for fixation in this area. This is established by insertion of a K-wire axially through the preserved plantar portion of the wing which allows proper positioning of the metatarsal head.

Dual mini locking plates will maintain stability and resist tension, shear, and bending forces. Bone grafting of the dorsal wing for existing defects also needs to be performed. Eccentric use of the compression slots can offer some compression through the medially applied plate.

Case #3A: Revision of Displaced Capital First Metatarsal Head Osteotomy with a Mini External Fixator

Additional Adjunctive Case

As an additional approach in a similar case, the patient was a 45-year-old NIDDM (non-insulin dependent diabetes mellitus) with loss of protective sensation from neuropathy. A double osteotomy was performed for hallux abductovalgus (HAV) to eliminate a chronic recurrent plantar ulceration. Her clinical appearance 2 weeks postoperatively was concerning for infection and radiographs showed displacement of the first metatarsal head (Figs. 3A.1 a, b and 3A.2 a, b). The patient was to be NWB after the initial procedure but began immediate WB postoperatively.

In this case, the hardware was removed and soft tissue and bone cultures were taken. Due to concern for infection, the osteotomies of the first metatarsal and proximal phalanx were again stabilized with a 0.062" K-wire (Fig. 3A.3). Due to her

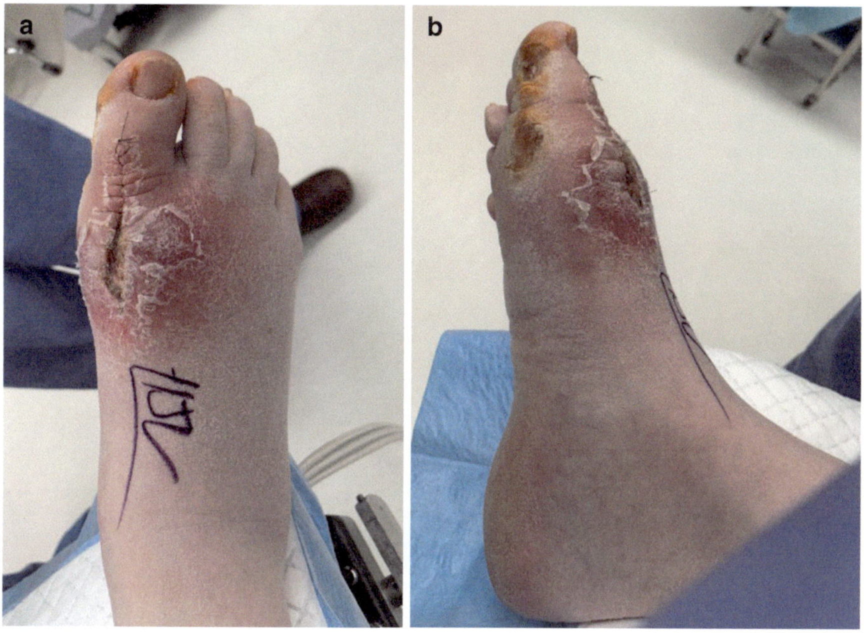

Fig. 3A.1 (**a**, **b**) Clinical appearance displays wound dehiscence and possible infection 2 weeks status post Austin-Akin osteotomy

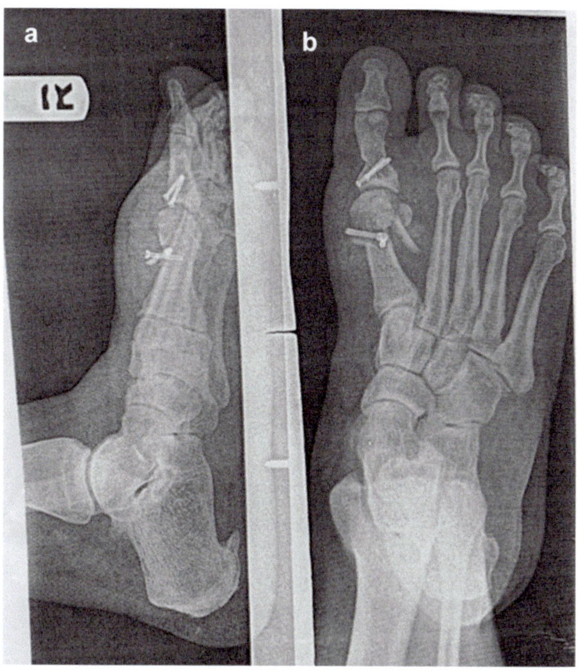

Fig. 3A.2 (**a**, **b**) Radiographs demonstrate fixation failure with displacement of the first metatarsal head

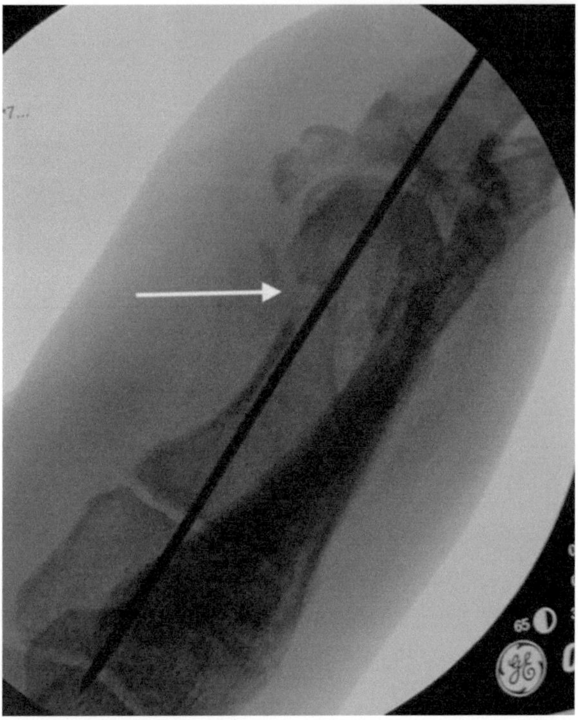

Fig. 3A.3 The joint was realigned, the osteotomy sites were stabilized, and the first metatarsal was brought out to length with K-wire fixation. The plantar cortex was used as reference for re-alignment of the first metatarsal

neuropathy, a mini-external fixator was applied and the wound closed at the capsular level (Fig. 3A.4a, b) [7, 8] Prior to closure, bone allograft chips were used to pack the defect in the dorsal wing of the osteotomy (Fig. 3A.5a, b). Vancomycin powder was utilized at the bone/capsule interface and closed (Fig. 3A.6). The remaining wound at the subcutaneous level was left open to heal by secondary intent utilizing negative pressure therapy (wound vacuum).

Ultimately, the intraoperative bone biopsy and culture were negative and infection was excluded. The patient was kept on NWB for 8 weeks and the fixator removed. Good consolidation and healing of the osteotomies were noted and the patient was placed in a CAM boot for further 4 weeks with initiation of first MPJ ROM. The patient had full healing of both osteotomies and returned to shoe wear protected by accommodating foot orthotic no further recurrence of re-ulceration occurred.

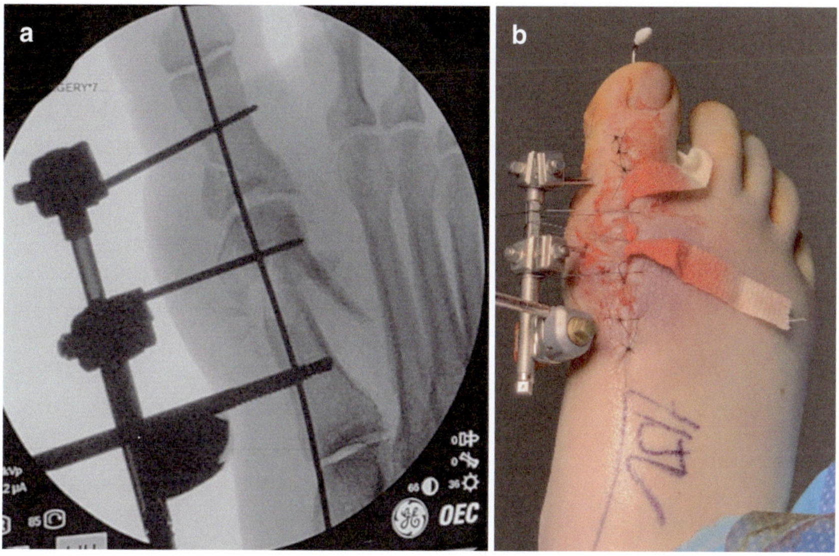

Fig. 3A.4 (**a**, **b**) Realignement of capital fragment with 0.062″ Intramedullary K-wire and mini external fixator

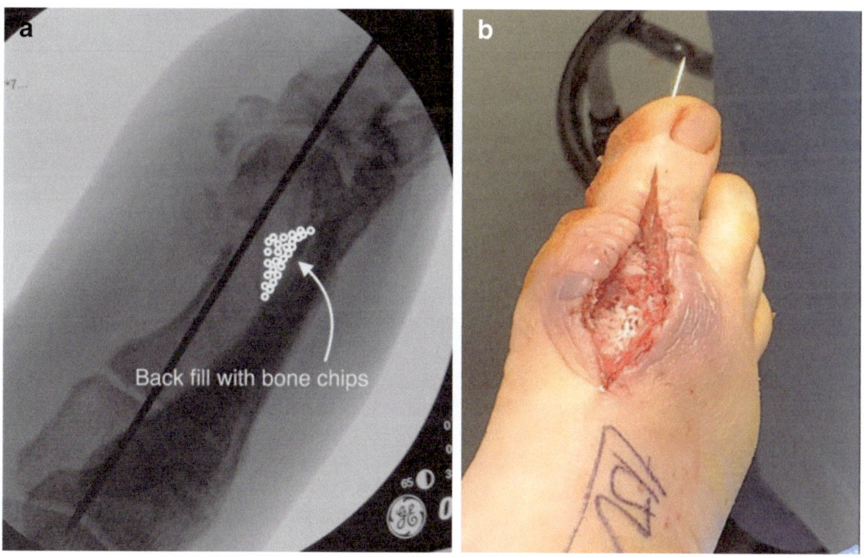

Fig. 3A.5 (**a**, **b**) Filling dorsal defect with allograft bone chips

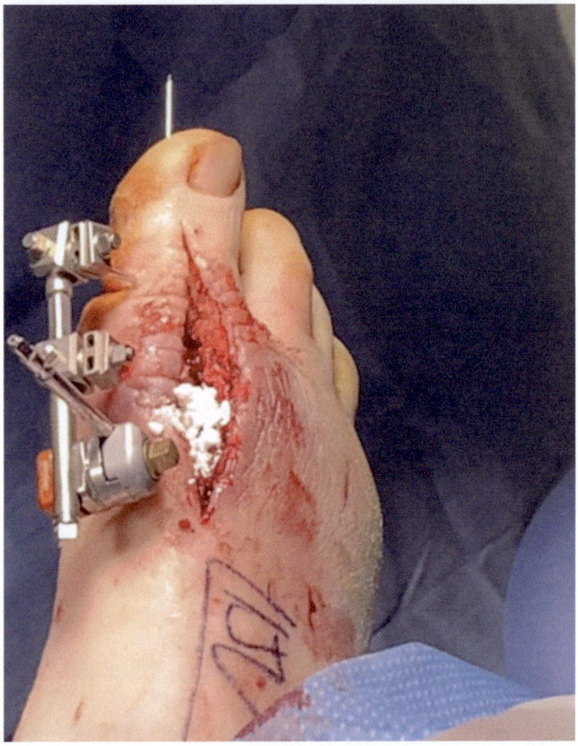

Fig. 3A.6 Closure of bone-capsule interphase over vancomycin powder

References

1. Sammarco GJ, Idusuyi OB. Complications after surgery of the hallux. Clin Orthop Relat Res. 2001;391:59–71.
2. Laughlin TJ. Complications of distal first metatarsal osteotomies. J Foot Ankle Surg. 1995;24(6):593–4.
3. Meisenhelder DA, Harkless LB, Patterson JW. Avascular necrosis after first metatarsal head osteotomies. J Foot Surg. 1984;23(6):429–35.
4. Shereff MJ, Yang QM, Kummer FJ. Extraosseous and intraosseous arterial supply to the first metatarsal and metarsophalangeal joint. Foot Ankle Int. 1987;8(2):81–93.
5. Seibert FJ, Fankhauser F, Elliott B, Stockenhuber N, Peicha G. External fixation in trauma of the foot and ankle. Clin Podiatr Med Surg. 2003;20(1):159–80.
6. Edwards WH. Avascular necrosis of the first metatarsal head. Foot Ankle Clin. 2005;10(1):117–27.
7. Schweinberger MH, Roukis TS. Salvage of the first ray with external fixation in the high-risk patient. Foot Ankle Spec. 2008;1(4):210–3.
8. Brandão RA, Weber JS, Larson D, Bull PE, Berlet GC, Hyer CF. New fixation methods for the treatment of the diabetic foot: beaming, external fixation, and beyond. Clin Podiatr Med Surg. 2018;35(1):63–76.

Case #4: Management of First Metatarsal Head Capital Osteotomy with Secondary Avascular Necrosis Utilizing a Fresh Frozen Femoral Head Allograft for Arthrodesis

4

Case Presentation

This is a 42-year-old Caucasian female who had her original procedure 1 year prior to presentation. Patient had a double osteotomy (Austin-Akin) performed with a seemingly uneventful course. She was discharged at 6 weeks postoperatively. She began to develop symptoms of pain and swelling at around 9 months postoperatively. She did not seek care or another opinion until 1 full year postoperatively. The patient when initially seen was antalgic, swollen about the first metatarsal phalangeal joint (MPJ) and had loss of hallux purchase. Patient stated she had not exhibited wound problems in the initial postoperative period.

Diagnosis and Assessment

Radiographs of dorsal plantar (DP), medial oblique (MO), and lateral views were taken of the right foot and revealed an Austin osteotomy with (2) 3.0 mm cannulated screws along with an Akin proximal phalangeal osteotomy with a staple for fixation [1, 2]. There was extensive destruction of the first metatarsal head with resultant shortening and elevation. The hallux was floating with no available purchase (Fig. 4.1a–c). The obvious concern was a differential of avascular necrosis (AVN) vs osteomyelitis [3]. Laboratory values noted a white blood cell (WBC) count of 7.2 μL and CRP 2.4 mg/L and sedimentation rate of 25 mm/h. A Tc99 Hexamethyl Propylene Amine Oxime (HMPAO), Ceretec scan, was performed initially which was equivocal for osteomyelitis [4, 5]. A bone biopsy and culture were then performed via a Jamshidi needle which resulted in no growth of bacteria. Pathologic histology was not indicative of osteomyelitis. This indicated a presumptive diagnosis of AVN [6–8].

H. J. Visser, *Challenges in Foot and Ankle Reconstructive Surgery*,
https://doi.org/10.1007/978-3-031-07893-4_4

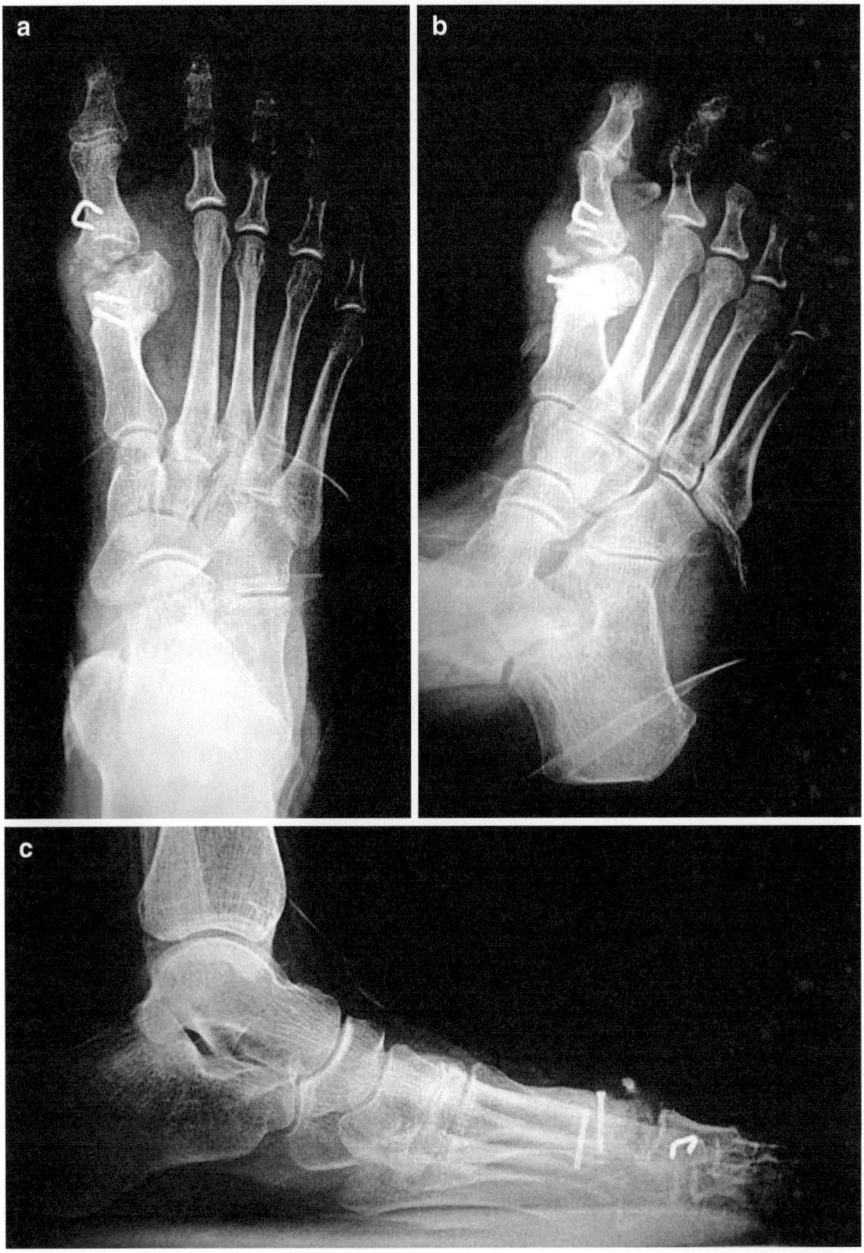

Fig. 4.1 (**a**–**c**) Pre-operative appearance, first metatarsal head, right foot; AVN vs osteomyelitis considered

Management

Management included complete resection of the first metatarsal head. The bony tissue was not viable, due to its avascular nature to allow a primary arthrodesis (Fig. 4.2a–c). A trephine was used to size the first metatarsal head that was resected

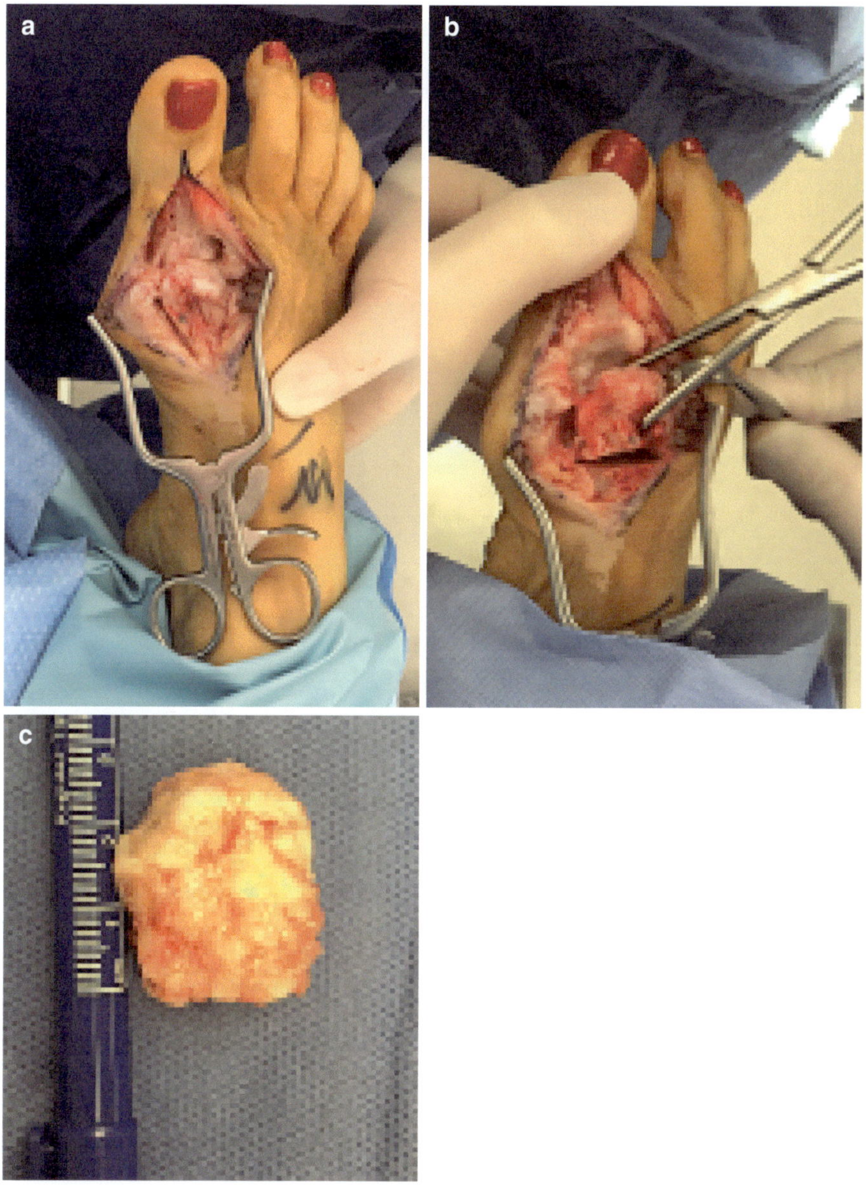

Fig. 4.2 (**a**) Avascular first metatarsal head, right. (**b**) Resection of avascular first metatarsal head at level of viable bone, right. (**c**) Resected avascular first metatarsal, right

(Fig. 4.3). This trephine was then used to harvest a cancellous plug from a fresh frozen femoral head allograft (Fig. 4.4). The allograft was prepared by fenestrating it with multiple 2.0 mm size drill holes. Bone marrow aspirate garnered from the metaphyseal area of the lower tibia was then utilized to soak the allograft (Fig. 4.5a and b) [9]. The graft was then inserted into the resected defect. The proximal phalangeal base and remaining first metatarsal were then prepared by curettage and fenestration with a 2.0 mm drill. A 0.062" Kirschner (K)-wire was then retrograded through the proximal phalanx out the distal tip of the hallux. The graft was then firmly placed in the resected area. The K-wire was then antigraded through the graft and the first metatarsal (Fig. 4.6). A 3.0 mm locking plate was applied as a bridge or buttress plate. Eccentric compression with non-locking screws in the compression slots of the locking plate were utilized at the proximal and distal margins; this allowed compression at the graft (Fig. 4.7). The remaining holes were filled with 3.0 mm locking screws (Fig. 4.8a–c).

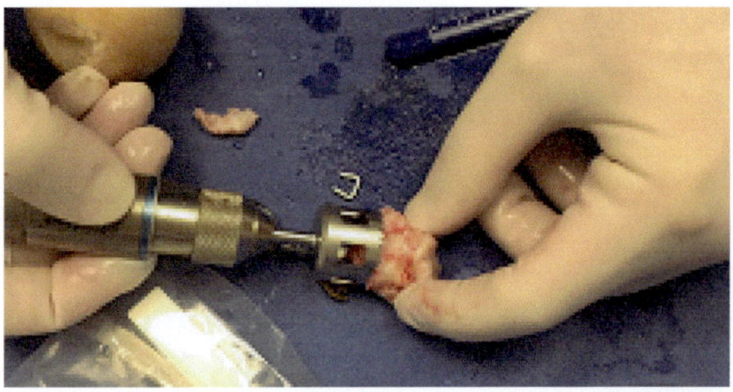

Fig. 4.3 Sizing resected first metatarsal head with trephine

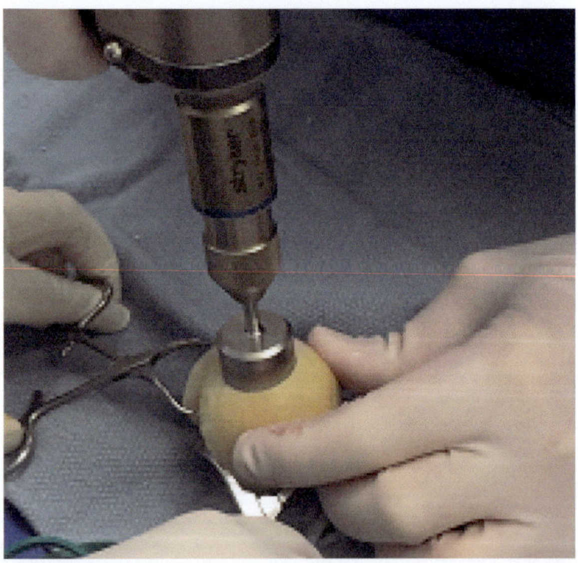

Fig. 4.4 Trephine plug from fresh frozen femoral head allograft matches resected first metatarsal head

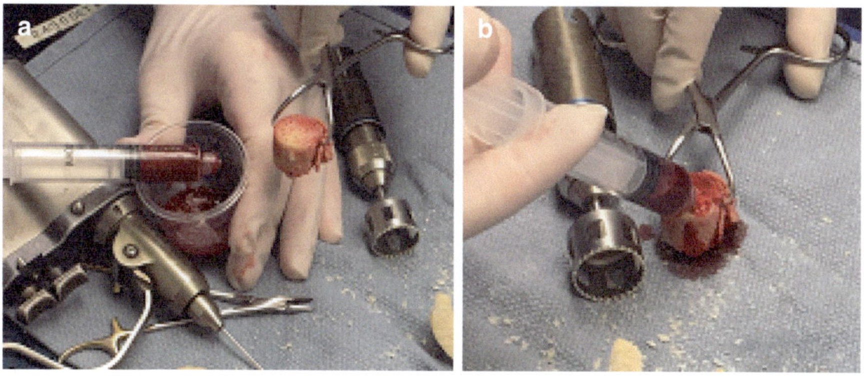

Fig. 4.5 (**a**, **b**) Soaking of femoral head allograft with bone marrow aspirate

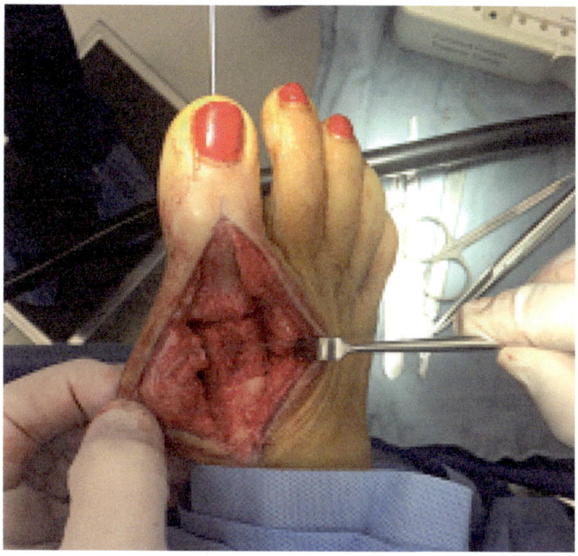

Fig. 4.6 Trephine measured allograft at resection site; 0.062″ K-wire positioning graft to the hallux

Outcome

The patient was kept on non-weight bearing (NWB) for 8 weeks and then began gradual weight bearing (WB) the next 3 weeks. The patient was then returned to shoe wear at 12 weeks postoperatively. The patient did extremely well and exhibited excellent interphalangeal joint (IPJ) range of motion. A solid arthrodesis was attained at the proximal and distal portion of the allograft.

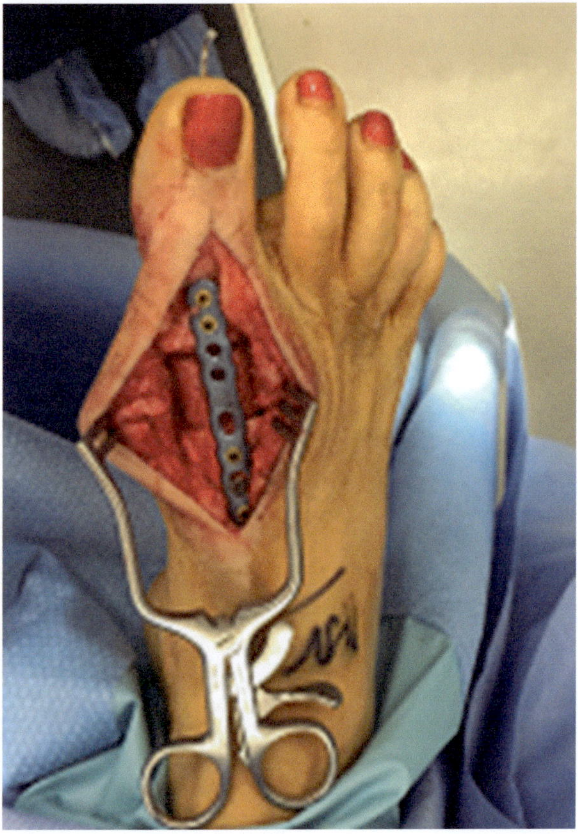

Fig. 4.7 Application of 3.0 mm locking plate, first MPJ, right

Clinical Pearls and Pitfalls

Utilization of a block, intercalary bone graft with resection of the first metatarsal head in some cases can be a challenging operation [10]. Re-establishing hallux length via ligament and capsular (ligamentotaxis) distraction is critical. This form of arthrodesis establishes stability to the altered windlass mechanism and protects the lateral metatarsals from lateral transference overload. The K-wire by using bending movement is extremely useful in stabilizing the graft prior to plate administration. It is also very helpful for positioning the graft and allowing proper position of the hallux. The graft, too, can be customized by using cup and cone reamers. The proximal phalanx is prepared with the cup and the distal portion of the graft with cone [11]. The proximal portion of the graft is prepared with the cup and the remaining proximal metatarsal with the cone. This allows for planal motion as the hallux is positioned with the K-wire. The graft was "dialed in." One must be aware that in every case despite clinical, laboratory and evaluations, infection, with the presence of bone destruction must be ruled out. Intercalary graft sizes must be kept to no

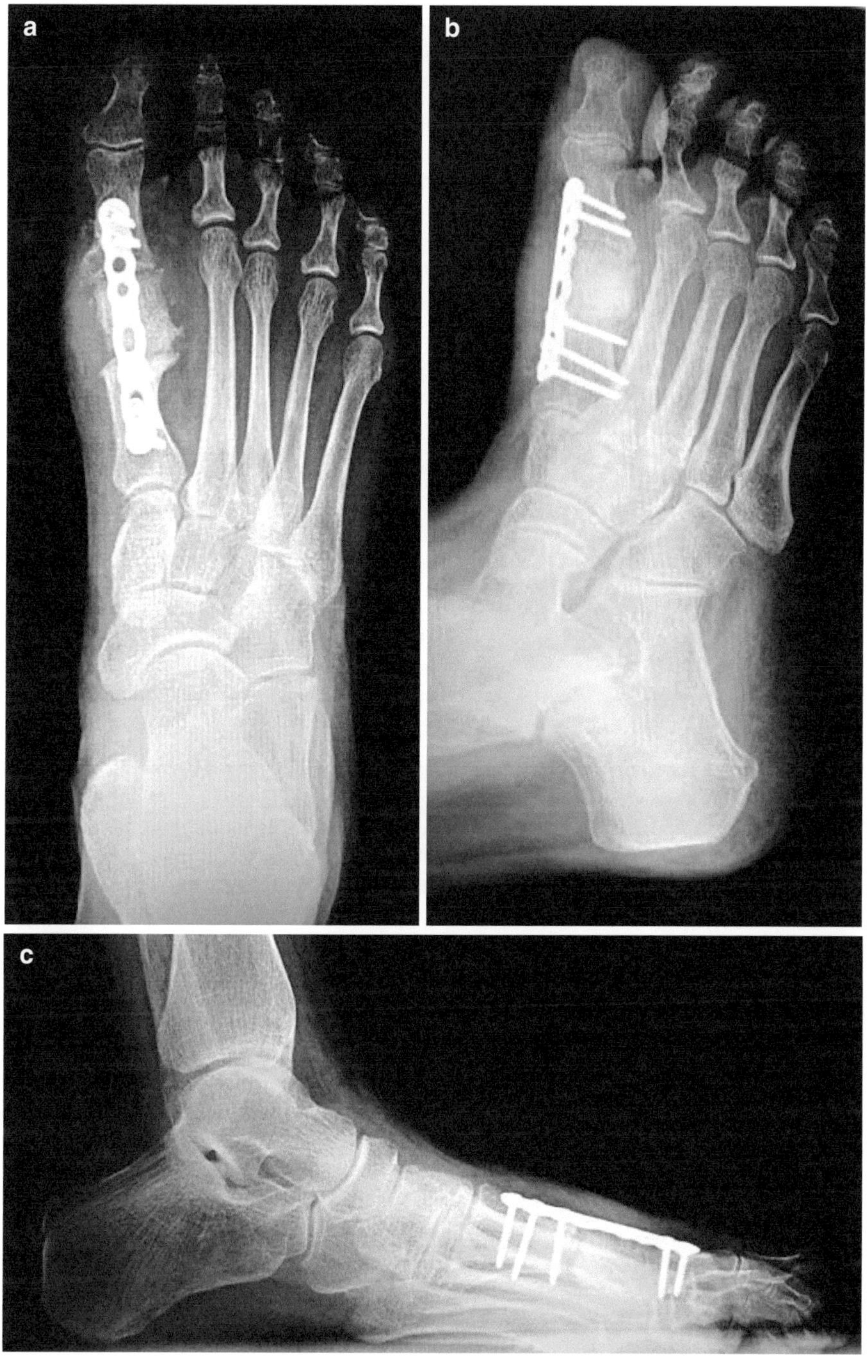

Fig. 4.8 (**a**–**c**) Post-operative view of femoral head allograft with restoration of hallux length and sagittal plane weight bearing

longer than 2.0 cm and preferable to 1.5 cm. Creeping substitution occurs at the proximal and distal portions of the allograft. The use of longer grafts can lead to collapse within the center portion. This then destabilizes the construct and leads to hardware loosening, failure, and nonunion.

References

1. Rigby RB, Fallat LM, Kish JP. Axial loading cross screw fixation for the Austin Bunionectomy. J Foot Ankle Surg. 2011;50(5):537–40.
2. Douthett SM, Plaskey NK, Fallat LM, Kish J. Retrospective analysis of the Akin osteotomy. J Foot Ankle Surg. 2018;57(1):38–43.
3. Weinraub GM, Meberg R, Steinberg JS. Vascular perfusion of the long dorsal arm versus chevron osteotomy: a cadaveric injection study. J Foot Ankle Surg. 2004;43(4):221–4.
4. Imhof H, Breitenseher M, Trattnig S, Kramer J, Hofmann S, Plenk H, Schneider W, Engel A. Imaging of avascular necrosis of bone. Eur Radiol. 1997;7(2):180–6.
5. Wilkinson SV, Jones RO, Sisk LE, Sunshein KF, Manen JW. Austin bunionectomy: postoperative MRI evaluation for avascular necrosis. J Foot Surg. 1992;31(5):469–77.
6. Filippi J, Briceno J. Complications after metatarsal osteotomies for hallux valgus: malunion, nonunion, avascular necrosis, and metatarsophalangeal osteoarthritis. Foot Ankle Clin. 2020;25(1):169–82.
7. Peterson DA, Zilberfarb JL, Greene MA, Colgrove RC. Avascular necrosis of the first metatarsal head: incidence in distal osteotomy combined with lateral soft tissue release. Foot Ankle Int. 1994;15(2):59–63.
8. Neary MT, Jones RO, Sunshein K, Van Manen W, Youngberg R. Avascular necrosis of the first metatarsal head following Austin osteotomy: a follow-up study. J Foot Ankle Surg. 1993;32(5):530–5.
9. Ayerza MA, Piuzzi NS, Aponte-Tinao LA, Farfalli GL, Muscolo DL. Structural allograft reconstruction of the foot and ankle after tumor resections. Musculoskelet Surg. 2016;100(2):149–56.
10. Myerson MS, Schon LC, McGuigan FX, Oznur A. Result of arthrodesis of the hallux metatarsophalangeal joint using bone graft for restoration of length. Foot Ankle Int. 2000;21(4):297–306.
11. Kundert H. Cup & cone reamers for arthrodesis of the first metatarsophalangeal joint. Oper Orthop Traumatol. 2010;22(4):431–9.

Case #5: Revision of a Silastic Flexible Hinged Implant Involving the First Metatarsophalangeal Joint with Arthrodesis Utilizing a Fresh Frozen Femoral Head Allograft

5

Case Presentation

This is a 52-year-old female who presented with pain and swelling around the second metatarsal phalangeal joint (MPJ) right foot for the past 6 months. She had a silastic flexible hinge implant arthroplasty of the first MPJ performed 3 years prior [1]. For 1 year, her postoperative course was uneventful. She denied a history of a wound problem or infection. She began to have second MPJ pain about a year after her surgery. She saw her operating surgeon who performed multiple corticosteroid injections and prescribed orthotics. She states that she noted improvement for a small period of time but the symptoms again worsened. She noted no problems with the first MPJ surgical site itself.

Diagnosis and Assessment

Evaluation clinically noted palpable pain about the dorsal second MPJ right but no significant plantar discomfort on palpation. X rays show a silastic flexible hinge implant at the first MPJ. The hinge appears intact and there were no signs of implant sinkage, engulfment, or fibrous dysplasia. There was significant resection of the first metatarsal head. The patient demonstrated subchondral collapse at the second MPJ consistent stage II Freiberg's infraction (Fig. 5.1) [2]. This was secondary to lateral transference overload generated by a cascade effect. This led to loss of the windlass mechanism which occurred as a result of bone resection and flexor hallucis brevis (FHB) detachment during implant arthroplasty.

H. J. Visser, *Challenges in Foot and Ankle Reconstructive Surgery*,
https://doi.org/10.1007/978-3-031-07893-4_5

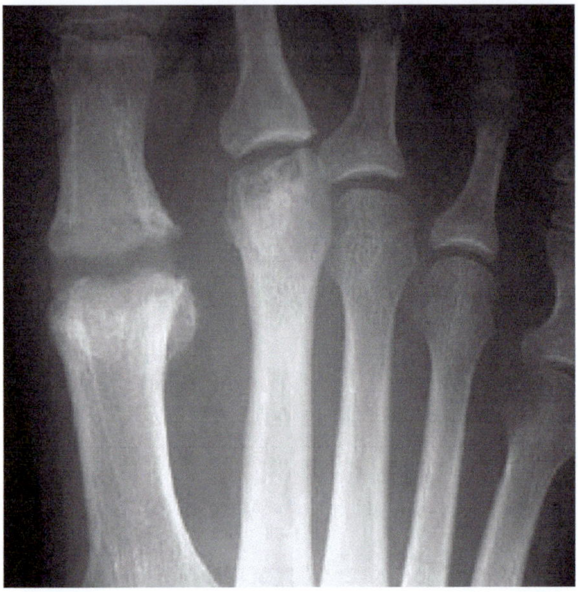

Fig. 5.1 Silastic flexible hinge implant arthroplasty first MPJ; Freiberg's infraction of second metatarsal head secondary to lateral transference

Management

The purpose of the operative procedure was to stabilize the first MPJ and thus the medial column by performing a bone block arthrodesis with removal of the implant [3, 4]. This would also help to re-establish the windlass mechanism [5]. The defect size to attain hallux length was 1 cm (Fig. 5.2a, b). The intercalary graft fits easily into the implant site as it contoured well to the resection site on the phalanx and metatarsal (Fig. 5.3). Dual-locking reconstruction plates were utilized to secure the graft and position the hallux (Fig. 5.4a, b) [6]. The allograft was prepared by fenestration using an 0.062 Kirschner (K)-wire and bone marrow aspirate from the calcaneus. No surgical procedure was performed on the second metatarsal head [7].

Outcome

The patient was kept on non-weight bearing (NWB) for nearly 9 weeks and then full weight bearing (WB) ensued. She returned to shoe wear at 12 weeks. The patient did reasonably well with no further pain occurring at the second metatarsal head. She did develop a fibrous nonunion at the distal interface of the allograft. Proximally, an arthrodesis occurred. Her residual discomfort did not warrant reoperation.

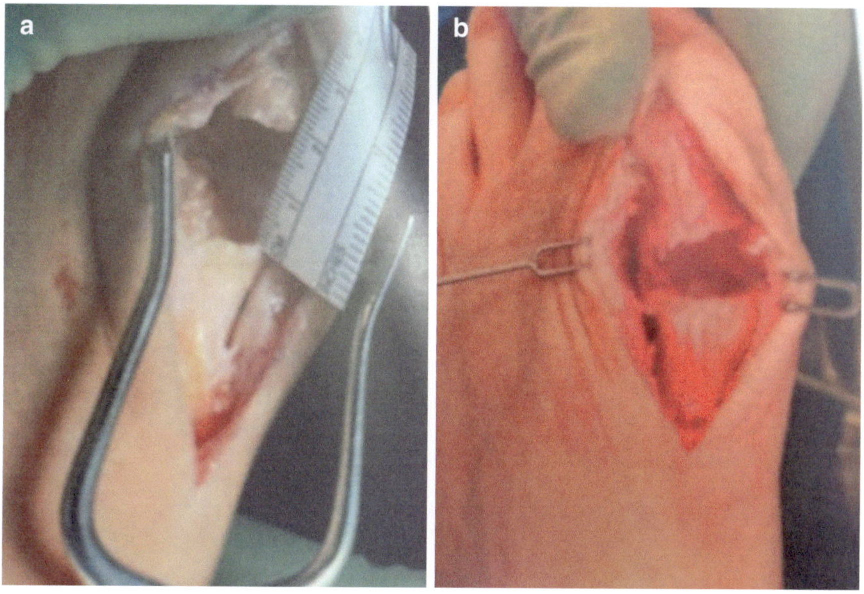

Fig. 5.2 (**a**, **b**) Measuring defect size post implant removal and canal debridement

Fig. 5.3 Insertion of intercalary allograft to attain hallux length, stablize first MPJ and hallux to the floor

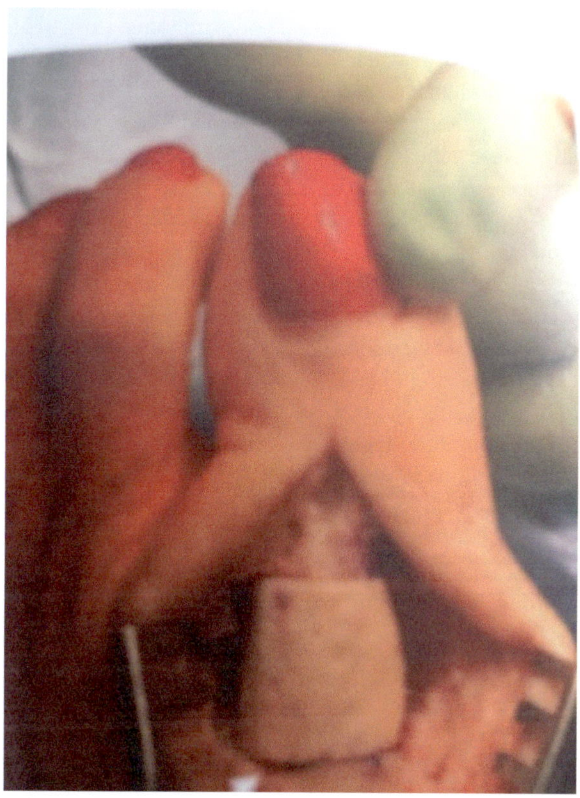

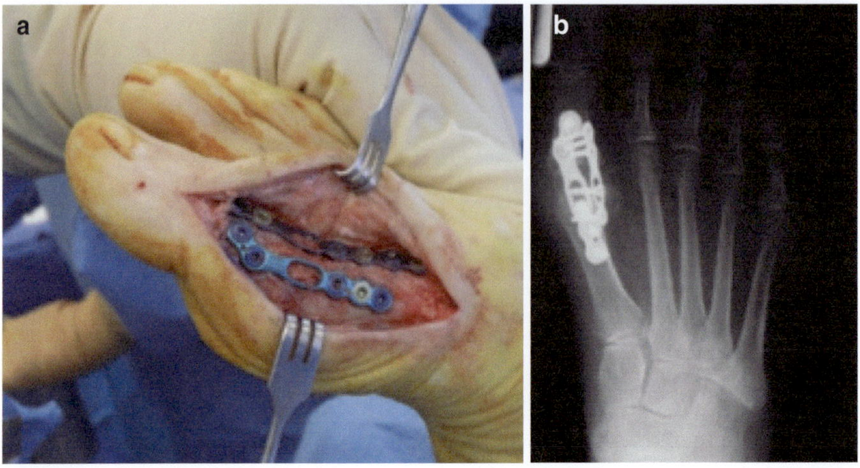

Fig. 5.4 (**a**, **b**) Internal fixation of intercalary allograft with dual locking plates; K-wire removed after plate fixation

Clinical Pearls and Pitfalls

Management of implant complications can be quite difficult. Often the implant, as was in this case, is not a cause of symptoms. Loss of stability and damage of windlass effect occur when the insertion of the FHB tendon becomes detached from the proximal phalanx. Also excessive resection of the metatarsal head leads to further destabilization. Once the first MPJ and the medial column are stable by arthrodesis, it then re-establishes the medial column stability and serves to prevent lateral transference or metatarsalgia. As was seen in this case, proper loading of the first MPJ after arthrodesis led to resolution of second MPJ symptoms despite persistent radiographic findings of a stage II Freiberg's infraction [8].

Another problem encountered is the scalloped intramedullary canals created by preparation for the implant. The endosteal bone of the remaining proximal phalangeal and first metatarsal cortical bone is all that remains. These must be prepared by "gentle" burring to stimulate bone bleeding. The canals must then be "back filled" tightly with bone allograft soaked in bone marrow aspirate. The graft incorporation must occur along these "thin" cortical edges and the graft interface. This can often lead to failure of arthrodesis. More recently, I have used trephine plugs from the calcaneus as autograft to fill the canals [9]. The trephine width matches the canal. The graft is then "press fitted" into the canal. Fortunately, if a "fibrous" nonunion occurs; it is often not painful and is relatively stable. Hardware loosening may occur as a result and require removal. Since the institution of trephine bone block autograft, nonunions and delayed unions have decreased significantly.

References

1. Granberry WM, Noble PC, Bishop JO, Tullos HS. Use of a hinged silicone prosthesis for replacement arthroplasty of the first metatarsophalangeal joint. J Bone Joint Surg. 1991;73(10):1453–9.
2. Talusan PG, Diaz-Collado PJ, Reach JS. Freiberg's infraction: diagnosis and treatment. Foot Ankle Spec. 2014;7(1):52–6.
3. Fujioka H, Doita M, Saura R, Mizuno SK. The long-term result of implant arthroplasty for hallux valgus deformity in rheumatoid arthritis. Ryumachi. 1999;39(3):561–7.
4. Hecht PJ, Gibbons MJ, Wapner KL, Cooke C, Hoisington SA. Arthrodesis of the first metatarsophalangeal joint to salvage failed silicone implant arthroplasty. Foot Ankle Int. 1997;18(7):383–90.
5. Barp EA, Jones NE, Prusa RD. Revision of failed first metatarsophalangeal joint implant. Clin Podiatr Med Surg. 2020;37(3):421–31.
6. Kitaoka HB, Holiday AD, Chao EY, Cahalan TD. Salvage of failed first metatarsophalangeal joint implant arthroplasty by implant removal and synovectomy: clinical and biomechanical evaluation. Foot Ankle Int. 1992;14(5):243–50.
7. Trnka H, Lara JS. Freiberg's infraction: surgical options. Foot Ankle Clin. 2019;24(4):669–76.
8. Mahieu C, Chaput A, Bouillet R. The treatment of rigid hallux using Swanson's silastic implant (single and double stem). Clinical radiological and podobarographic review with a 16-year maximum follow-up. Acta Orthop Belg. 1992;58(3):314–24.
9. Kindred KB, Wavrunek MR, Blacklidge DK, Wadehra A. First metatarsophalangeal joint distraction arthrodesis with Bicortical calcaneal autograft. J Foot Ankle Surg. 2020;59(3):568–76.

Case #6: Management of Stage 3 Hallux Limitus Deformity with Acellular Dermal Allomatrix for Resurfacing of the First Metatarsal Head

6

Case Presentation

This is a 56-year-old Caucasian male who presents with a long history of a painful first MPJ (metatarsal phalangeal joint). The patient states that he injured his joint while playing basketball in high school. He stated it took 3-months to fully recover from the injury. He had become symptomatic about 5-years prior to evaluation. Orthotics with the first ray extension (Mayo) and also use of graphite insole helped initially [1]. He also noted the joint had been injected with corticosteroids on three prior occasions at yearly intervals [2]. This gave him some relief but states the third injection, 1-year prior, lasted about 2-months.

Diagnosis and Assessment

Clinically, the patient had restricted first MPJ motion with 10° (degrees) of dorsiflexion (DF) and 5° of plantarflexion (PF). There was crepitus noted on ROM (range of motion). Radiographs showed a stage 3 hallux limitus deformity (Fig. 6.1). On the dorsal plantar (DP) view, there was approximately 2mm of joint space with asymmetric narrowing. Large proliferative osteophytes noted medial and lateral on the metatarsal head were also present. Subchondral sclerosis and erosions were exhibited (Fig. 6.2a). The first metatarsal head was asymmetric on the lateral view and noted a large dorsal osteophyte. There was dorsal spurring at the base of the proximal phalanx. Joint mice (ossicles) were present within the dorsal confines of the joint. The metatarsal head retained most of its concentricity (Fig. 6.2b) [3].

H. J. Visser, *Challenges in Foot and Ankle Reconstructive Surgery*,
https://doi.org/10.1007/978-3-031-07893-4_6

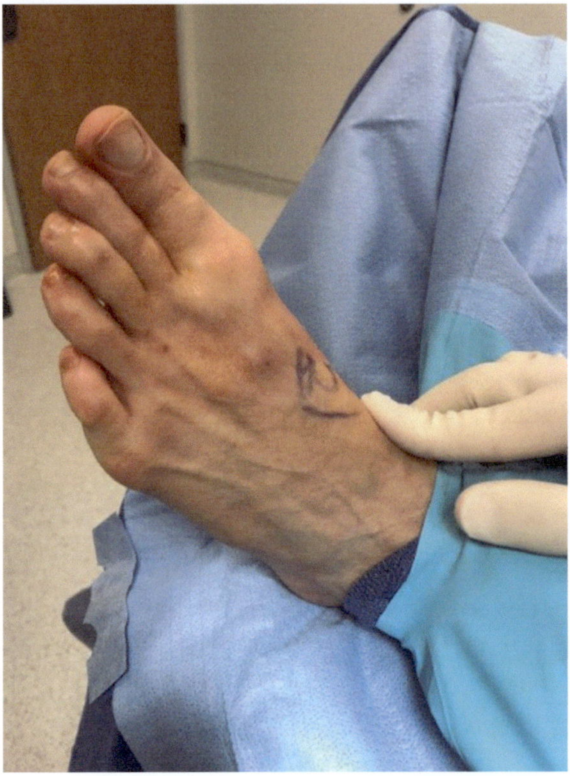

Fig. 6.1 Clinical appearance of hallux rigidus deformity

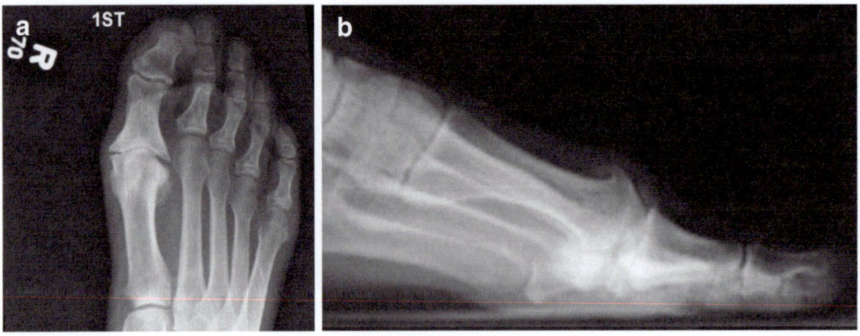

Fig. 6.2 (**a**, **b**) DP view displays assymetric joint space narrowing with osteophyte formation as well as subchondral bone sclerosis; Dorsal spurring of the proximal phangeal base and first metatarsal head as seen on the lateral view

Management

The first MPJ was approached with a dorsal curvilinear incision (Fig. 6.3). A cheilectomy was performed removing dorsal osteophytes and medial lateral proliferative bone from the first metatarsal head [4]. The loose joint ossicles (joint mice) were

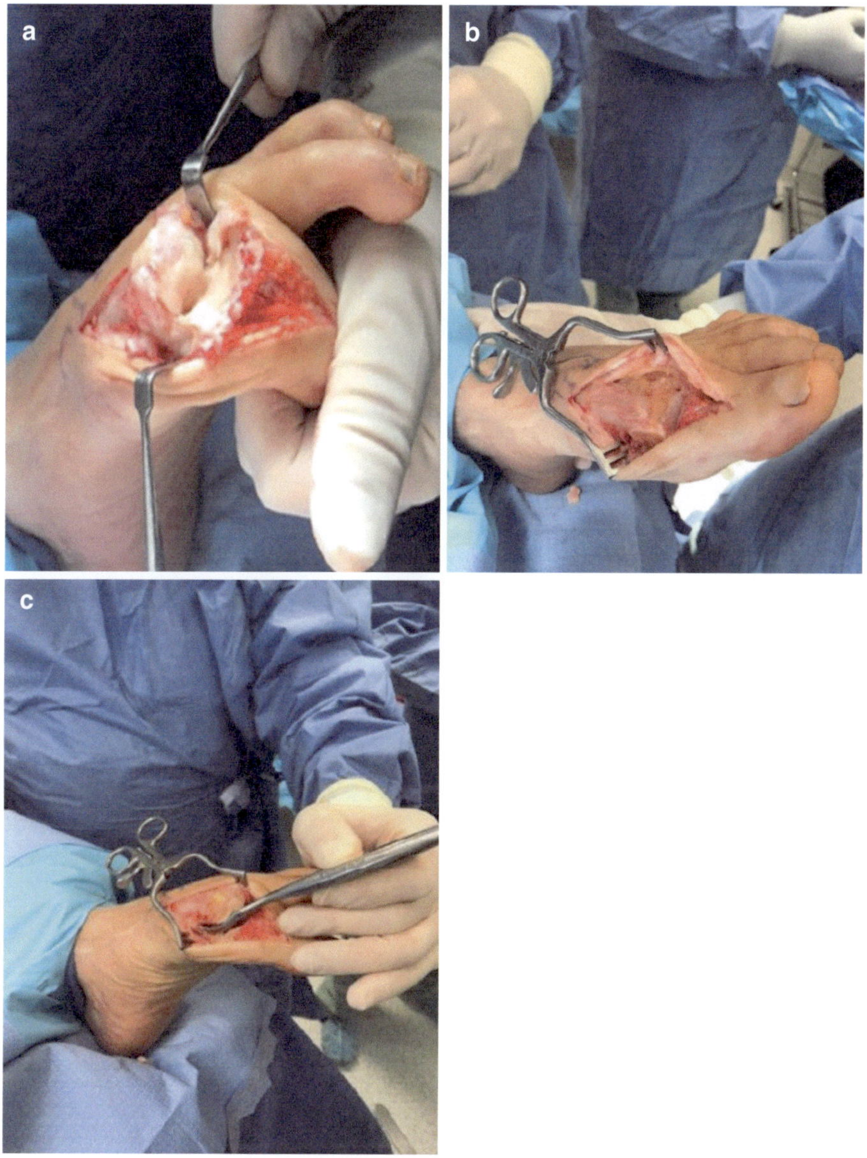

Fig. 6.3 (**a**) Large proliferative osteophytes and loose body ossicles presentwithin the joint; (**b**) Cheilectomy of the first metatarsal head was performed; (**c**) A McGlamry elevator was used to release the plantar adhesions and free the sesamoid apparatus

easily removed. A rongeur was used to remove peripheral spurring from the base of the proximal phalanx. The remaining cartilage of the first metatarsal head was removed with a power oscillating burr, a McGlamry elevator was used to free the sesamoid apparatus (Fig. 6.4a–c). The oscillating burr was used to preserve the subchondral bone plate. Subchondral drilling was performed to provide a vascular bed for the dermal allograft (Fig. 6.4d–f). This served to help maintain the articular geometry of the joint. Mini suture anchors were placed dorsal and plantar and medial and lateral consisting four points of fixation on the first metatarsal head. A 3.3 mm allomatrix graft was then secured to the prepared metatarsal head [5]. The remaining proximal phalangeal base was left with its remaining native hyaline and fibrocartilage.

Outcome

The patient was then placed in a CAM (controlled ankle motion) boot and began weight bearing (WB) at tolerance. At 2-weeks, the sutures were removed and active ROM (range of motion) was begun at the first MPJ. The patient was then transitioned to shoe wear at 4-weeks. The patient did exceedingly well and was ambulating completely pain free at 3-months. At 1.5–year follow-up, he remained pain free.

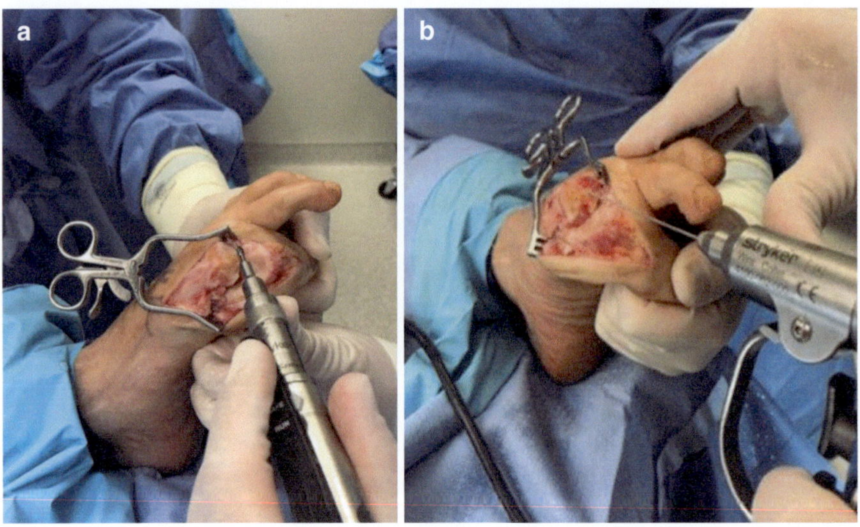

Fig. 6.4 (**a**) All remining cartilage was removed with a rotary burr. (**b**) The metatarsal head was prepared by fenestration of the subchondral bone to provide a vascular bed. (**c**) Four points of fixation were established with mini anchors medial, lateral, plantar, and dorsal on the metatarsal head. (**d**–**f**) 3.3 mm Allomatrix graft secured over the metatarsal head

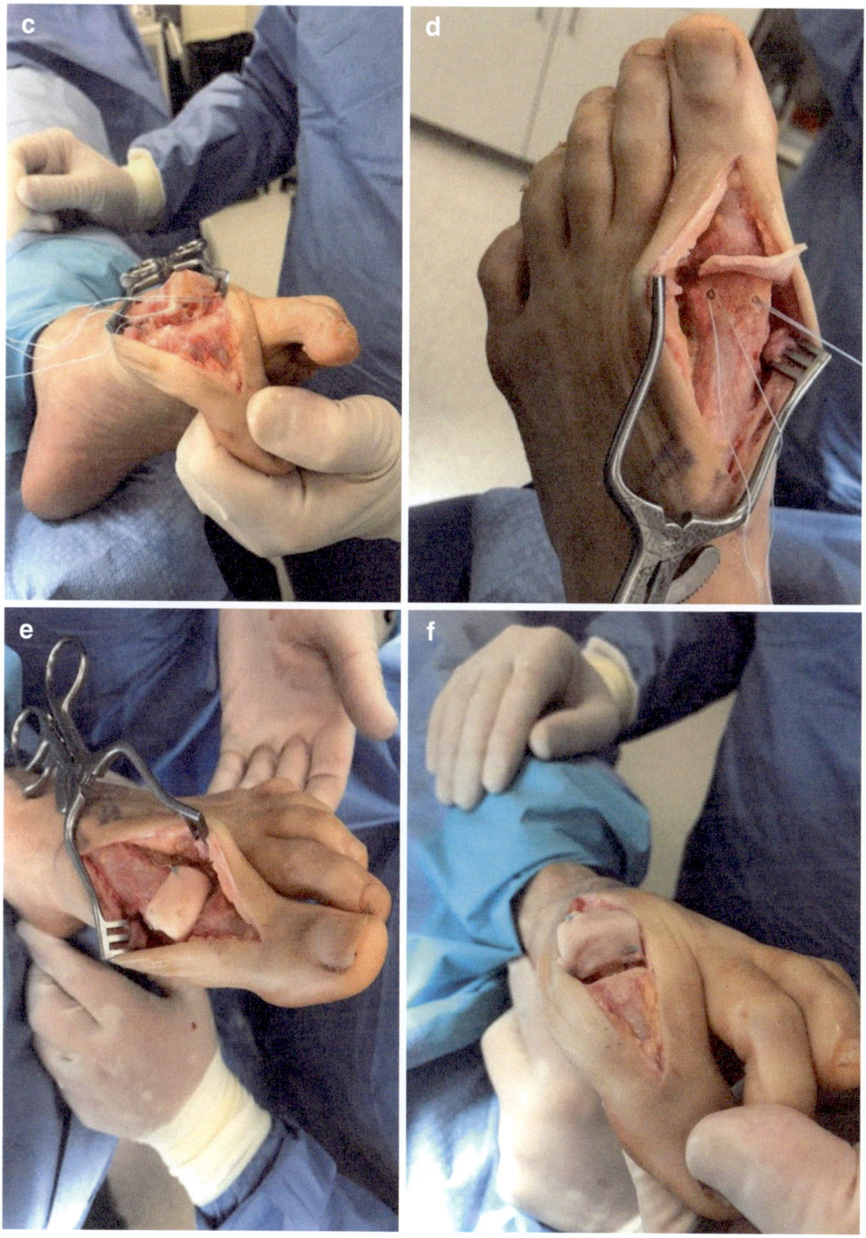

Fig. 6.4 (continued)

Clinical Pearls and Pitfalls

Utilization of acellular dermal matrix (ADM) as a form of interpositional arthroplasty is a newer technique to address the troublesome stage III joint in hallux limitus [6]. Traditional cheilectomy is utilized but with advanced stages of joint destruction, outcomes have been variable. The combination of proximal phalangeal (Moberg) and first metatarsal osteotomies (Youngswick) have not shown evidence of superiority as compared to cheilectomy alone. The utilization of implant arthroplasty and arthrodesis are certainly options but represent joint destructive procedures. Although resurfacing can include the proximal phalangeal side, I have found monopolar resurfacing of the metatarsal head itself to be adequate.

ADM provides a three-dimensional biocompatible non-cytotoxic matrix that retains its chemical properties. It allows for revascularization and cellular repopulation. It contains growth factors fibroblast growth factor (BFGF), platelet-derived growth factor (PDGMFbb), transforming growth factor (TBFn), and bone macrophage protein 2 (BMD2). The result is incorporation and formation of a biologic bioscaphold [7].

Case #6A: Interpositional Capsular Autograft for a Failed Silastic Flexible Hinged Implant Involving the First Metatarsophalangeal Joint

As another approach, a painful La Porta designed silastic implant was removed [8, 9]. The hinge was destroyed and the source of pain occurred at the resected edges of the proximal phalanx and metatarsal created impingement (Fig. 6A.1a–c). In this case, an interpositional arthroplasty with a U-shaped capsulotomy flap was performed (Fig. 6A.2a–g). Prior to securing the flap to the plantar first metatarsal head with mini anchors, the canals were filled with ADM after canal preparation with a burr to stimulate endosteal bleeding (Fig. 6A.3a–c)

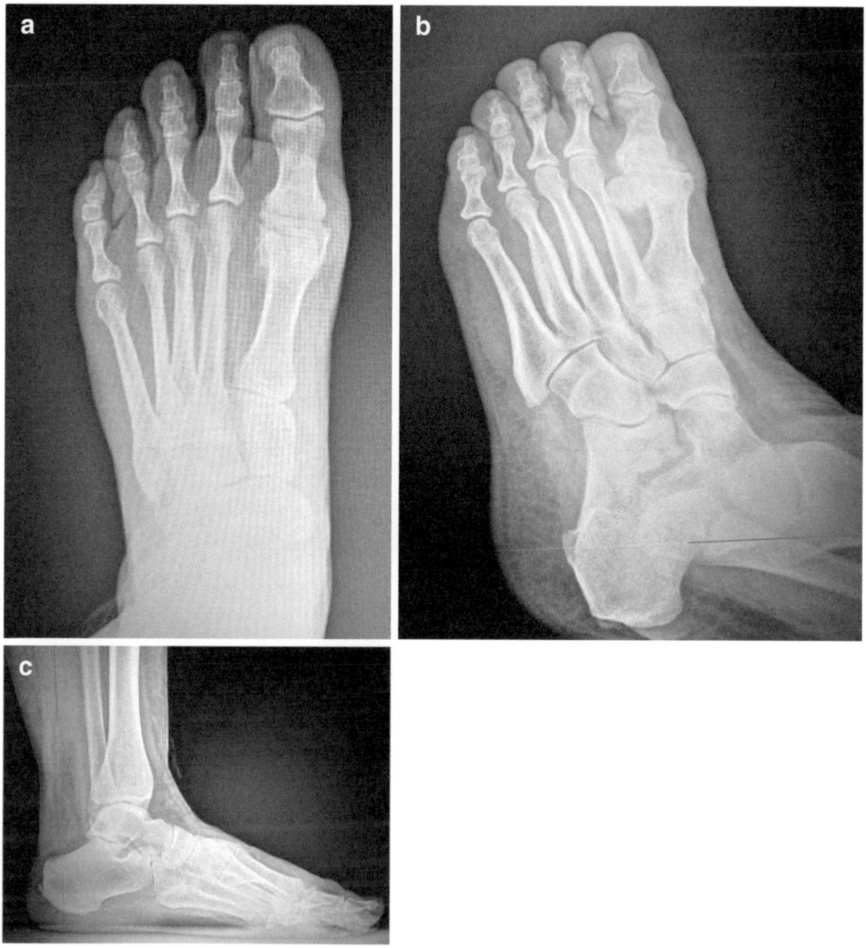

Fig. 6A.1 Preoperative radiographs (**a**) indicated implant breakage (**b**) loss of hallux length (**c**) and purchase of hallux

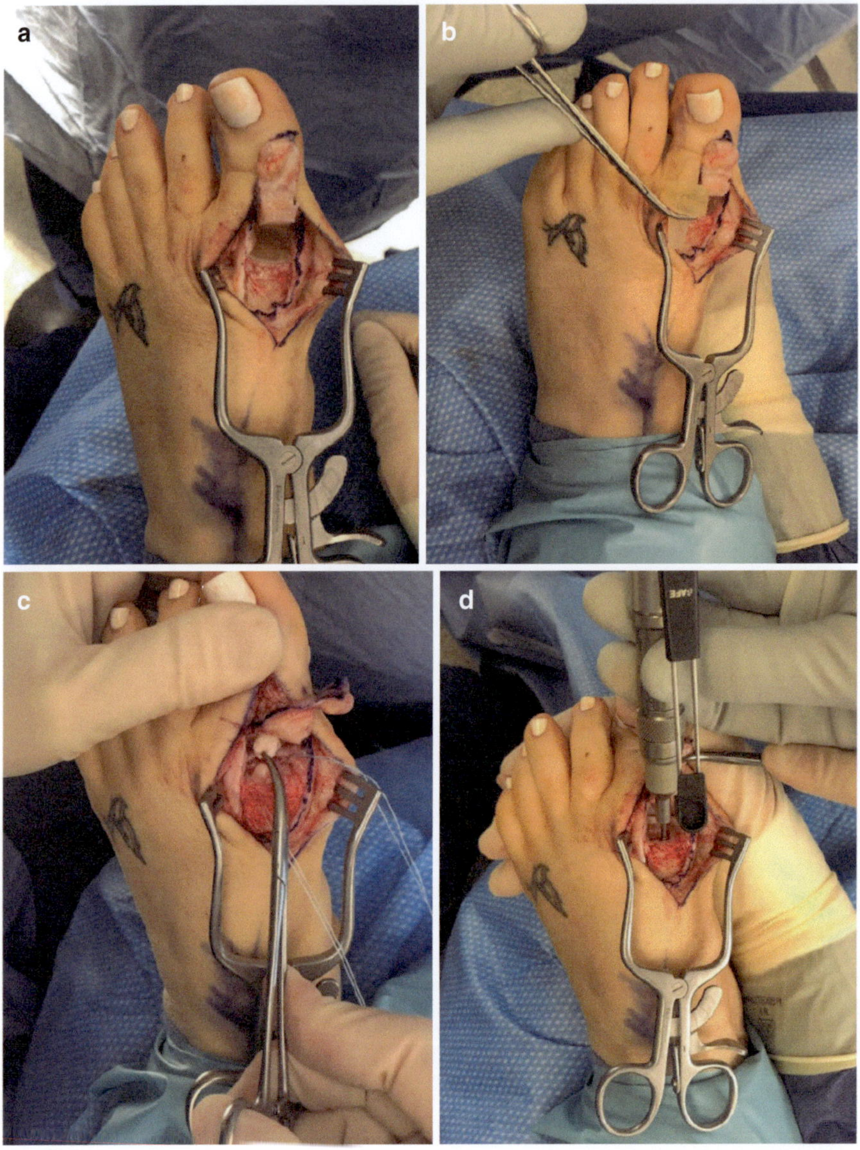

Fig 6A.2 (**a**) Creation of proximal capsular flap from first metatarsal, left. (**b**) Mobilization of plantar plate, left. (**c**) Mobilization of FHL, left. (**d**) Preparation of intramedullary canals. (**e**) Suture anchors secured to plantar first metatarsal. (**f**) Incorporating plantar plate to FHL prior to capsular autograft suture. (**g**) Interposition of proximal capsular autograft

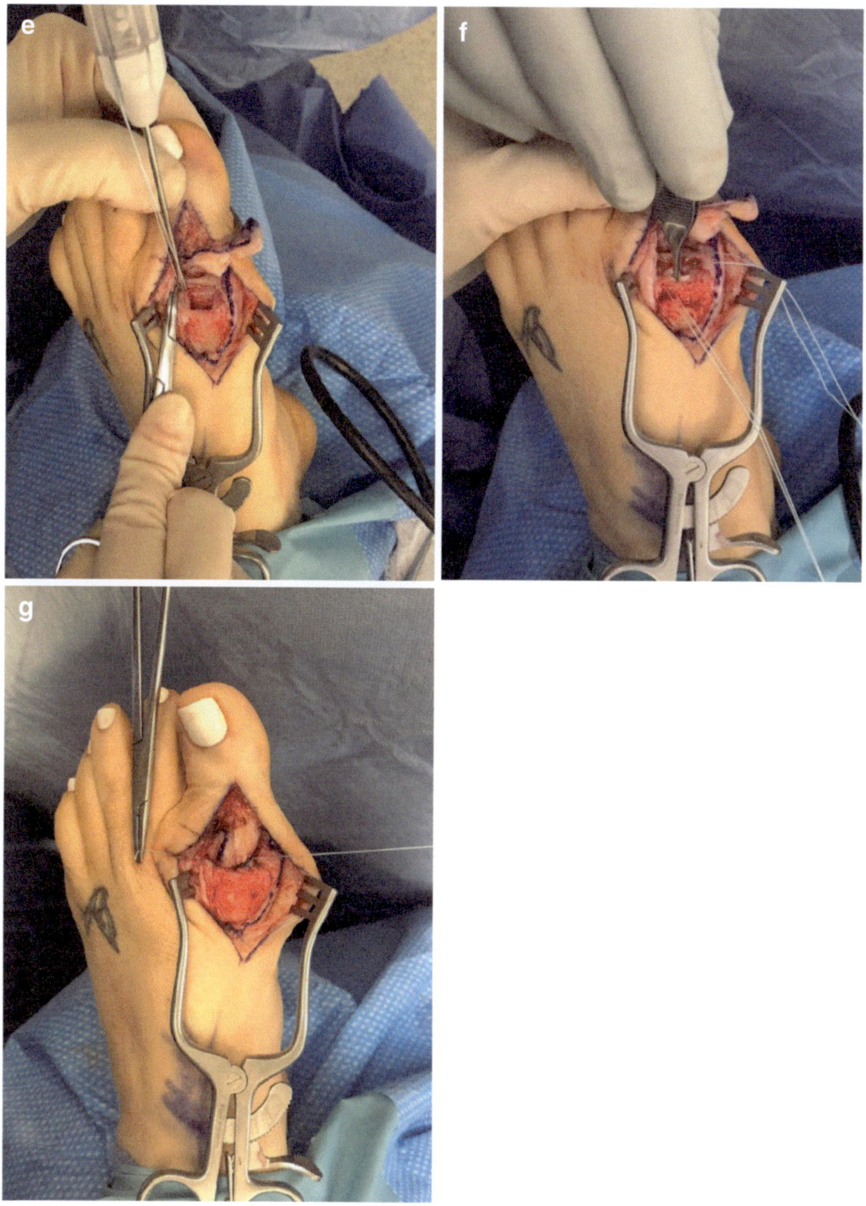

Fig. 6A.2 (continued)

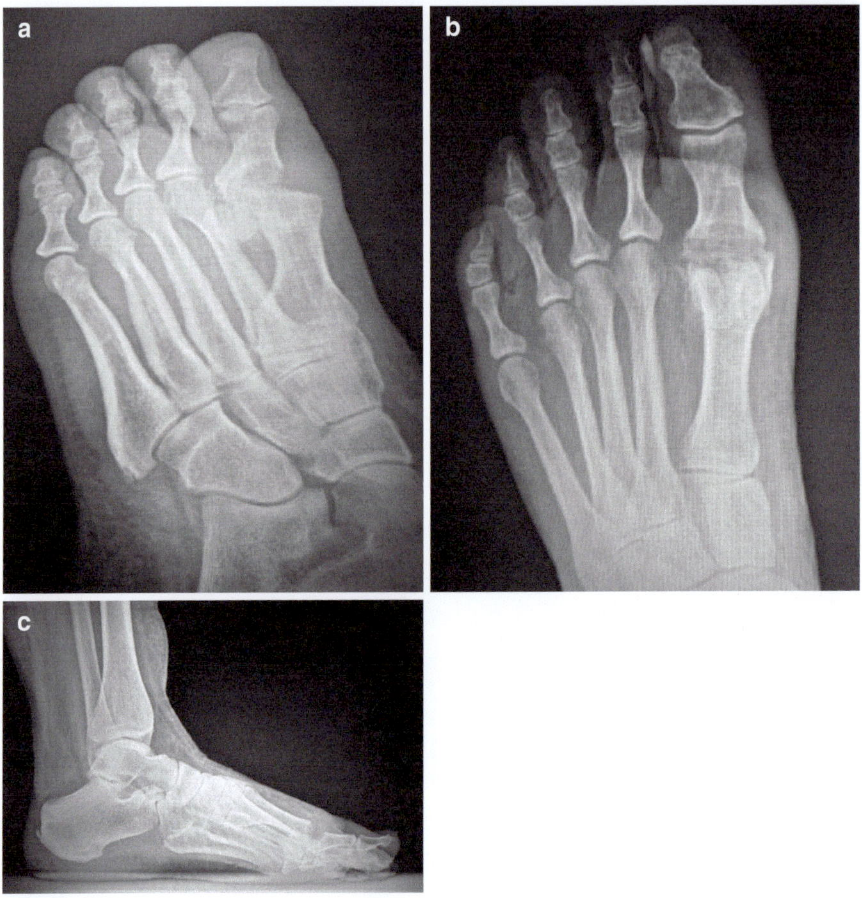

Fig. 6A.3 Post operative radiographs (**a**, **b**) indicating restoration of joint space, (**c**) hallux length and realignment in the sagittal plane

References

1. Chan F, Bowlby MA, Christensen JC. Medial column biomechanics: nonsurgical and surgical implications. Clin Podiatr Med Surg. 2019;37(1):39–51.
2. Kunnasegaran R, Thevendran G. Hallux Rigidus: nonoperative treatment and orthotics. Foot Ankle Clin. 2015;20(3):401–12.
3. Hamid KS, Parekh SG. Clinical presentation and management of Hallux Rigidus. Foot Ankle Clin. 2015;20(3):391–9.
4. Lam A, Chan JJ, Surace MF, Vulcano E. Hallux rigidus: how do I approach it? World J Orthop. 2017;8(5):364–71.
5. Lee J, So E, Logan DB. Conversion of first metatarsophalangeal joint arthrodesis to Interpositional arthroplasty with acellular dermal matrix for first ray ulceration: a case report. J Foot Ankle Surg. 2020;59(3):634–7.

6. Hollawell S, Moen R, Coleman M, Carson M. Osteochondral fresh allograft transfer to address osteochondral defect of the first metatarsal head in early hallux Limitus. J Foot Ankle Surg. 2021;60(1):157–62.
7. Hyer CF, Granata JD, Berlet GC, Lee TH. Interpositional arthroplasty of the first metatarso-phalangeal joint using a regenerative tissue matrix for the treatment of advanced hallux rigidus: 5-year case series follow-up. Foot Ankle Specialist. 2012;5(4):249–52.
8. Dobbs B. LaPorta great toe implant. Long-term study of its efficacy. J Am Podiatry Assoc. 1990;80(7):370–3. [insert in alternative case during discussion of laPorta]
9. Farnworth C, Haggard S, Nahmias MC, Dobbs B. The LaPorta great toe implant. A preliminary study of its efficacy. J Am Podiatry Assoc. 1986;76(11):625–30.

Case #7: Management of Brachymetapody with Multiple Metatarsal Osteotomies and Autograft

7

Case Presentation

This is a 37-year-old white female presents with a history of congenital shortening of her digits (toes) 3 and 4, right foot [1]. She did not seek medical treatment until she began to develop forefoot pain. This occurred as nucleated intractable plantar keratosis (IPK) sub second and fifth metatarsal of the left foot. She had them debrided professionally and wore custom made orthosis for the past 4 years. She opted for surgical correction for this reason. She was also very interested in establishing a normal appearing foot.

Diagnosis and Assessment

Clinically, the patient noted IPKs involving the sub second and fifth metatarsal heads of the left foot [2]. She had considerable shortening of the third and fourth digits [3]. Right foot radiographs noted hypoplasia of the third and fourth metatarsals with normal proximal, middle, and distal phalangeal length. Her remaining joint structures were biomechanically normal (Fig. 7.1a, b).

Management

Due to the presence of two congenitally hypoplastic metatarsals (brachymetapody), a decision was made to shorten metatarsals 2 and 5 by removing cylindrical wedges of 5 mm of bone [4]. This was determined by measurement of preoperative radiographs. An osteotomy was then created at the distal metaphyseal diaphyseal junction (neck) of metatarsals 3 and 4. The 5 mm wedges were then inserted into the

H. J. Visser, *Challenges in Foot and Ankle Reconstructive Surgery*,
https://doi.org/10.1007/978-3-031-07893-4_7

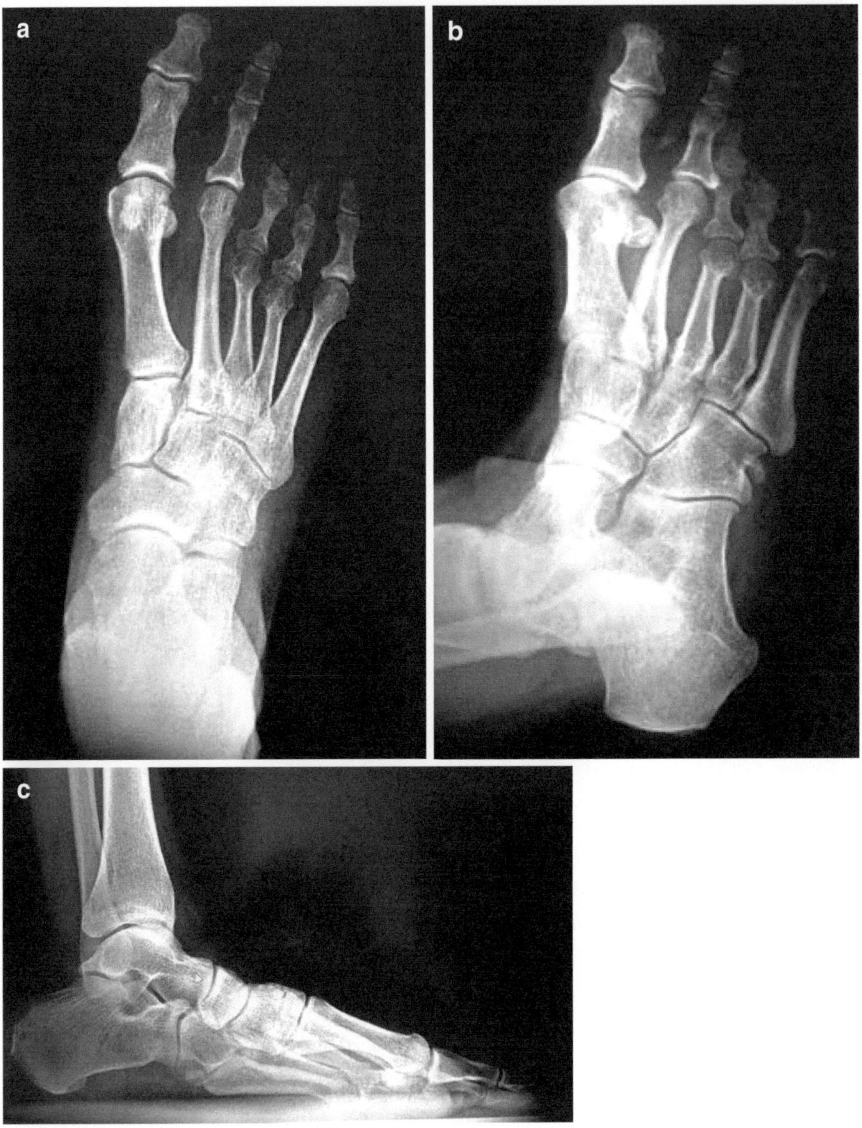

Fig. 7.1 (**a–c**) Presence of congenitally short third and fourth metatarsals, right foot, demonstrating brachymetapody

created metatarsal osteotomies 3 and 4 [5]. They were then stabilized with 0.045 Kirschner (K)-wires. The "donor" site metatarsal osteotomies were then fixated with mini plates and 2.0 mm cortical screws. Upon completion the parabola was restored. The second digit still appeared overly long and was managed with a proximal phalanx head resection and subsequent arthrodesis. The first metatarsal was left intact (Fig. 7.2a, b).

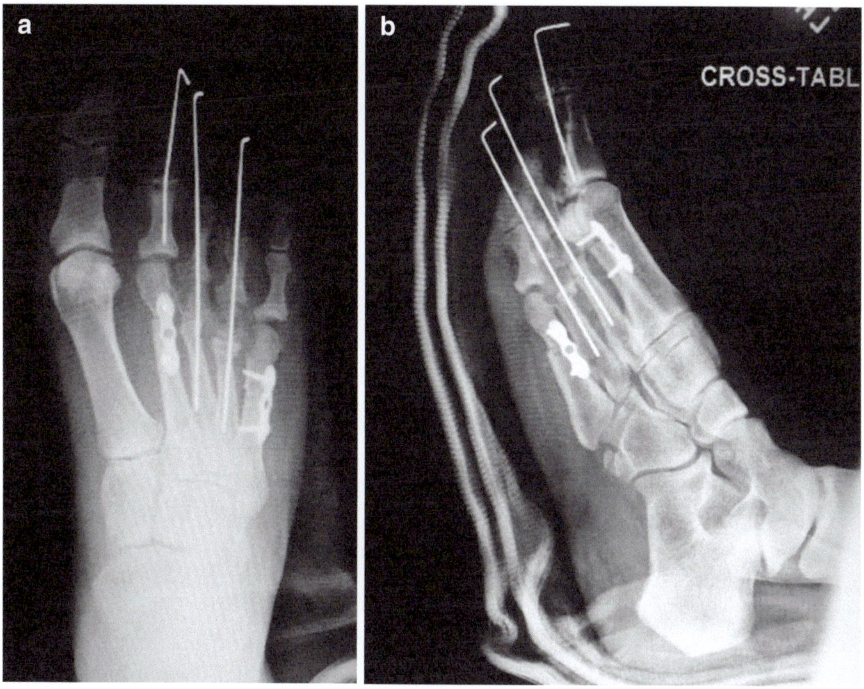

Fig. 7.2 (**a**, **b**) Post-operative shortening; by resection of cylindrical autografts metatarsal 2 and 5; insertion of cylindrical autografts into metatarsals 3 and 4 to gain length; further shortening of the second toe with second PIPJ arthrodesis to restore digital symmetry

Outcome

Postoperatively the patient was kept at NWB for 8 weeks. ROM (range of motion) exercises to the ankle and subtalar joint (STJ) began at 2 weeks. K-wires were removed at 6 weeks (Fig. 7.3a–c). The patient then began WB (weight bearing) in a boot and transitioned to shoe wear at 10 weeks. She did extremely well with healing of the osteotomies and attained solid graft incorporation. She was happy with the cosmetic result and the IPKs resolved.

Clinical Pearls and Pitfalls

Although much has been written about the condition of brachymetatarsia [6, 7] where there is hypoplasia of one metatarsal there is little for consideration of two metatarsals (brachymetapody). In this condition, distraction osteogenesis with a mini external fixator is not a viable option [8]. This is due to the proximity of both metatarsals and violation of blood supply needed for corticotomy distraction histogenesis. A one-stage distraction grafting also poses significant risk to the neurovascular structures.

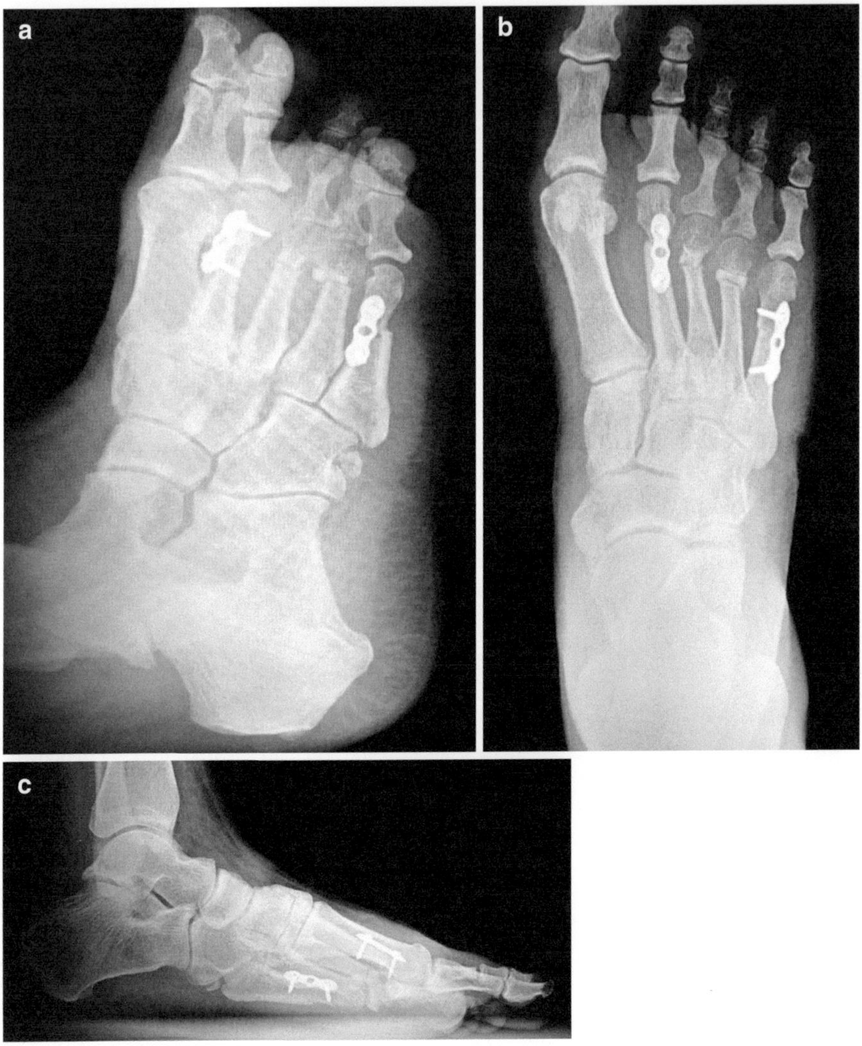

Fig. 7.3 (**a**–**c**) Post-operative at 6 months

Although a chevron type shortening first metatarsal osteotomy can be considered in some cases, it is best to maintain relative length and maintain the windlass mechanism. This serves to protect the adjacent lateral metatarsals. In cases where the digits cosmetically still look asymmetric or overly long, a resection arthroplasty with arthrodesis of the proximal phalanx is a good option. This is more effective than adjusting the osteotomy or graft interposition sites.

References

1. Rampal V, Giuliano F. Forefoot malformations, deformities and other congenital defects in children. Orthop Traumatol Surg Res. 2019;106(1):S115–23.
2. Mann RA, DuVries HL. Intractable plantar keratosis. Orthop Clin North Am. 1973;4(1):67–73.
3. Burger EB, Hovius SER, Burger BJ, Van Nieuwenhoven CA. The Rotterdam foot classification: a classification system for medial polydactyly of the foot. J Bone Joint Surg Am. 2016;98(15):1298–306.
4. Mahan KT. Brachymetapody: case report of surgical correction. J Foot Surg. 1991;30(2):125–32.
5. Biggs EW, Brahm TB, Efron BL. Surgical correction of congenital hypoplastic metatarsals. J Am Podiatr Assoc. 1979;69(4):241–4.
6. Shecaira AP, Fernandes RMP. Brachymetatarsia: one-stage versus two-stage procedures. Foot Ankle Clin. 2019;24(4):677–87.
7. Bartolomei FJ. Surgical correction of brachymetatarsia. J Am Podiatr Assoc. 1990;80(2):76–82.
8. Wilusz PM, Van P, Rupp GR. Complications associated with distraction osteogenesis for the correction of brachymetatarsia: a review of five procedures. J Am Podiatr Assoc. 2007;97(3):189–94.

8 Case #8: Management of Severe Congenital Hallux Varus and Digital Adductus Deformity with 1st Metatarsophalangeal Arthrodesis, Metatarsal Head Resection, and Closed Digital Osteoclasis

Case Presentation

This is a 72-year-old Caucasian female who presents with severe long-standing congenital hallux varus deformity with significant digital adductus and flexus to her right foot. The patient has a history of hypertension and associated cardiovascular disease. A stent was placed in her coronary ascending artery about 3 years prior. She was stable and well managed on Aspirin therapy. Otherwise, the patient was healthy and had no history of rheumatoid arthritis. The patient was quite astonishingly able to function with this severe deformity in open-toed sandals. She was originally from Southern Florida and did not have to wear closed shoe wear for any extended period. She then moved to St. Louis, Missouri to be close to her children. In this temperate climate, she was now forced to wear closed-toed shoes and was unable to tolerate them. Also, her daughter, upon seeing her foot deformity, was aghast and sought medical care.

Diagnosis and Assessment

Right foot radiographs were taken and severe deformity was noted at the digital, midfoot, and rearfoot level. The dorsoplantar view noted severe hallux varus without an associated malleus [1]. The first metatarsophalangeal joint (MPJ) was dislocated in a medial and plantar position (dislocato adductoflexus). The lesser digits, 2–5, were severely adducted (subluxed) at their respective MPJ with proximal interphalangeal joint (PIPJ) contractures (Fig. 8.1a). The lateral view noted significant hallux flexus. There was significant peritalar subluxation of subtalar joint (STJ) with severe midfoot collapse noted by the presence of a navicular-medial cuneiform fault and associated forefoot supinatus (thinning of the tarsus) (Fig. 8.1b).

H. J. Visser, *Challenges in Foot and Ankle Reconstructive Surgery*,
https://doi.org/10.1007/978-3-031-07893-4_8

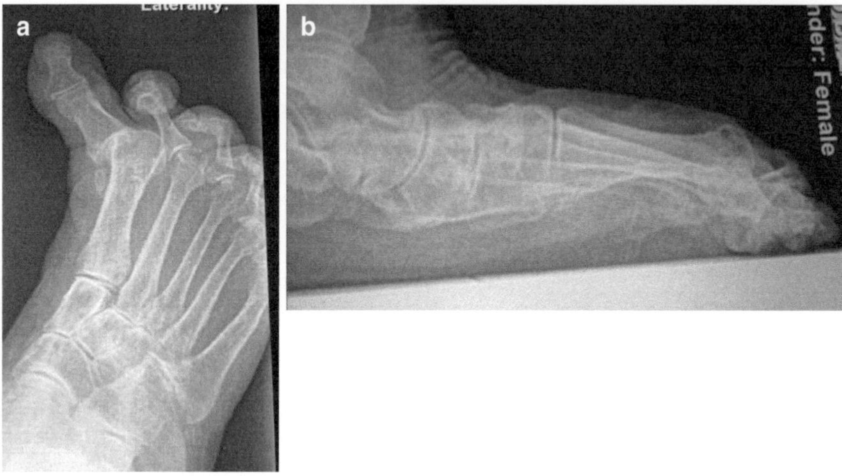

Fig. 8.1 (**a**) Pre-operative congenital hallux varus with secondary digital dislocato adducto flexus of MPJ's 2–5, right foot. (**b**) Peritalar subluxation with presence of forefoot supinatus

Management

Due to her severe varus deformity and associated arthrosis, the first MPJ arthrodesis was performed to stabilize that joint [2]. Metatarsal head resections were performed to correct digital deformity. There were no associated plantar callosities clinically. The lesser digits were stabilized by "closed osteoclasis" and percutaneous 0.062″ Kirschner wire stabilization (Fig. 8.2a–d) [3]. The patient and family did not want rearfoot and subtalar joint correction due to her age. Their aim was simply to allow her to wear closed shoe wear.

The patient was permitted to weight bear in a CAM boot with crutch assistance. Weight bearing being primarily concentrated to the heel. She also used a walker for assistance. At 3 weeks, she was able to bear full weight. The K-wires were removed at 6 weeks and she was then able to transition to shoe wear. She was sent to physical therapy for gait training. The opposite foot was performed 2 months later (Fig. 8.3a, b). After recovery, she was casted for accommodative orthotics for her flatfoot deformity.

Outcome

The patient did quite well with no associated wound problems. She was able, in rapid order, to wear traditional closed shoe wear. As she was not highly ambulatory, accommodation with foot orthotics was adequate for her flatfoot deformity which she states was painful only with increased activity.

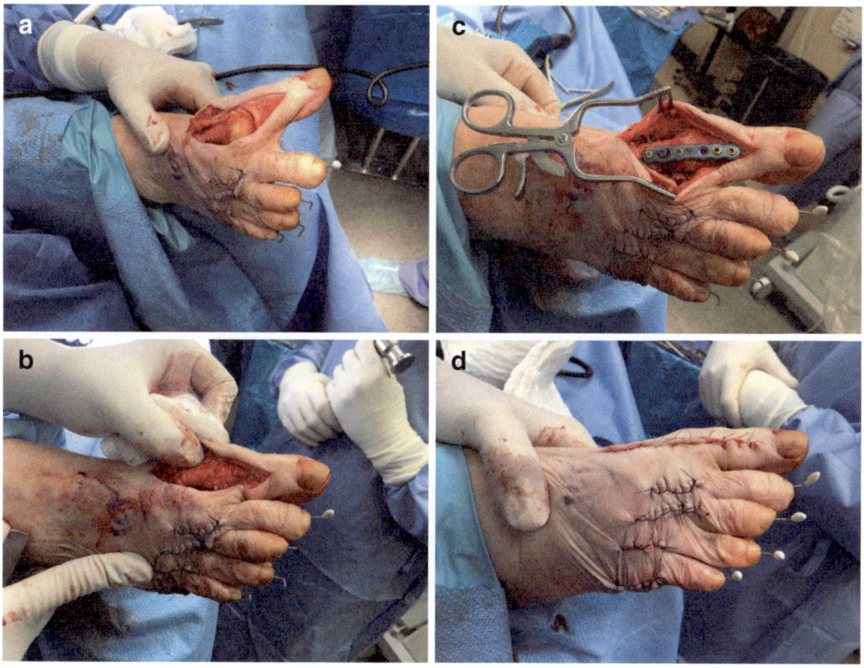

Fig. 8.2 (**a**) Intraoperative hallux varus; Digits aligned to remaining met shafts with 0.062″ k-wire. (**b**) Preparation and reduction of first MPJ, right foot (**c**) first MPJ arthrodesis with 3.0 mm locking plate. (**d**) Post-operative appearance first MPJ arthrodesis, pan metatarsal head resection with alignment to metatarsal shafts with 0.062″ K wires, closed digital osteoclasis performed on digits 2–5 prior to K wire fixation

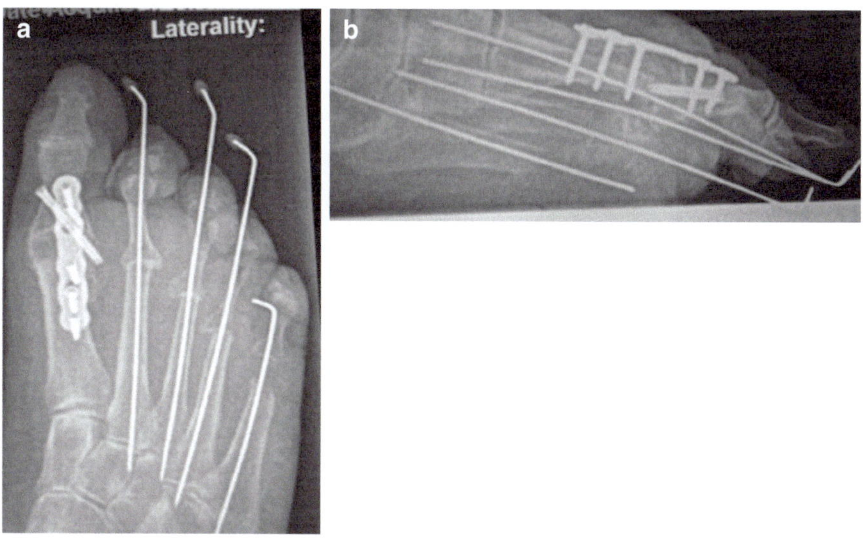

Fig. 8.3 (**a** and **b**) Post-operative alignment

Clinical Pearls and Pitfalls

This represents a very interesting case of severe forefoot deformity that was ignored for years with no prior history of surgery. On first appearance, review clinically and radiographically indicated the possibility of rheumatoid arthritis. Systemic Lupus Erythematosus (SLE) is known to cause significant joint destabilization by synovitis damaging the periarticular capsuloligamentous structures [4]. It does not cause joint destruction or erosions and the patient's MPJ deformities could simulate this. However, her serology was negative.

Long-standing congenital hallux varus can progress to a complete dislocation as can be seen in this patient. Once the tibial sesamoid is dislocated medial to the first metatarsal head, it creates a significant intrinsic imbalance making the abductor hallucis and medial head of the flexor hallucis brevis powerful deforming forces [5]. The adductor hallucis muscle is incapable of countering this force. The long digital flexor (FDL) then, due to its oblique pull created by the peritalar subluxation, is able to pull the digits plantarward (flexus) to overcome the elevated supinated midfoot and maintain floor contact.

Closed osteoclasis where the digits are manually corrected by forcibly plantarflexing the digits at the PIPJ avoids an open arthrodesis [6, 7]. An open digital procedure places further stress on the digital vessels where a proximal metatarsal head resection has been performed. The closed manipulation ruptures the plantar PIPJ capsuloligamentous structures and may fracture at the proximal phalangeal neck in osteopenic bone. Occasionally, the plantar skin at the PIPJ level may tear by being forced and manipulated into a straightened and corrected position. This easily heals by secondary intent. No attempt should be made to suture this if it occurs.

References

1. Abousayed M, Kwon JY. Hallux claw toe. Foot Ankle Clin. 2013;19(1):59–63.
2. Shim JS, Lim TK, Koh KH, Lee DK. Surgical treatment of congenital hallux varus. Clin Orthop Surg. 2014;6(2):216–22.
3. Graney C, Thorud JC, Murdoch D. Osteoclasis for the treatment of recalcitrant diabetic forefoot ulceration: a case study. Int J Lower Extrem Wounds. 2017;16(1):51–5.
4. Stewart S, Brenton-Rule A, Dalbeth N, Aiyer A, Frampton C, Rome K. Foot and ankle characteristics in systemic lupus erythematosus: a systematic review and meta-analysis. Semin Arthritis Rheum. 2018;48(5):847–59.
5. Bancroft LW, Anderson RB. Radiologic case study. Traumatic dislocation of the tibial sesamoid of the hallux. Orthopedics. 2010,33(9):618.
6. Nash WJ, Al-Nammari S, Khan WS, Pengas IP. Surgical management of the forefoot in patients with rheumatoid arthritis—a review article. Open Orthop J. 2015;9(1):78–83.
7. Jaakkola JI, Mann RA. Managing foot and ankle problems in RA: early treatment should focus on prevention and palliative care. J Musculoskelet Med. 2005;22(1):30–6.

Case #9: Rheumatoid and Psoriatic Forefoot Deformity: First MPJ Arthrodesis, Metatarsal Head Reduction with Hoffman Incision and Closed Digital Osteoclasis

9

Case Presentation

A 58-year-old female presents with a long-term history of rheumatoid and psoriatic arthritis. She remembers being diagnosed at the age of 8. She is currently on Enbrel and 10mg of prednisone daily. She has extremely painful plantar callosities and states that she walks primarily on her heels due to the pain. Her ambulation is greatly limited due to her foot pain. She has had no major joint surgeries but has had multiple surgeries on her hands. She was on oral vitamin D3.

Diagnosis and Assessment

Her physical examination noted good vascular perfusion distally with her dorsalis pedis and posterior tibial pulses being 2/4 bilaterally. Neurologically, there were no deficits noted. Dermatologically, she demonstrated large psoriatic plaques affecting the dorsum of the foot and extensively covering her lower legs (Fig. 9.1a). She had nucleated callosities located plantar to the metatarsal heads 2–5. The metatarsal heads were palpable directly under the skin (Fig. 9.1b). She has severe rigid hammertoe deformities with complete destruction and dislocation of the metatarsophalangeal joints (MPJs). On her radiographs, the right foot notes severe lesser MPJ and digital deformity and a relatively rectus first MPJ (Fig. 9.2a–c). The left foot, however, shows similar lesser MPJ and digital deformity involvement, but there is also a severe hallux abductovalgus deformity with complete dislocation of the first MPJ (Fig. 9.3a–c).

H. J. Visser, *Challenges in Foot and Ankle Reconstructive Surgery*,
https://doi.org/10.1007/978-3-031-07893-4_9

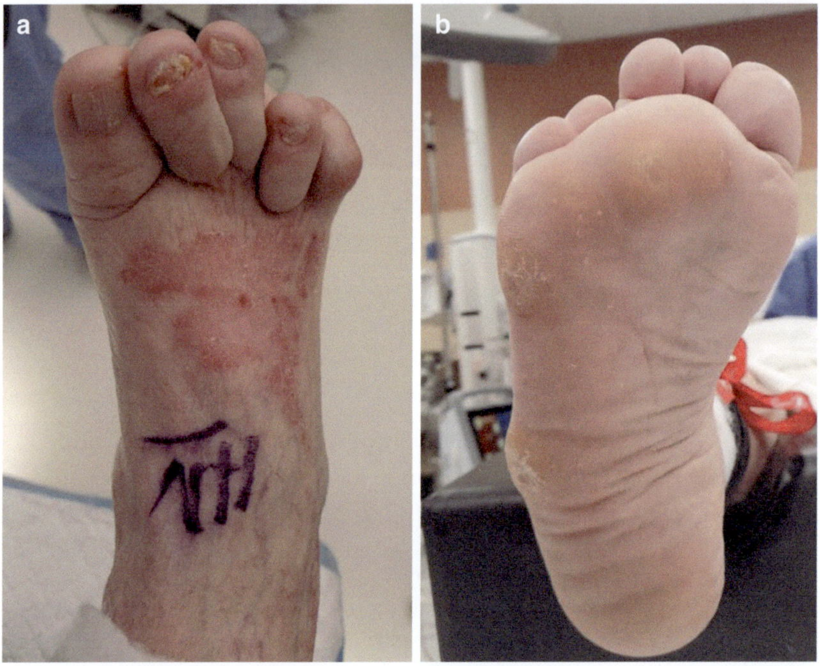

Fig. 9.1 (**a**) Severe dorsal psoriatic plaque formation over the dorsal right foot. (**b**) Severe plantar metatarsal head lesions due to MPJ dislocation from combined rheumatoid arthritis and psoriatic arthritis, right foot

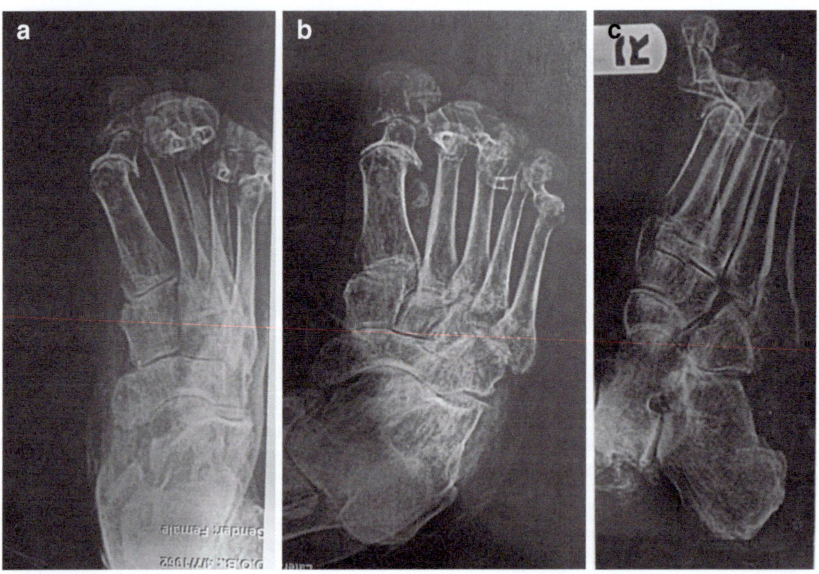

Fig. 9.2 (**a–c**) First MPJ and lesser MPJ involvement secondary to rheumatoid arthritis and psoriatic arthritis, right foot

Management

The procedure chosen was a modified Hoffmann procedure which utilizes a plantar approach for resection of metatarsal heads 2–5 (Fig. 9.4a–d) [1]. This approach was chosen in order to avoid the extensive area of psoriatic plaque involvement of the dorsum of the foot. A dorsal first MPJ approach was used to perform the first MPJ arthrodesis. The plaques did not extend into this area (Fig. 9.4d). The right foot involved curettage and drilling of the remaining subchondral bone and application of a dorsal locking plate and lag screw for fixation (Fig. 9.5a). The left foot was done 8 weeks later and required a planal form of first MPJ arthrodesis to realign the

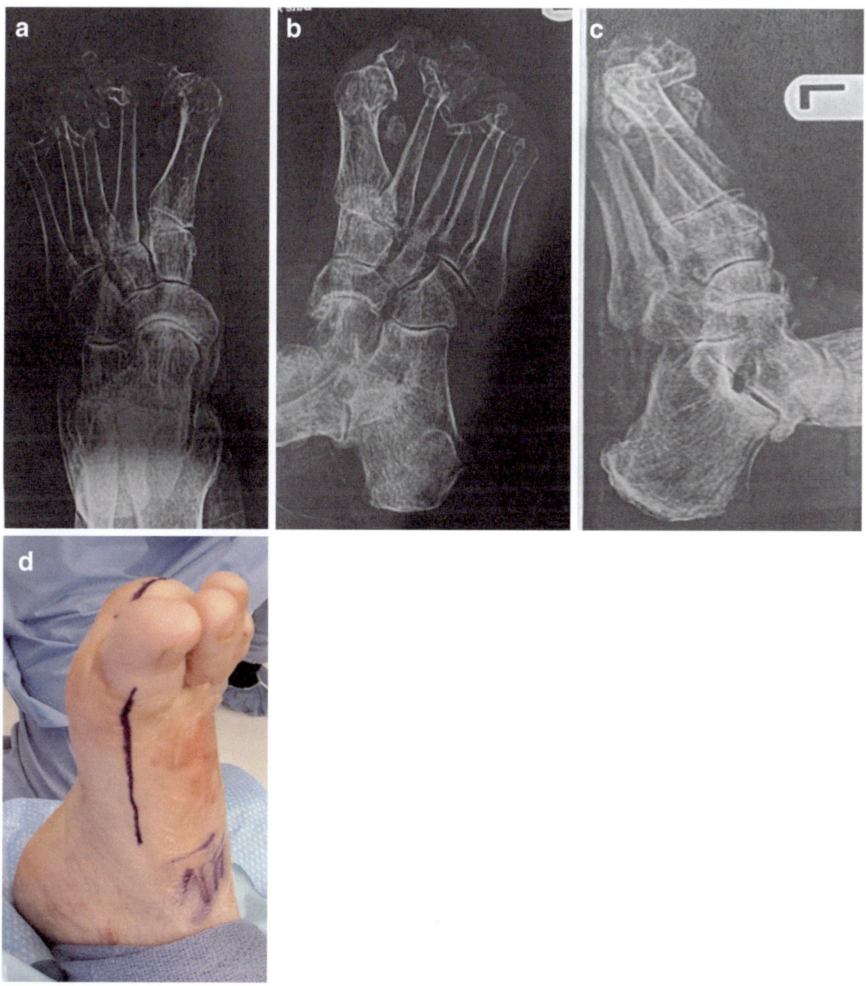

Fig. 9.3 (**a–c**) Severe destruction first MPJ and lesser MPJs; Note hypoplastic proximal phalanx, created by premature growth plate closure and to juvenile state of inflammatory disease state. (**d**) Dorsal first MPJ approach avoiding dorsal dermatological plaque formation

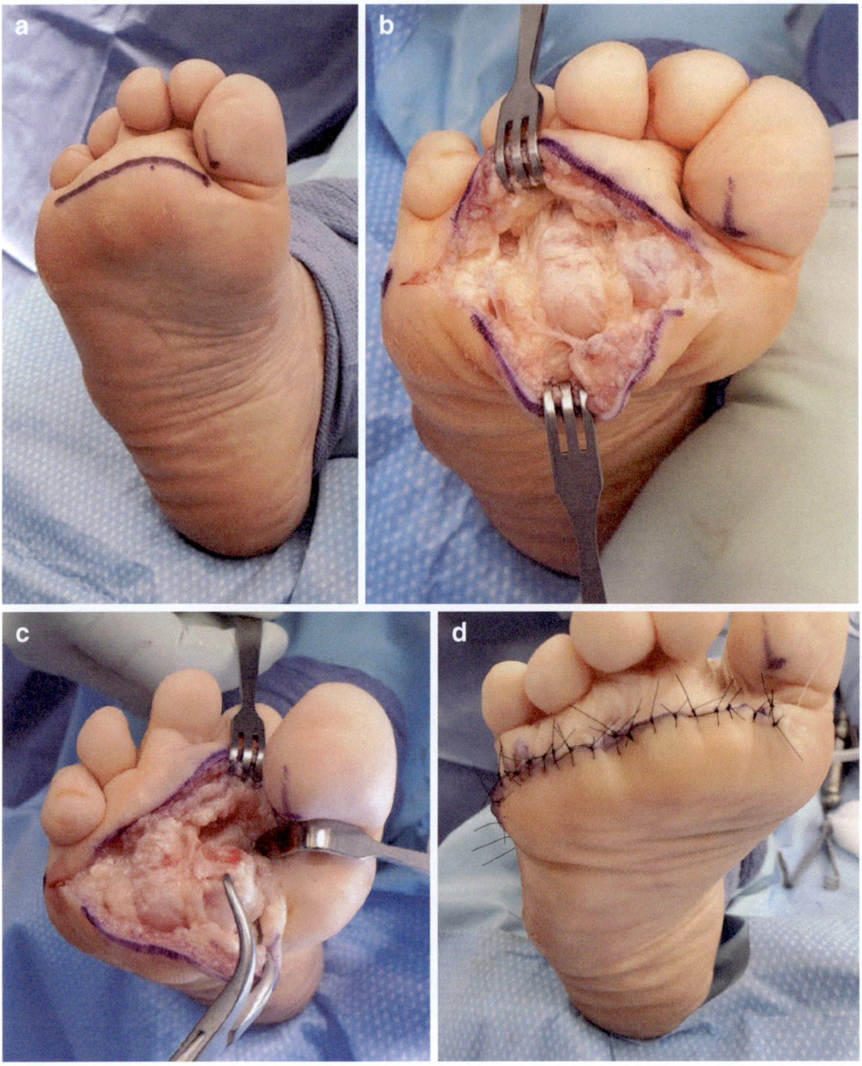

Fig. 9.4 (**a**) Plantar Hoffman incision. (**b**) Exposure of metatarsal heads plantarly. (**c**) Resection of metatarsal heads for forefoot arthroplasty. (**d**) Final closure of plantar incision

severely dislocated first MPJ (Fig. 9.5b). A locking plate and 0.062" K-wire fixation was utilized here. The hammertoes were managed by closed osteoclasis (Fig. 9.6a–c). She was allowed to ambulate with a walker in a postoperative shoe with weight bearing being focused to the heel. Something she had done for most of her life. Sutures were left for 3 weeks. She returned to normal shoe wear at 6 weeks. As the Enbrel and corticosteroids were not stopped as strictly per her rheumatologist, careful monitoring of wound status and signs of infection were mandatory [2].

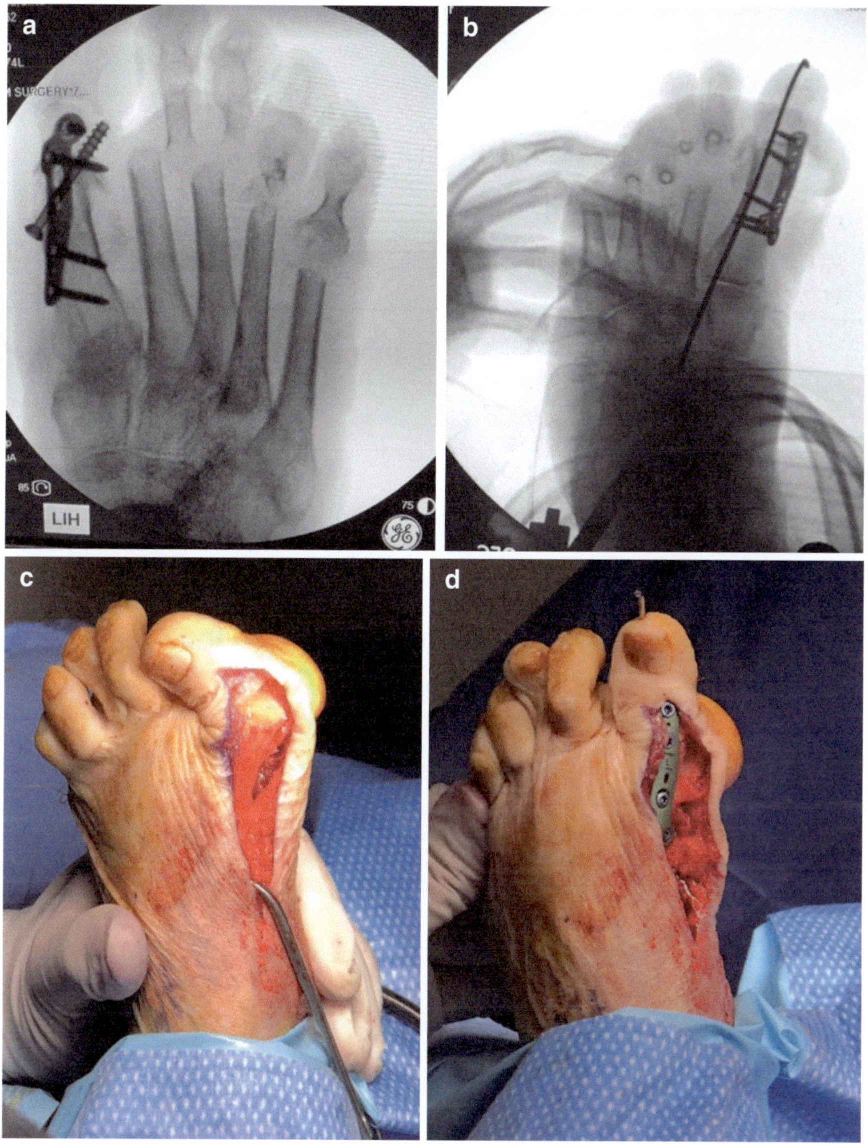

Fig. 9.5 (**a**) First MPJ arthrodesis, right foot with forefoot arthroplasty; (**b–d**) first MPJ arthrodesis, left foot with forefoot arthroplasty

Outcome

The patient had the right foot performed initially. Surprisingly, she had no wound issues. The left foot, however, had an issue with a wound dehiscence of the distal portion of the first MPJ incision. There were no signs of infection, however, the

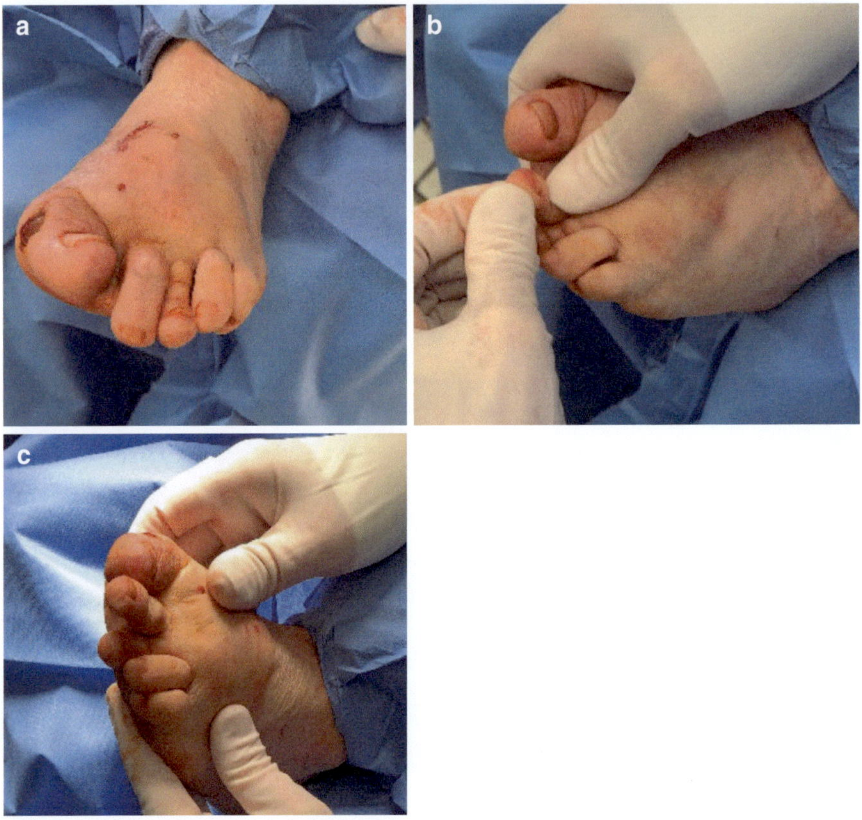

Fig. 9.6 (**a**) appearance of hammer toes 2–5 (**b**) closed osteoclasis technique for correction of hammer toe deformity (**c**) post osteoclasis correction of the second digit, left foot

locking plate and screws were exposed due to a full-thickness dehiscence. Removal of internal fixation was required at this time. This led to a nonunion, but it ended as a painless arthrofibrosis. The wound healed completely.

Clinical Pearls and Pitfalls

In this case, the rheumatoid arthritis foot is complicated by superimposed psoriatic arthritis and dermatologic conditions that can pose a tangled challenge [3]. It is quite rare to see a patient manifest this degree of deformity with rheumatoid and psoriatic arthritis, thanks to advances in pharmacologic agents such as DMARDs (disease modifying anti-rheumatic drugs) and biologic response modifiers (BRM).

In this case, a plantar (Hoffmann) approach was utilized to avoid the extensive plaque formation due to her psoriatic skin condition [4]. Incisions involving plaques greatly increase the risk of infection. It can also produce the problematic Koebner phenomenon [5]. Plaques carry very high levels of bacteria. The plantar approach allows easy access to the metatarsal heads. It is an approach many surgeons are uncomfortable with. Initial subcutaneous dissection is performed to capsule. In this case, there was no subcutaneous tissue but just dermal skin. All further dissection at the capsular level is longitudinal. Resection of the metatarsal heads requires careful palpation. With metatarsal declination, the resection site can be quite deep in the soft tissue and may require fluoroscopic assistance [6].

Management of hallux valgus was a difficult issue on the left foot. Due to her juvenile involvement, she had an extremely small, atrophic proximal phalanx. This was secondary to premature growth plate closure created by her inflammatory disease state. Her hallux was completely dislocated and positioned on the lateral aspect of the first metatarsal head. Cup and cone reamers couldn't be used due to her severe osteopenia. A planal approach was chosen which involves resecting bone to allow soft tissue shortening primarily on the metatarsal side to realign the hallux. It is advantageous at this point to use an intramedullary K-wire to position the joint in anatomic alignment. A locking plate was then utilized. A lag screw proves ineffective here due to bone quality. The K-wire must be retained to assist the locking plate. The locking slot in the plate can offer some form of joint compression.

Concerning hammertoes, the amount of dissection if an arthrodesis is chosen can challenge the neurovascular structures. Thus, a manual osteoclasis is performed. This is accomplished by "manual force" to straighten the digit.

References

1. Hoffmann P. An operation for severe grades of contracted or clawed toes. 1911. Clin Orthop Relat Res. 1997;340:4–6.
2. Wang AS, Armstrong EJ, Armstrong AW. Corticosteroids and wound healing: clinical considerations in the perioperative period. Am J Surg. 2013;206(3):410–7.
3. Saini R, Shupack JL. Psoriasis: to cut or not to cut, what say you? Dermatol Surg. 2003;29(7):735–40.
4. Hugar DW, Gucfa CV. Pan metatarsal head resections: the Hoffman procedure. J Am Podiatr Assoc. 1974;64(12):983–6.
5. Alolabi N, White CP, Cin AD. The Koebner phenomenon and breast reconstruction: psoriasis eruption along the surgical incision. Can J Plast Surg. 2011;19(4):143–4.
6. McGlamry ED, Bernbach M. (1986) Panmetatarsal head resections: plantar approach. In: McGlamry ED, editor. Surgery of the foot and leg. Tucker, GA: Doctors Hospital Podiatric Education and Research Institute. 1986;p. 156–60.

Case #10: Fat Pad Augmentation with Acellular Dermal Allomatrix Involving Submetatarsal Heads 2 and 3

10

Case Presentation

This is a 52-year-old Caucasian female who presents with chronic submetatarsal head metatarsalgia 2 and 3 of the right foot. The patient gives a history of injections of corticosteroids plantarly for capsulitis. She has no significant medical issues.

Diagnosis and Assessment

On manual exam, there was noted atrophy of the plantar fat pad involving the sub second and third metatarsal head location. She did not have associated hammertoe deformity. Her plantar plate was intact with a negative Lachman test [1]. Radiographically, the metatarsal parabola was preserved.

Management

Due to the fact that there were no significant biomechanical considerations, a fat pad augmentation procedure with an acellular dermal matrix was chosen. A transverse incision was made just distal to the metatarsal heads 2 and 3. A plantar condylectomy was performed. A parachute technique was utilized securing the acellular dermal matrix subcutaneously [2]. It was placed directly over the metatarsal head capsular surfaces. It was secured with a 2.0 vicryl stitch. A 3.3mm allomatrix dermal graft was chosen (Fig. 10.1a–d). The patient was kept non-weight bearing for 3 weeks on a knee walker. The sutures were removed and full weight bearing was initiated.

H. J. Visser, *Challenges in Foot and Ankle Reconstructive Surgery*,
https://doi.org/10.1007/978-3-031-07893-4_10

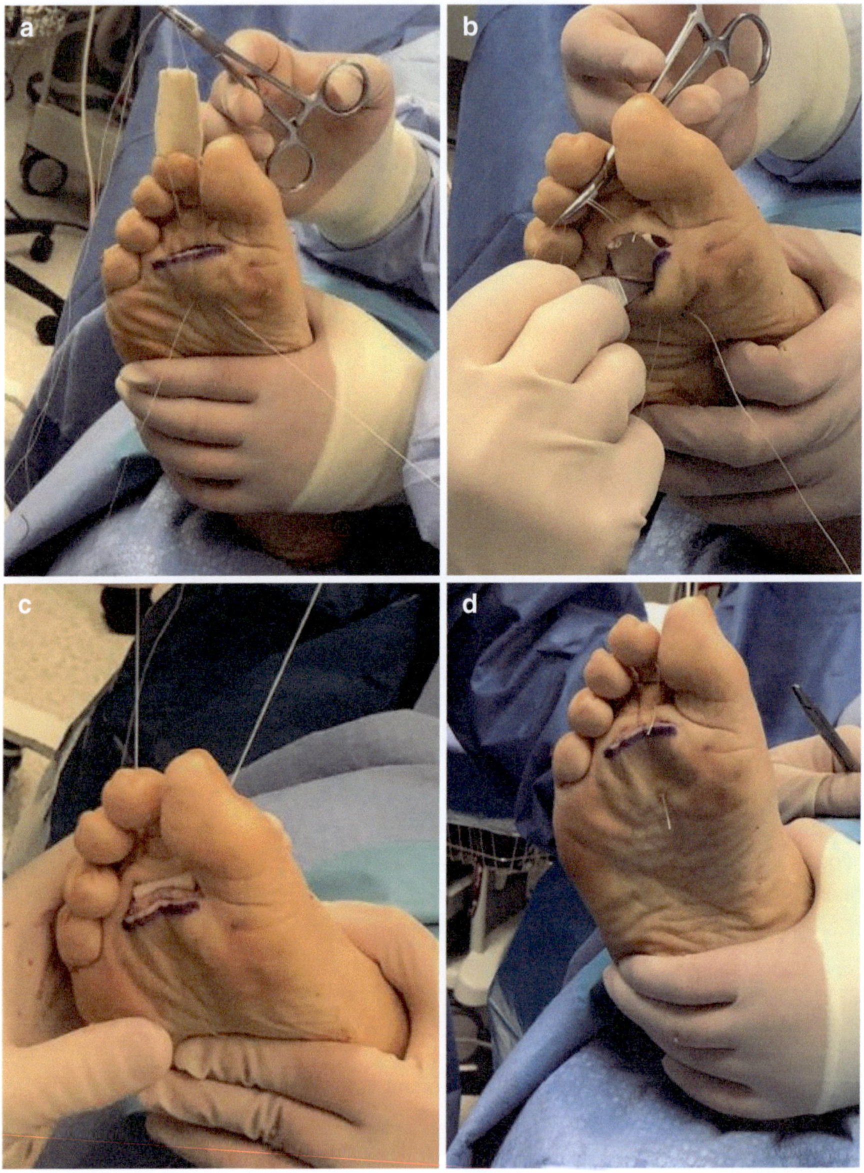

Fig. 10.1 (**a**) 3.3 mm acellular dermal matric secured with 2-0 vicryl; subcutaneous plantar pouch created over capsules of metatarsal heads 2 and 3, right foot. (**b**) Parachute technique to pull allograft into subcutaneous pocket. (**c**) Securing acellular dermal matric graft; Positioning by tension of proximal 2-0 vicryl stitch. (**d**) Complete resurfacing of plantar metatarsal heads as a form of plantar fat pad augmentation; (all four images) Parachute technique utilizing 3.3 mm acellular dermal matrix dermal allograft

Outcome

The patient did very well postoperatively. There was a complaint for the first 3 months of some induration and tenderness. This subsequently resolved. She had full restoration of function and returned to full activity at 4 months.

Clinical Pearls and Pitfalls

Chronic plantar metatarsalgia with fat pad atrophy is a complex condition [3, 4]. The use of fat pad augmentation with an acellular dermal matrix should only be used when there are no significant biomechanical abnormalities [2]. It can be considered, however, when the said deformities are corrected [5].

Use of a plantar condylectomy allows a flat surface over the convex plantar metatarsal head prominence. A careful incision of the plantar plate should be done with care to resecure it with mini sutures. However, there is a risk of a floating toe due to the loss of internal cubic content. Thus, this should only be done if deemed clinically necessary. Thus, only the prominent portion of the condyle should be resected.

Creation of a subcutaneous pocket to pull the graft into position is done with manual digital manipulation at the capsular level. The allomatrix is tagged with 2.0 vicryl stitches at all four corners. The proximal portion is then pulled through like a "parachute" utilizing the two proximal sutures. The distal sutures are then tensioned distally over the metatarsal heads and then secured distal to the incision. This provides proper tension and fills the created subcutaneous pocket. Thus, this serves to restore plantar metatarsal head protection by padding the weight-bearing surfaces of the metatarsal heads.

References

1. Bergeron MC, Ferland J, Malay DS, Lewis SE, Burkmar JA, Giovinco NA. Use of metatarsophalangeal joint dorsal subluxation in the diagnosis of plantar plate rupture. J Foot Ankle Surg. 2019;58(1):27–33.
2. Rocchio TM. Augmentation of atrophic plantar soft tissue with an acellular dermal allograft: a series review. Clin Podiatr Med Surg. 2009;26(4):545–57.
3. Jahss MH, Kummer F, Michelson JD. Investigations into the fat pads of the sole of the foot: heel pressure studies. Foot Ankle. 1992;13(5):227–32.
4. Quirk R. Metatarsalgia Aust Fam Phys. 1996;25(6):863–5.
5. Baron ME, Minteer DM, Gusenoff BR, & Gusenoff JA. (2020);Patient selection for pedal soft tissue augmentation. Aesthet Surg J Open Forum. 2(3): ojaa031.

Part II

The Varus Foot and Ankle

Case #11: Reconstruction of the Lateral Foot Column due to Loss of the Cuboid and Anterior Calcaneus Secondary to Gunshot Trauma with Hemi-Fibular Strut Graft and Reattachment of the Peroneus Brevis Tendon

11

Case Presentation

This a 35-year-old Caucasian male with a progressive adductovarus foot deformity (Fig. 11.1). He gives a history of sustaining a shotgun wound to his left foot, the anterior calcaneus, and cuboid were destroyed. The patient was treated with wound care and debridement of shrapnel. There was no attempt to restore the lateral column of the foot or analyze the peroneus brevis tendon. The patient progressed over a year's time into a severe adductovarus deformity. There was significant gait instability.

Diagnosis and Assessment

The initial radiographs noted loss of the cuboid and the anterior calcaneus by the shotgun blast (Figs. 11.1 and 11.2a, b). There was also complete detachment of the peroneus brevis at its insertion point at the fifth metatarsal base. The peroneus longus was also damaged at the cuboid level. The loss of the lateral column and peroneus brevis/longus function led to an unstable adductovarus foot deformity. The unopposed function of the tibialis posterior muscle accelerated and accentuated the deformity.

Management

The first step included reconstructing the lateral column of the foot. This involved a hemi-fibular autograft which served to re-established lateral column length and correct the forefoot adductus [1]. The peroneus brevis was then reattached to the fifth

H. J. Visser, *Challenges in Foot and Ankle Reconstructive Surgery*,
https://doi.org/10.1007/978-3-031-07893-4_11

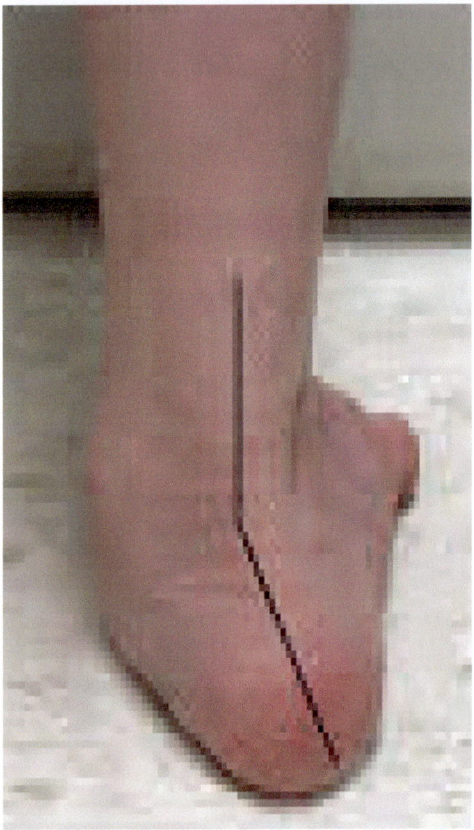

Fig. 11.1 Progressive adducto varus deformity right foot secondary to shotgun injury

metatarsal base using a turn-down technique. The peroneus longus was then inserted into the peroneus brevis tendon [2]. The recurring subtalar joint varus was addressed with an STJ arthrodesis to attempt to create 3° of heel valgus [3]. A fractional lengthening of the tibialis posterior at the myotendinous junction was performed to weaken and re-establish balance about the midfoot (Fig. 11.3) [4].

Outcome

The patient did reasonably well overall. Despite the STJ arthrodesis, however, persistent heel inversion was present. The talocalcaneal angle remained convergent. There was still some persistent heel varus with full weight bearing. He has tolerated it adequately at this juncture, but the need for a calcaneal osteotomy to reduce the calcaneal varus may be needed in the future.

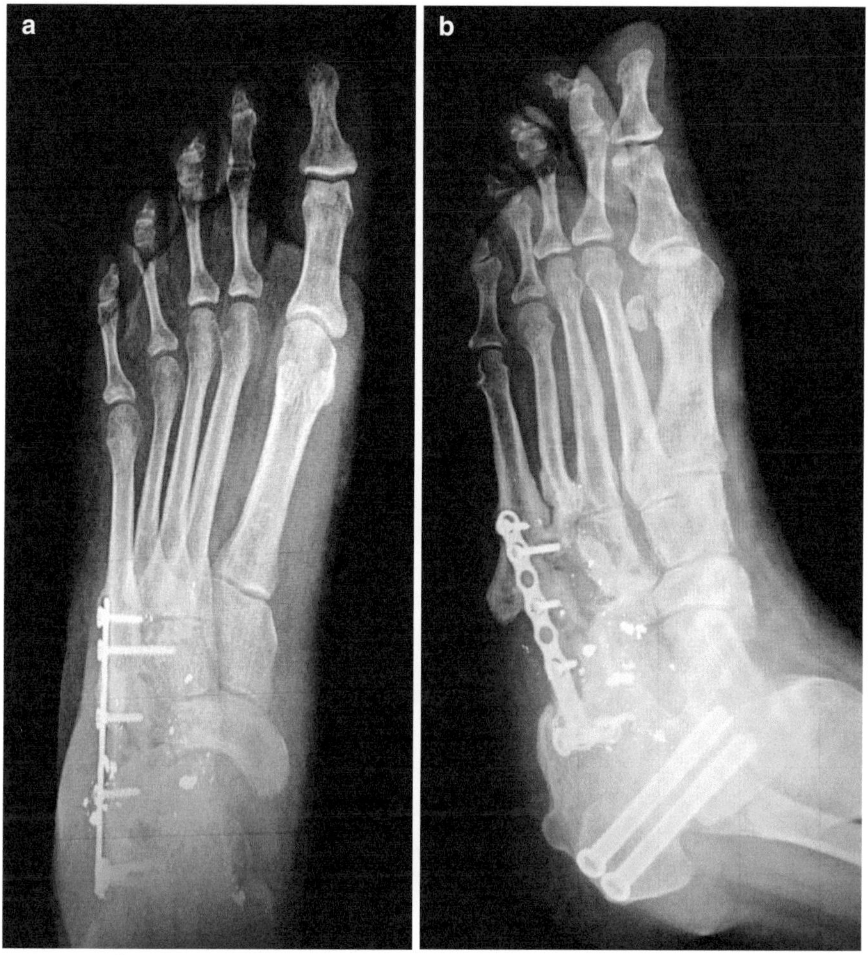

Fig. 11.2 (**a**) Restoration of anterior calcaneal cuboid lateral column with fibular hemi autograft and 3.0 mm locking plate. (**b**) Note residual shrapnel

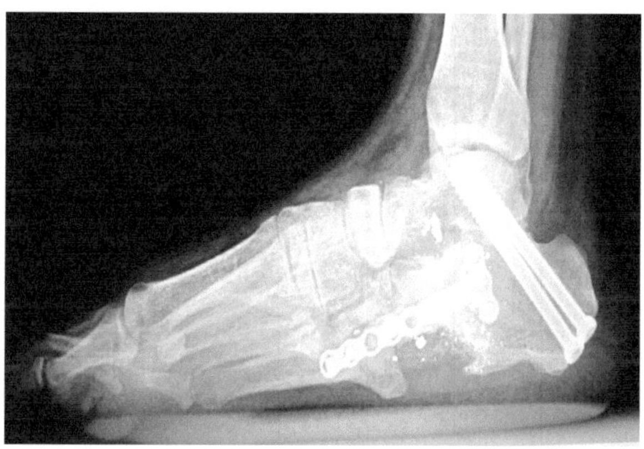

Fig. 11.3 Re-establishment of the midfoot and rearfoot with STJ arthrodesis. This serves to stabilize the rearfoot to the recontructed lateral column

Clinical Pearls and Pitfalls

Loss of function of the oblique midtarsal joint (OMTJ) axis as well as the peroneus brevis/longus tendon function can lead to significant subtalar varus instability. Also, the longitudinal midtarsal joint (LMTJ) axis is allowed to progress into end range adduction and inversion demonstrated at the talonavicular (TN) joint level. This was seen in this case. The issue at hand is that the midfoot and STJ developed a rapid and fixed varus deformity. To address this, an autograft was needed to restore the defect and establish lateral column length. This allowed forefoot adduction and varus to be corrected. The anterior portion of the fibula was used and thus the remaining fibula was left intact as well as the peroneal pulley. Slots were created in the remaining calcaneus and fifth metatarsal base and the fibular autograft used as a strut [5]. Re-establishing muscle balance is critical. This was attained by reattaching the peroneus brevis and longus, as well as, weakening its antagonist, the tibialis posterior by a myotendinous lengthening. A tenotomy or tenectomy is also a consideration. In this case, the peroneus brevis was found retracted to the level of the fibular tip. A turn-down of the tendon was performed. This technique cuts the tendon in half into an anterior and posterior portion and stops 2 cm short of the end of the retracted tendon. The anterior half is then turned down toward the styloid process. This "doubles" its length. The "kink point" was reinforced with suture and tapered. The subtalar joint was rigid and not reducible. An arthrodesis was chosen rather than a calcaneal osteotomy to provide better stability.

References

1. Mendicino RW, Leonheart E, Shromoff P. Techniques for harvesting autogenous bone graft of the lower extremity. J Foot Ankle Surg. 1996;35(5)
2. Li S, Myerson MS. Failure of surgical treatment in patients with Cavovarus deformity: why does this happen and how do we approach treatment? Foot Ankle Clin. 2019;24(2):361–70.
3. Zide JR, Myerson MS. Arthrodesis for the cavus foot: when, where, and how? Foot Ankle Clin. 2013;18(4):755–67.
4. Altuntas AO, Dagge B, Chin TY, Palamara JE, Eizenberg N, Wolfe R, Graham HK. The effects of intramuscular tenotomy on the lengthening characteristics of tibialis posterior: high versus low intramuscular tenotomy. J Child Orthop. 2011;5(3):225–30.
5. Paley D. Principles of deformity correction. Berlin: Springer-Verlag; 2002.

12 Case #12: Loss of Peroneus Brevis Tendon Insertion Secondary to Failed Surgery of the Epimetaphyseal Styloid Process with Subsequent Development of Adductovarus Deformity

Case Presentation

This is a 30-year-old Caucasian female who originally sustained an epimetaphyseal fracture of the fifth metatarsal styloid process, left foot. She has three separate attempts at open reduction, internal fixation (ORIF) of the fracture. It ultimately went on to a nonunion with extensive fragmentation. She presented clinically with an extreme adductovarus deformity that was flexible and reducible. Radiographs on the medial oblique and lateral views showed extensive fragmentation of the styloid process (Fig. 12.1a, b, c). On the anterior–posterior view of the ankle, there was relative extreme varus of the subtalar joint (STJ) and adduction of the midtarsal joint (MTJ). The ankle joint itself was anatomically stable indicated by maintained tibiotalar congruity. The foot demonstrated extreme medial displacement relative to bisection of the tibia.

Diagnosis and Assessment

There were two main issues. The first was the extensive fragmentation of the styloid process from the three prior surgeries. The concern here was osteomyelitis vs avascular necrosis. There were no issues with prior wound healing according to the patient's history. The second was the extreme, but very flexible and reducible adductovarus deformity created by the loss of function of the peroneus brevis secondary to detachment.

H. J. Visser, *Challenges in Foot and Ankle Reconstructive Surgery*,
https://doi.org/10.1007/978-3-031-07893-4_12

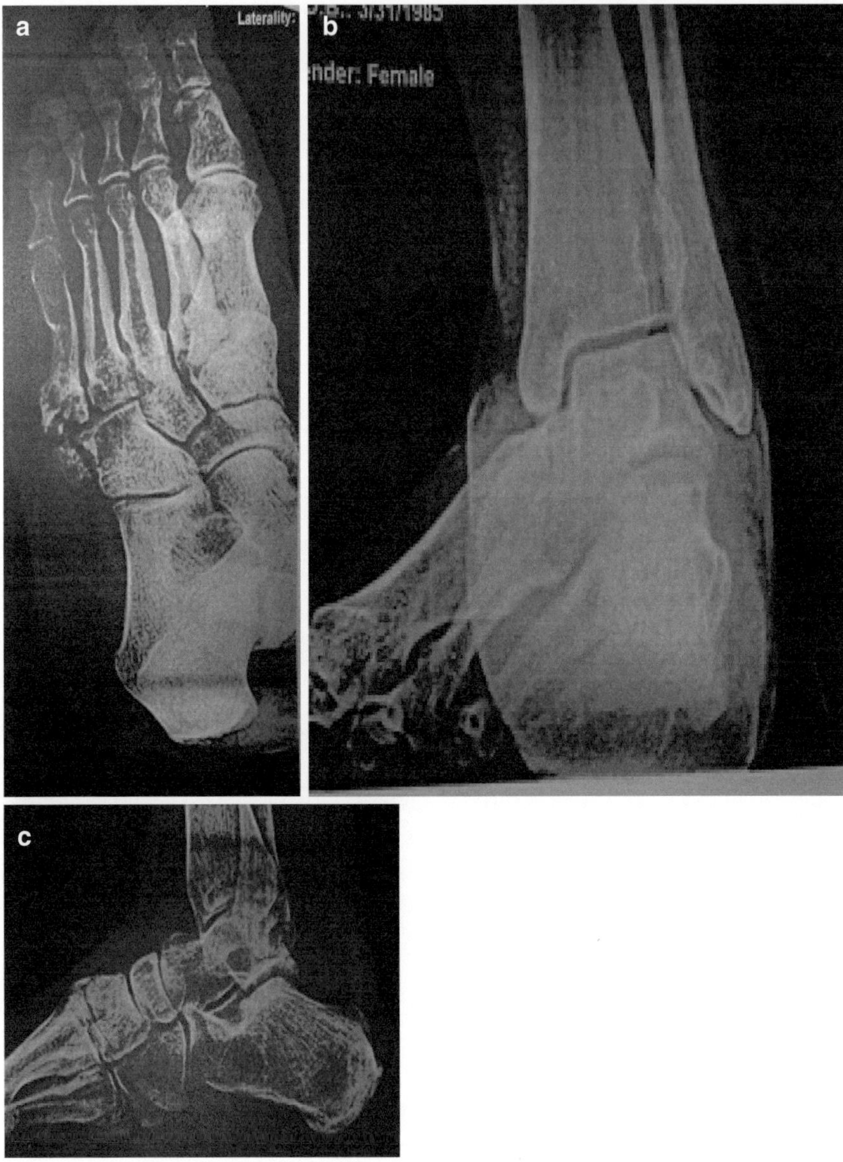

Fig. 12.1 (**a**) Epi-metaphyseal AVN from prior ORIF attempts, left foot. (**b**) Flexible adducto varus deformity accentuated by weight bearing, left foot (**c**) Flexible anterior cavus deformity created by loss of peroneus brevis function

Management

The first step was to resect the fragmented styloid process and send the bone for intraoperative frozen section (Fig. 12.2) [1]. With the results not indicating osteomyelitis, an arthrodesis was created between the remaining diaphyseal remnant of the fifth metatarsal and it's coinciding fourth metatarsal base with two 2.5 headless screws (Fig. 12.3a, b). The peroneus longus was then transferred to the cuboid with an interference screw with the foot in full plantarflexion and abduction (Fig. 12.4a, b) [2]. The peroneus brevis was then transferred to the peroneus longus just distal to

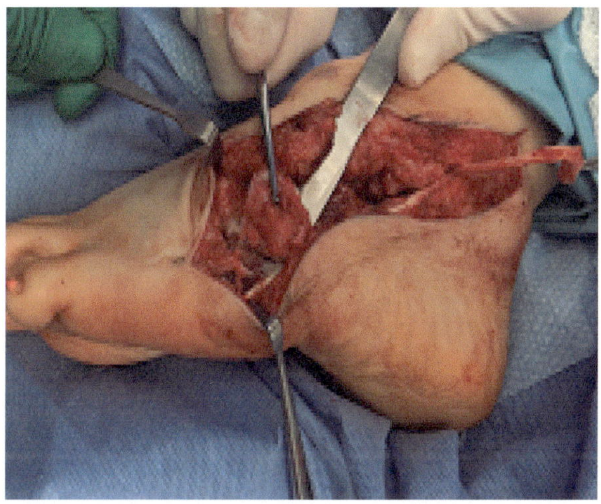

Fig. 12.2 Resection of avascular necrotic styloid process fifth metatarsal, left foot

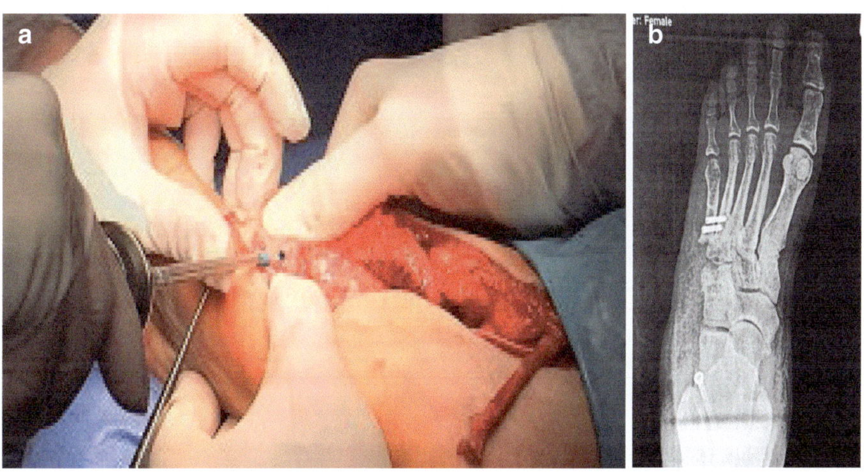

Fig. 12.3 (**a**) Arthrodesis remaining fifth metatarsal diaphysis to fourth metatarsal. (**b**) Arthrodesis of fourth and fifth metararsals with 2.5 mm headed screws

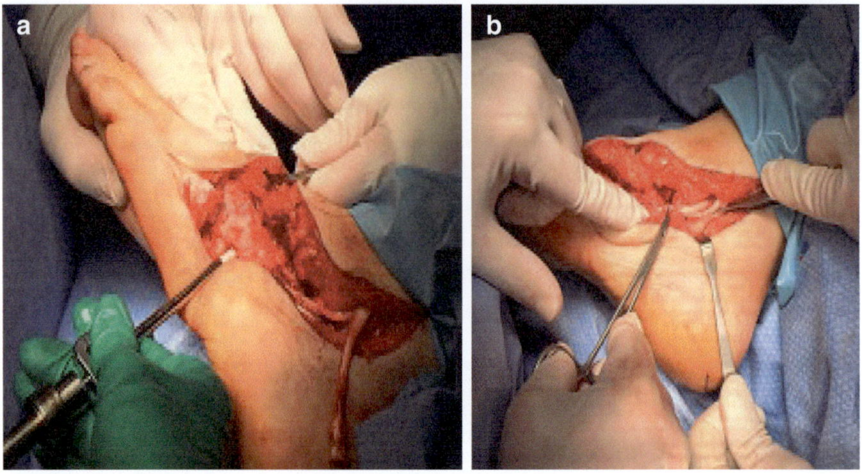

Fig. 12.4 (**a**) Isolation of peroneus longus and brevis tendons. (**b**) Peroneus longus transfer to cuboid with interference screw

Fig. 12.5 Transfer of peroneus brevis to longus

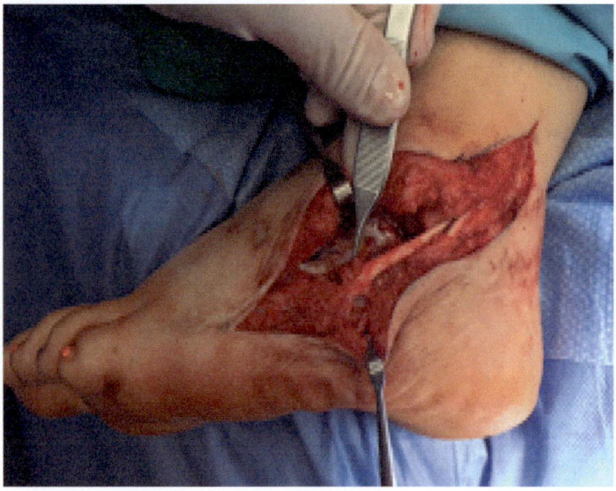

the retrofibular groove (Fig. 12.5). The tibialis posterior was tenotomized at its myotendinous junction [3]. The subtalar joint underwent an arthrodesis. It was placed in 3 degrees of valgus (Fig. 12.6a, b).

Outcome

The patient sustained a good result. She maintained a plantigrade foot. There was some mild residual adductus but the heel maintained valgus position. The arthrodesis between the metatarsal diaphyseal shafts did not go on to a full fusion. It, however, remained stable and did not act as a source of pain.

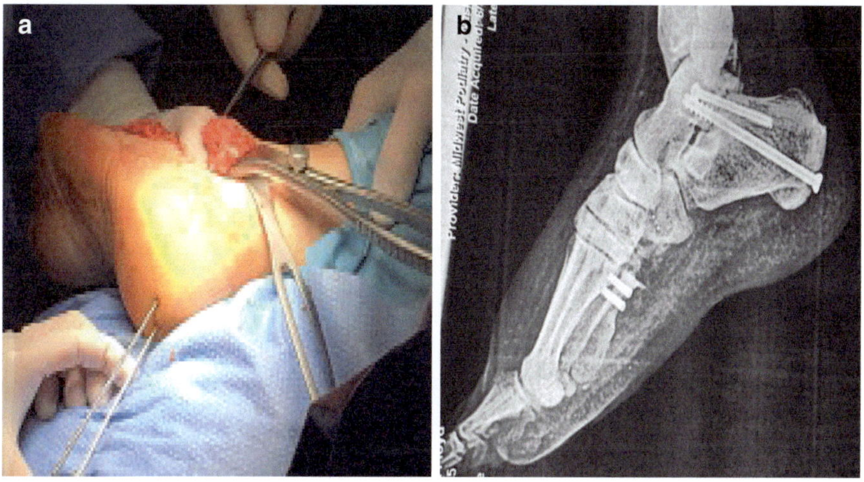

Fig. 12.6 (**a**) Arthrodesis of subtalar joint. (**b**) Post-operative fourth and fifth metatarsal and subtalar joint arthrodesis

Clinical Pearls and Pitfalls

Loss of insertional function of the peroneus brevis can lead to deformity whose significance is tied to overall STJ and MTJ flexibility. In this case, the patient demonstrated an extremely flexible foot (arthrochalasis multiplex congenita) [4]. The degree of deformity (adductovarus) with dynamic weight bearing was severe.

Transfer of the peroneus longus to the cuboid and the transfer more proximally of the peroneus brevis in the peroneus longus attempts to re-establish midfoot and rearfoot stability [2]. This new "lever arm" however can't mimic the brevis insertion to the styloid process. Thus, weakening its antagonist, the tibialis posterior, is quite essential. The subtalar joint was stabilized with an arthrodesis [5]. "Re-balancing" was not thought to be adequate enough to offset varus forces. With the outcome, certainly a double arthrodesis including the talonavicular joint (TNJ) may have led to a better overall result although the patient was satisfied.

Concerning "resecting" the styloid process vs creating a replica such as a fresh frozen donor, I did not feel an osseous allograft of this size would actually heal. In most case scenarios, they undergo collapse [6].

References

1. Monaco SJ, Manway JM, Burns PR. Utility of fresh frozen section analysis in foot and ankle surgery: a pilot study. J Foot Ankle Surg. 2016;55(4):874–6.
2. Marsland D, Stephen JM, Calder T, Amis AA, Calder JDF. Strength of interference screw fixation to cuboid vs Pulvertaft weave to peroneus brevis for tibialis posterior tendon transfer for foot drop. Foot Ankle Int. 2018;39(7):858–64.

3. Altuntas AO, Dagge B, Chin TY, Palamara JE, Eizenberg N, Wolfe R, Graham HK. The effects of intramuscular tenotomy on the lengthening characteristics of tibialis posterior: high versus low intramuscular tenotomy. J Child Orthop. 2011;5(3):225–30.
4. Hass J, Hass R. Arthrochalasis multiplex congenita; congenital flaccidity of the joints. J Bone Joint Surg Am. 1958;40-A(3):663–74.
5. Moss M, Radack J, Rockett M. Subtalar arthrodesis. Clin Podiatr Med Surg. 2004;21(2):179–201.
6. Bowes J, Buckley R. Fifth metatarsal fractures and current treatment. World J Orthop. 2016;7(12):793–800.

Case #13: Two-Staged Allograft Reconstruction of the Peroneal Tendon with Subsequent Adductovarus Foot Deformity Utilizing a Hunter Rod for Loss of Gliding Function of the Peroneal Groove

13

Case Presentation

This is a 43-year-old Caucasian male who presents with a history of prior operations for peroneal tendon split tears involving both the peroneus brevis and longus tendons of the left foot and ankle. The patient was referred for a second opinion and was told he would need an isolated Dwyer calcaneal osteotomy. On examination, he demonstrated an adductovarus deformity in relaxed calcaneal stance position (RCSP) (Fig. 13.1a). A peak-a-boo heel sign was noted when viewing from the front (Fig. 13.1b). There was significant pain with ambulation. He also related feeling very unstable and noted that his ankle gave way on numerous occasions. He had 0/5 peroneal strength and the subtalar joint on maximal eversion could only attain 5 degrees of varus. The forefoot adduction at the midtarsal joint (MTJ) was reducible to a rectus neutral position (Fig. 13.1).

Diagnosis and Assessment

Radiographs show a subtle cavovarus deformity (Fig. 13.2a–d). The patient also had prior surgery for a Jones-type stress fracture of the fifth metatarsal (Fig. 13.2). MRI imaging showed extensive tendinosis of both the peroneus brevis and longus tendons. But they remained intact. There was no fatty infiltration noted involving the peroneal musculature. The compared symmetry of the peroneal musculature of the contralateral leg was similar (Fig. 13.1b). The patient thus demonstrated an adductocavovarus foot deformity secondary to combined peroneal dysfunction (Fig. 13.1a).

H. J. Visser, *Challenges in Foot and Ankle Reconstructive Surgery*,
https://doi.org/10.1007/978-3-031-07893-4_13

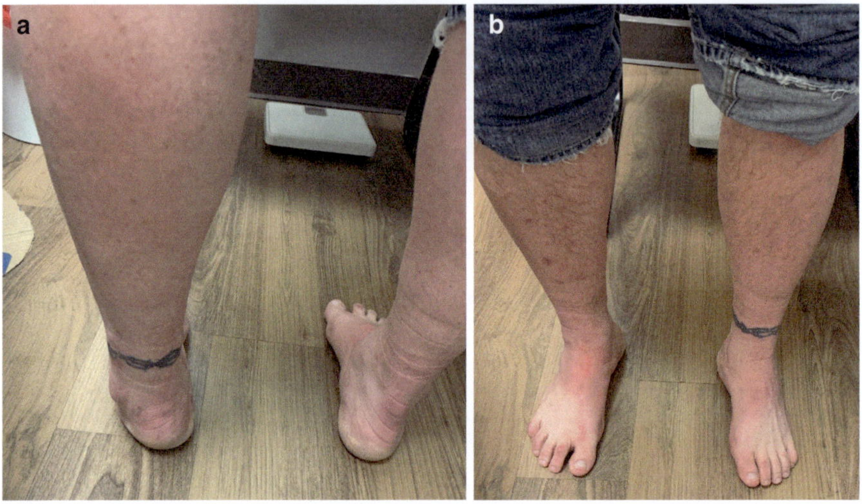

Fig. 13.1 (**a**) Subtle cavovarus foot deformity secondary to peroneal tendon dysfunction. (**b**) Peek a boo heel sign subtle cavovarus, left foot

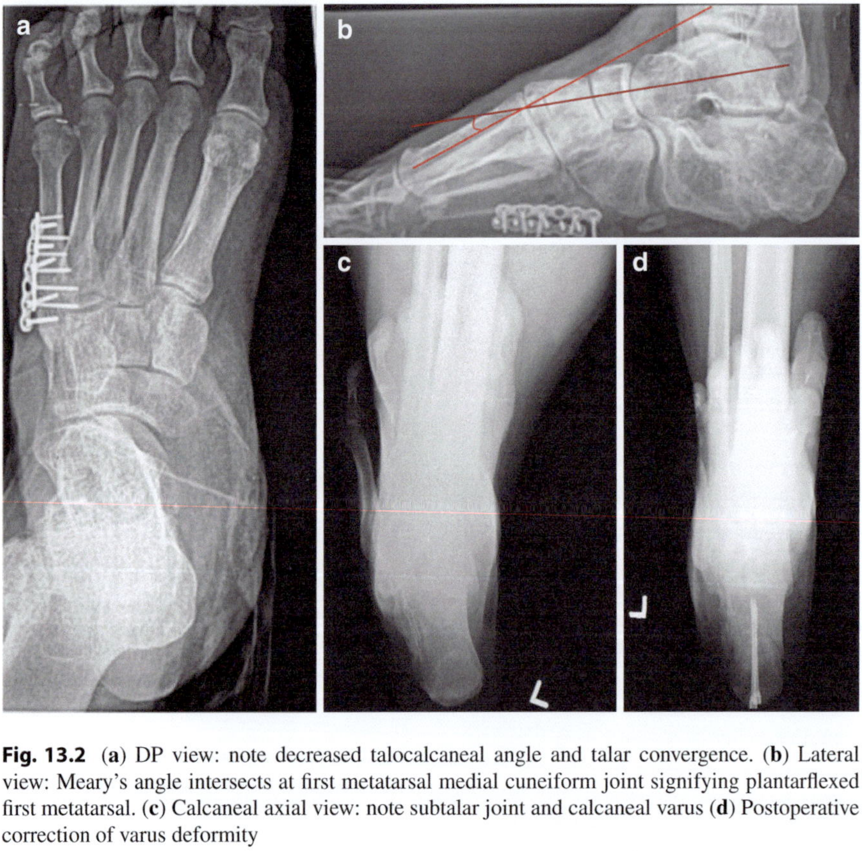

Fig. 13.2 (**a**) DP view: note decreased talocalcaneal angle and talar convergence. (**b**) Lateral view: Meary's angle intersects at first metatarsal medial cuneiform joint signifying plantarflexed first metatarsal. (**c**) Calcaneal axial view: note subtalar joint and calcaneal varus (**d**) Postoperative correction of varus deformity

Management

A two-stage procedure was discussed. The first stage involved addressing the stenosis and tendinosis of the peroneal tendons. This served as the etiology of their dysfunction. Both tendons demonstrated tendinosis secondary to prior surgery (Fig. 13.3a).

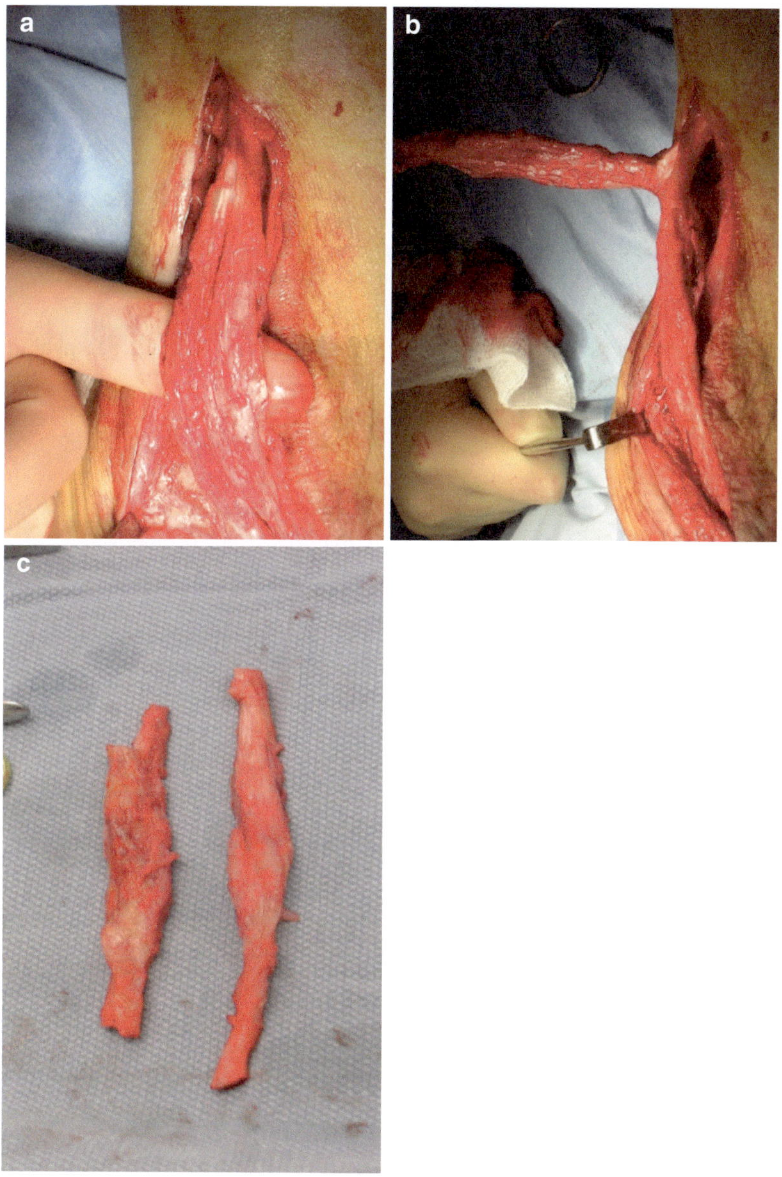

Fig. 13.3 (**a**) Advanced stenosis of peroneus brevis and longus tendons. (**b**) Stenosis of peroneal tendons retro malleolar groove. (**c**) Excised stenotic peroneus longus and brevis tendons

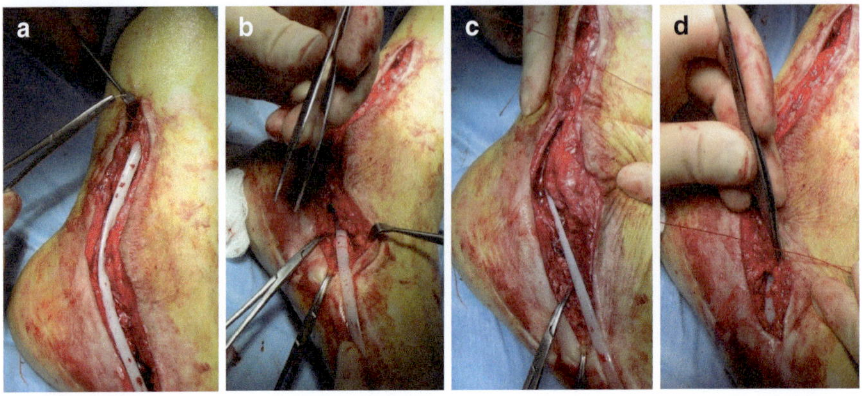

Fig. 13.4 (**a**) Stage 1: Insertion of 6 mm silicone Hunter Rod to recreate peroneal groove. (**b**) 6 mm Hunter Rod in peroneal tunnel. (**c**) Proximal aspect of Hunter rod with anastomosis of peroneus longus and brevis tendons. (**d**) Distal securement of Hunter rod to fifth metatarsal bone

This led to chronic fibrosis, tendinopathy, and stenosis involving the peroneal tunnel and retrofibular groove.

Intraoperatively, the peroneal musculature was responsive to stimulation. It retracted when the peroneal muscles were pulled with an Alice clamp. The peroneal tendons themselves were excised, but a portion of the proximal stump was left intact (Fig. 13.3c). A 6 mm hunter rod (silicone) was placed in the peroneal tunnel (Fig. 13.4a and b) [1, 2]. Anastomosis proximally was performed to the peroneus brevis and longus remaining proximal stumps (Fig. 13.4c). Distally, it was secured to the fifth metatarsal styloid process with a suture anchor (Fig. 13.4d). A Dwyer calcaneal osteotomy was also performed to address the heel varus (Fig. 13.5a–c) [3]. Lengthening of the tibialis posterior tendon was performed at the myotendinous junction [4, 5]. The patient was kept non-weight bearing for 6 weeks. At 6 weeks, a second-stage procedure was performed that involved removal of the Hunter rod and insertion of a tendon allograft [2]. It was retrieved proximally and attached to a tibialis anterior allograft [6]. It was then drawn through the "recreated' 'peroneal tunnel and attached with a suture anchor at the fifth metatarsal base (Fig. 13.6a–c). The allograft was then tensioned in maximal plantarflexion and eversion. It was secured proximally to the peroneal tendon stumps. This was via the Pulvertaft technique (Fig. 13.7a–c) [7]. The patient was then kept non-weight bearing for another 4 weeks and then full weight bearing in a CAM boot for 4 more weeks.

Outcome

The patient had an acceptable result. He, however, did continue to demonstrate mild residual adductovarus. Overall, peroneal muscle strength was 3/5 and the patient had about 3 degrees of heel varus that maintained residual deformity. He was prescribed an Arizona brace and functioned well. He did not have further surgery. His pain was completely relieved despite the residual deformity.

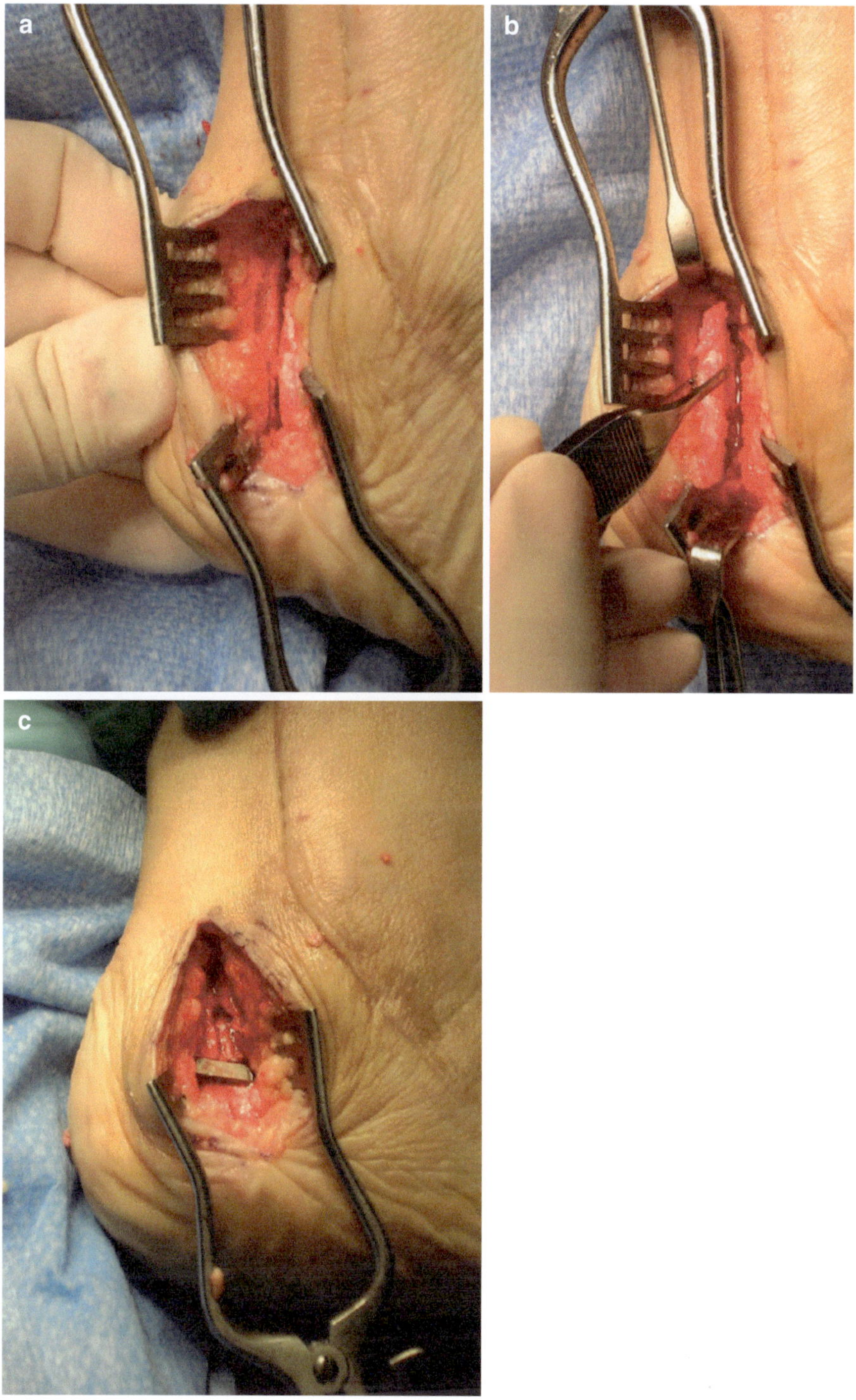

Fig. 13.5 (**a, b, c**) Dwyer calcaneal osteotomy

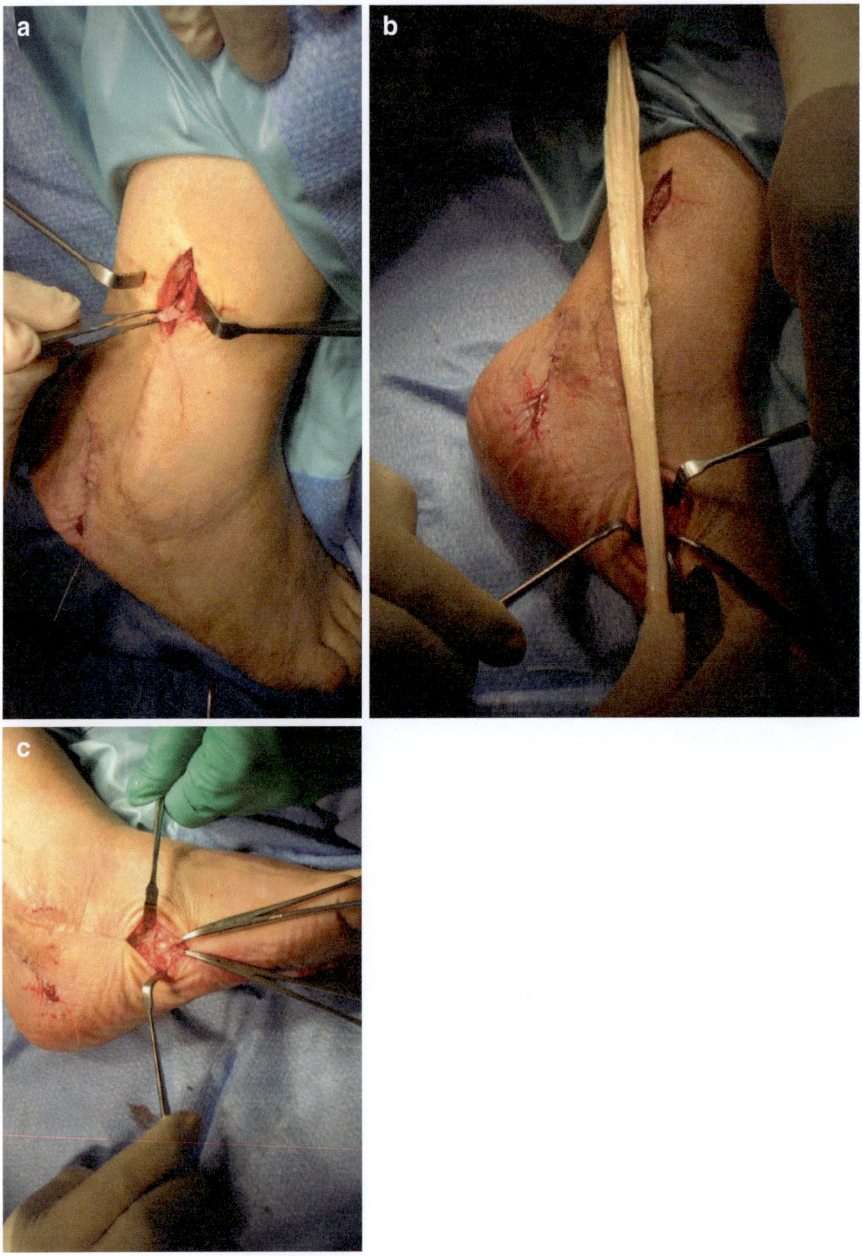

Fig. 13.6 (**a**) Stage 2: Retrieval of Hunter rod at proximal anastamosis. (**b**) Tibialis anterior allograft. (**c**) Exposure of Hunter rod distally to fifth metatarsal base

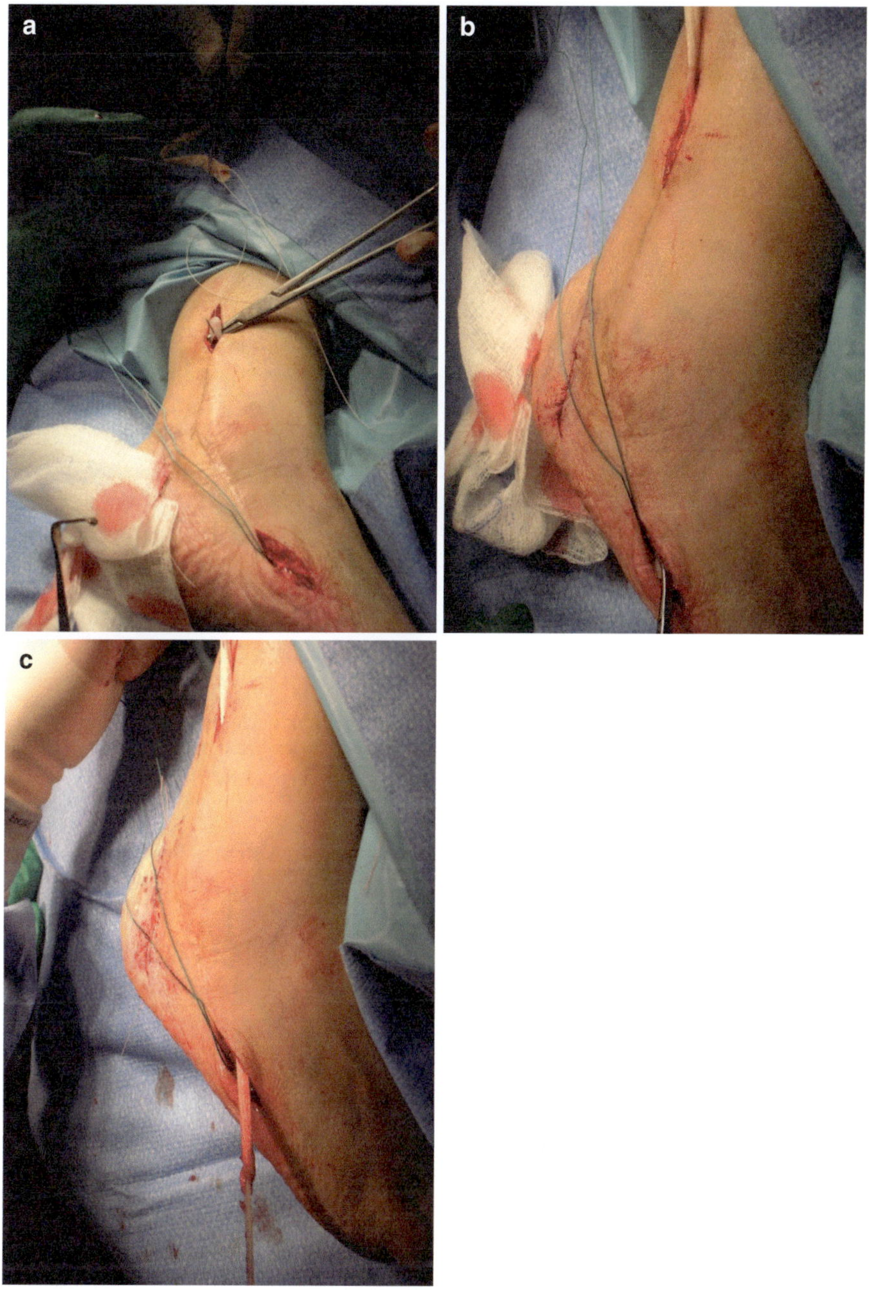

Fig. 13.7 (**a**) Attachment of contoured tibial anterior allograft to proximal silicon rod. (**b**) Drawing allograft through newly created peroneal tunnel by pulling silicon rod distally. (**c**) Distal allograft secured to fifth metatarsal base. Proximal allograft tensioned by Pulvertaft technique to proximal peroneal longus and brevis tendon with ankle joint in maximal plantarflexion and eversion

Clinical Pearls and Pitfalls

Peroneal dysfunction secondary to fibrosis, tendinopathy, and stenosis creates a significant problem for functional ambulation [8, 9]. Despite "intact" tendons, they are, as in this case, "cables in cement" and, thus, are not functional. Establishing residual peroneal muscle function is critical. Determination of muscle function is by two sources. Muscle reactivity, MRI findings, and intraoperatively. Fibrosis and fatty infiltration on MRI is one finding that can be used. Clinical comparison of muscle bulk by comparison of both of the lower legs for symmetry is another. This two-stage procedure utilizing a silicone rod is unique [1, 2, 10]. It serves to create a tunnel that can allow gliding function for the replacement allograft [10]. Correction of structural varus deformity (heel varus) and weakening of its antagonist, the tibialis posterior, is paramount. I have more recently resorted to tendon resection rather than myotendinous lengthening [5]. Further stabilization of the STJ may need to include arthrodesis. Despite this, the main issue that remains is established muscle strength. This is determined by its overall remaining functionality of the peroneal musculature, tendon length, and proper tension. Adjunctive bracing at the ankle level may be needed.

References

1. Wapner KL, Taras JS, Lin SS, Chao W. Staged reconstruction for chronic rupture of both peroneal tendons using Hunter rod and flexor hallucis longus tendon transfer: a long-term followup study. Foot Ankle Int. 2006;27(8):591–7.
2. Raikin SM, Schick FA, Karanjia HN. Use of a Hunter rod for staged reconstruction of peroneal tendons. J Foot Ankle Surg. 2016;55(1):198–200.
3. Tennant JN, Carmont M, Phisitkul P. Calcaneus osteotomy. Curr Rev Musculoskelet Med. 2014;7(4):271–6.
4. Kim BS. Reconstruction of Cavus foot: a review. Open Orthop J. 2017;11:651–9. https://doi.org/10.2174/1874325001711010651.
5. Altuntas AO, Dagge B, Chin TY, Palamara JE, Eizenberg N, Wolfe R, Graham HK. The effects of intramuscular tenotomy on the lengthening characteristics of tibialis posterior: high versus low intramuscular tenotomy. J Child Orthop. 2011;5(3):225–30.
6. Mook WR, Parekh SG, Nunley JA. Allograft reconstruction of peroneal tendons: operative technique and clinical outcomes. Foot Ankle Int. 2013;34(9):1212–20.
7. Hashimoto T, Thoreson AR, An KN, Amadio PC, Zhao C. Comparison of step-cut and Pulvertaft attachment for flexor tendon raft: a biomechanics evaluation in an in vitro canine model. J Hand Surg Eur. 2012;37(9):848–54.
8. Davda K, Malhotra K, O'Donnell P, Singh D, Cullen N. Peroneal tendon disorders. EFORT Open Rev. 2017;2(6):281–92.
9. Redfern D, Myerson M. The management of concomitant tears of the peroneus longus and brevis tendons. Foot Ankle Int. 2004;25(10):695–707.
10. Hunter JM, Salisbury RE. Flexor-tendon reconstruction in severely damaged hands. A two-stage procedure using a silicone-dacron reinforced gliding prosthesis prior to tendon grafting. J Bone Joint Surg Am. 1971;53(5):829–58.

Case #14: One Stage Allograft for Dual Peroneal Tendon Ruptures and Subsequent Adductovarus foot Deformity

14

Case Presentation

This is a 57–year-old Caucasian male who gives no history of significant medical problems. 7 months prior, the patient sustained a "twisting" injury to his left foot and ankle [1, 2]. He was a ballroom dancing instructor and injured the foot while dancing. He felt a large "pop" which, immediately, was symptomatic. He then developed ecchymosis, edema, and pain. Over a relatively short time span (4 weeks), the pain resolved but his edema persisted. Some 6 months post injury he began to notice a "change" in the shape of his foot (Fig. 14.1a and b). It appeared to curve inward. He also noted that during gait, he walked more to the outside of his foot.

Diagnosis and Assessment

An MRI was performed and showed rupture of both peroneal tendons. The brevis at the retrofibular groove and the longus at the cuboid notch. Due to a relatively early diagnosis, the foot primarily exhibited calcaneal varus with only mild midfoot adduction on radiographs (Fig. 14.2a and b). The tibialis anterior did not exhibit a significant supinatory force about the talonavicular joint (TNJ) (long midtarsal joint axis) or the first ray. Thus, the designed approach was to excise the ruptured peroneal tendons and replace them with a tendon allograft (peroneus brevis) in a single-staged procedure [3, 4].

H. J. Visser, *Challenges in Foot and Ankle Reconstructive Surgery*,
https://doi.org/10.1007/978-3-031-07893-4_14

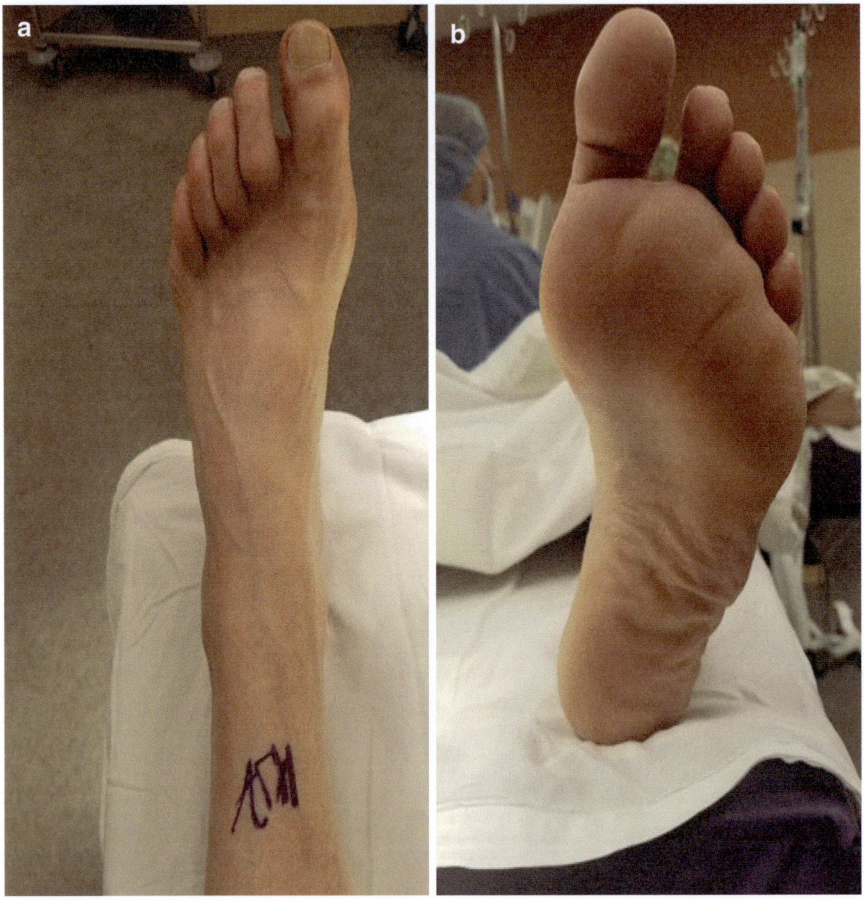

Fig. 14.1 (**a**) Subtle change of forefoot adduction. (**b**) Subtle change of calcaneal varus

Management

An initial Dwyer-type calcaneal osteotomy was performed which included removing a 1 cm wedge and also allowing about 6 mm of lateral translation (Fig. 14.3a and b) [5]. The peroneal tendons were identified and found to be ruptured (Fig. 14.4a). They exhibited extensive tendinosis. The locations of rupture were as described by the MRI. Both tendons were excised. The allograft was placed proximally into both the remaining tendon stumps of the peroneus brevis and longus muscles (Fig. 14.4b and c). The decision for utilization of an allograft was based on muscle reactivity [3, 6, 7]. Distal traction with an Alice clamp produced active contracture of the peroneal musculature. The end of the allograft was secured to the fifth metatarsal base with a suture anchor. Tensioning proximally occurred by a Pulvertaft technique with the ankle maximally plantarflexed and everted (Fig. 14.4d) [8]. The tibialis posterior

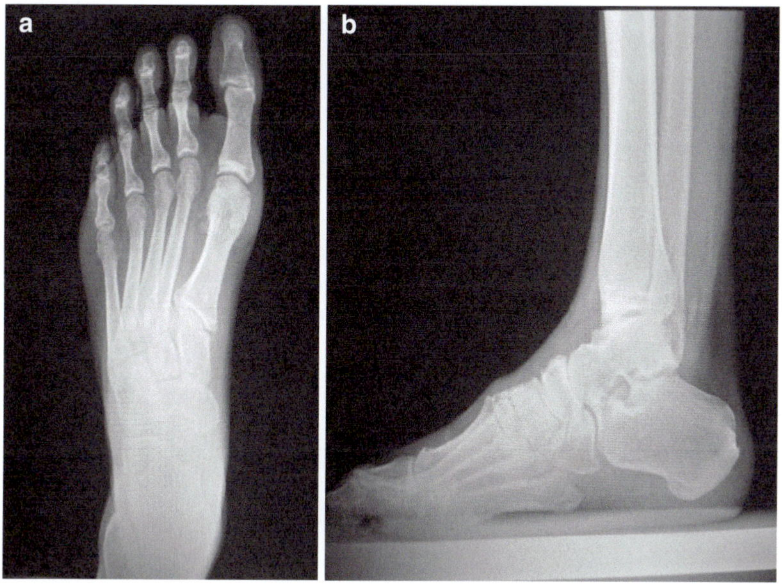

Fig. 14.2 (**a**) Talar convergence, midfoot adduction at talonavicular joint. (**b**) Anterior cavus, left foot

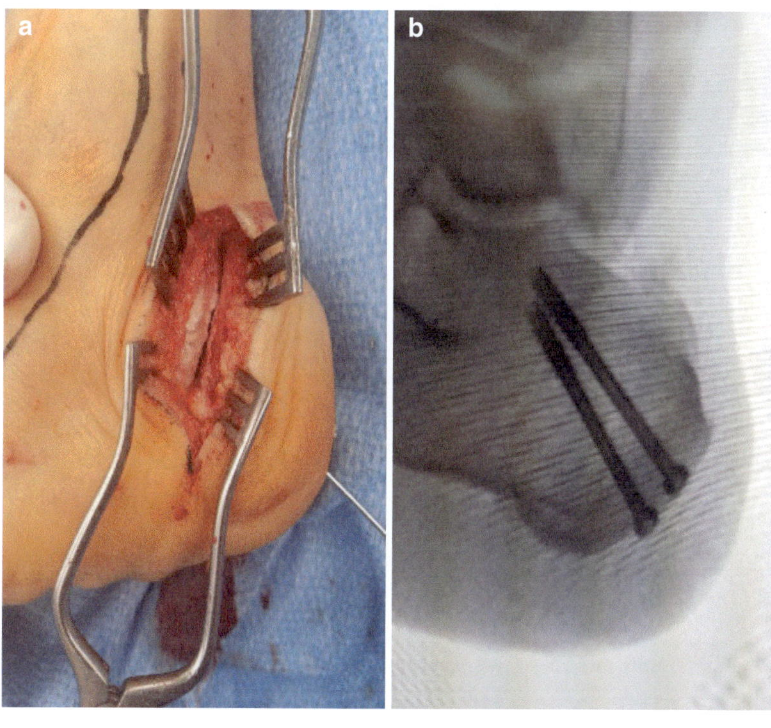

Fig. 14.3 (**a**) Dwyer calcaneal osteotomy. (**b**) Lateral translation of calcaneal tuber

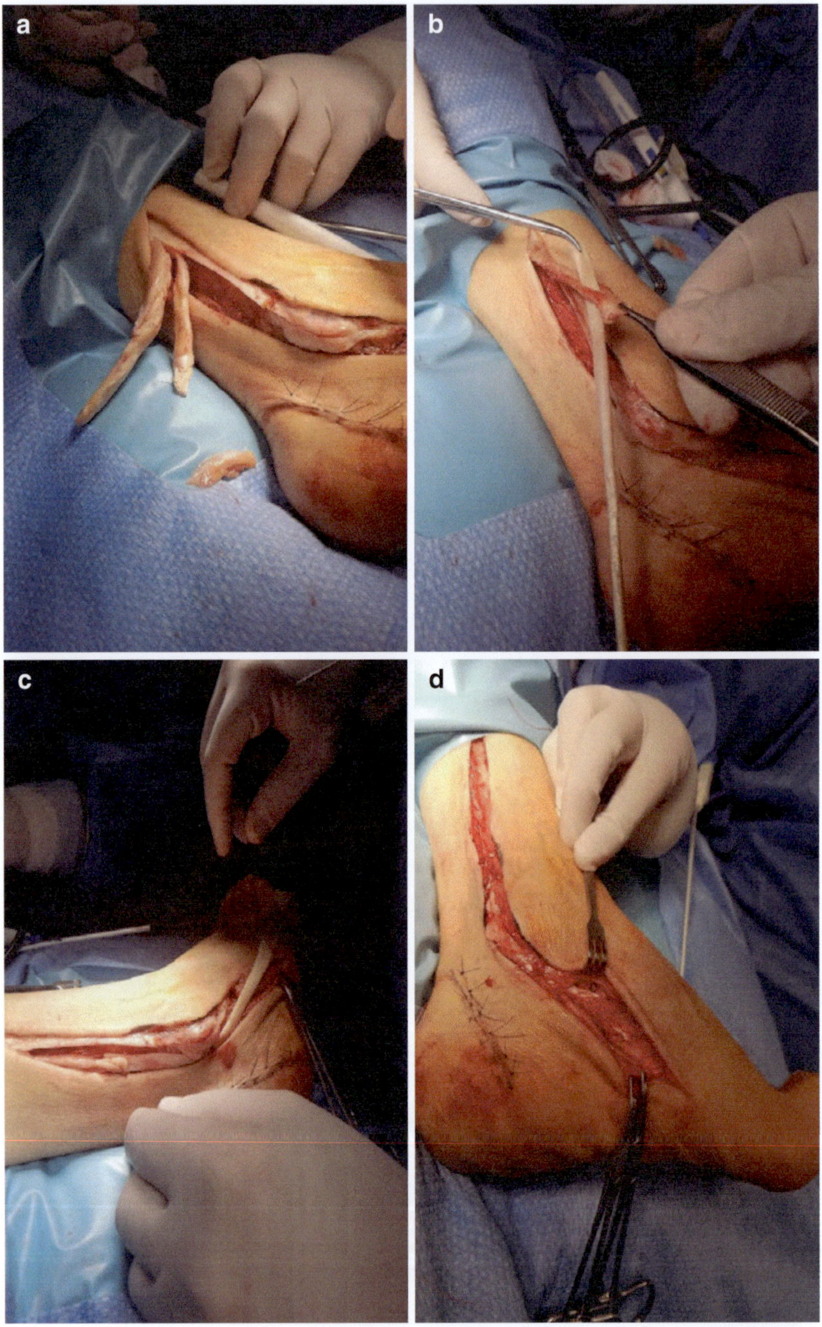

Fig. 14.4 (**a**) Advanced tendinosis and rupture of both the peroneus longus and brevis tendons. (**b**) Insertion of one stage peroneus brevis allograft proximally into tendon, secured to peroneus longus. (**c**) Course of peroneal allograft in retrofibular groove. (**d**) Securing peroneus brevis allograft distally to the fifth metatarsal base with suture anchor. Integrating allograft proximally to peroneus brevis and longus stumps with Pulvertaft technique; maximal ankle joint plantarflexion and eversion

then underwent a tenectomy of cm above the retromalleolar groove [9]. The patient was kept non-weight bearing for 6 weeks. He was then placed in a weight bearing CAM boot for a further 4 weeks. He then began exercise to increase range of motion and peroneal strengthening at 8 weeks post op.

Outcome

The patient progressed very well. He was back to dancing and serving as an instructor at 3.5 months. He slowly progressed to his full level of activity by 6 months. His foot remained stable. He demonstrated 2° of heel valgus. His peroneal strength was 4/5 during a final physical exam.

Clinical Pearls and Pitfalls

In this instance, a rupture of both tendons occurred due to a rather incidental injury [3, 5]. However, their state of attrition led to the impending rupture. Clinically, he initially noted pain which then rapidly became painless. Often resolution of pain gives a false sense of security. Release of traction by tendon rupture is the source of that security. The danger is the patient feels he has recovered from a sprain.

Having not had prior surgery at the peroneal tendon site, a one-stage procedure with allograft is a good option [3, 4]. The sheath and gliding mechanism are preserved. One-stage performance depends solely on peroneal muscle strength [3, 7, 10]. This is best determined clinically and intraoperatively [3]. Certainly, any event that leads to significant edema and ecchymosis should make the physician suspicious of a more significant injury.

References

1. Wind WM, Rohrbacher BJ. Peroneus longus and brevis rupture in a collegiate athlete. Foot Ankle Int. 2001;22(2):140–3.
2. Verheyen CP, Bras J, van Dijk CN. Rupture of both peroneal tendons in a professional athlete. A case report. Am J Sports Med. 2000;28(6):897–900.
3. Redfern D, Myerson M. The management of concomitant tears of the peroneus longus and brevis tendons. Foot Ankle Int. 2004;25(10):695–707.
4. Ousema PH, Nunley JA. Allograft replacement for peroneal tendon tears. Techniq Foot Ankle Surg. 2010;9(2):72–5.
5. Tennant JN, Carmont M, Phisitkul P. Calcaneus osteotomy. Curr Rev Musculoskelet Med. 2014;7(4):271–6.
6. Krause JO, Brodsky JW. Peroneus brevis tendon tears: pathophysiology, surgical reconstruction, and clinical results. Foot Ankle Int. 1998;19(5):271–9.
7. Silver RL, de la Garza J, Rang M. The myth of muscle balance. A study of relative strengths and excursions of normal muscles about the foot and ankle. J Bone Joint Surg Br. 1985;67(3):432–7.
8. Hashimoto T, Thoreson AR, An KN, Amadio PC, Zhao C. Comparison of step-cut and Pulvertaft attachment for flexor tendon graft: a biomechanics evaluation in an in vitro canine model. J Hand Surg Eur. 2012;37(9):848–54.

9. Altuntas AO, Dagge B, Chin TY, Palamara JE, Eizenberg N, Wolfe R, Graham HK. The effects of intramuscular tenotomy on the lengthening characteristics of tibialis posterior: high versus low intramuscular tenotomy. J Child Orthop. 2011;5(3):225–30.
10. Stamatis ED, Karaoglanis GC. Salvage options for peroneal tendon ruptures. Foot Ankle Clin. 2014;19(1):87–95.

Case #15: Flexor Digitorum Longus Transfer to the Fifth Metatarsal for Dual Loss of Peroneal Tendon and Muscle Function and Subsequent Adductovarus Foot Deformity

15

Case Presentation

This is a 60-year-old female who presented with a history of developmental anterior lateral left foot and ankle pain. She demonstrated no prior history of injury. She relates that she "was born" with relatively high arched feet. She was concerned that her left foot seemed to have even a higher arch and that she felt very unstable. She also noted it worsened considerably with weight bearing. She also had significant pain and discomfort with any form of increased activity. She then sought medical care but no presumptive diagnosis was made. Due to her worsening symptoms, 9 months after her initial medical evaluation an MRI was performed [1].

Diagnosis and Assessment

The MRI related a rupture of the peroneus brevis at the calcaneal peroneal tubercle [2]. There was also an advanced peroneus longus tendinopathy with a high grade tear inferior to the cuboid. There were also noted small areas of fibrosis and fatty infiltration of the peroneal musculature [1].

In a relaxed calcaneal stance position, the left foot demonstrated a severe adductovarus deformity (Fig. 15.1a–e). This was accentuated secondary to antagonist pull of the tibialis posterior muscle. The dorsal-plantar X-ray shows convergence of the talus with forefoot adduction (Fig. 15.2a). The CORA (center of rotation of angulation) was at the talonavicular joint. The lateral view shows a "bullet hole" sign due to extreme talar abduction and calcaneal inversion (closed kinetic chain supination) (Fig. 15.2b) [3]. The anterior-posterior view of the ankle shows the foot was medial to the ankle joint axis. There were no signs of talar incongruity (Fig. 15.2c). The

H. J. Visser, *Challenges in Foot and Ankle Reconstructive Surgery*,
https://doi.org/10.1007/978-3-031-07893-4_15

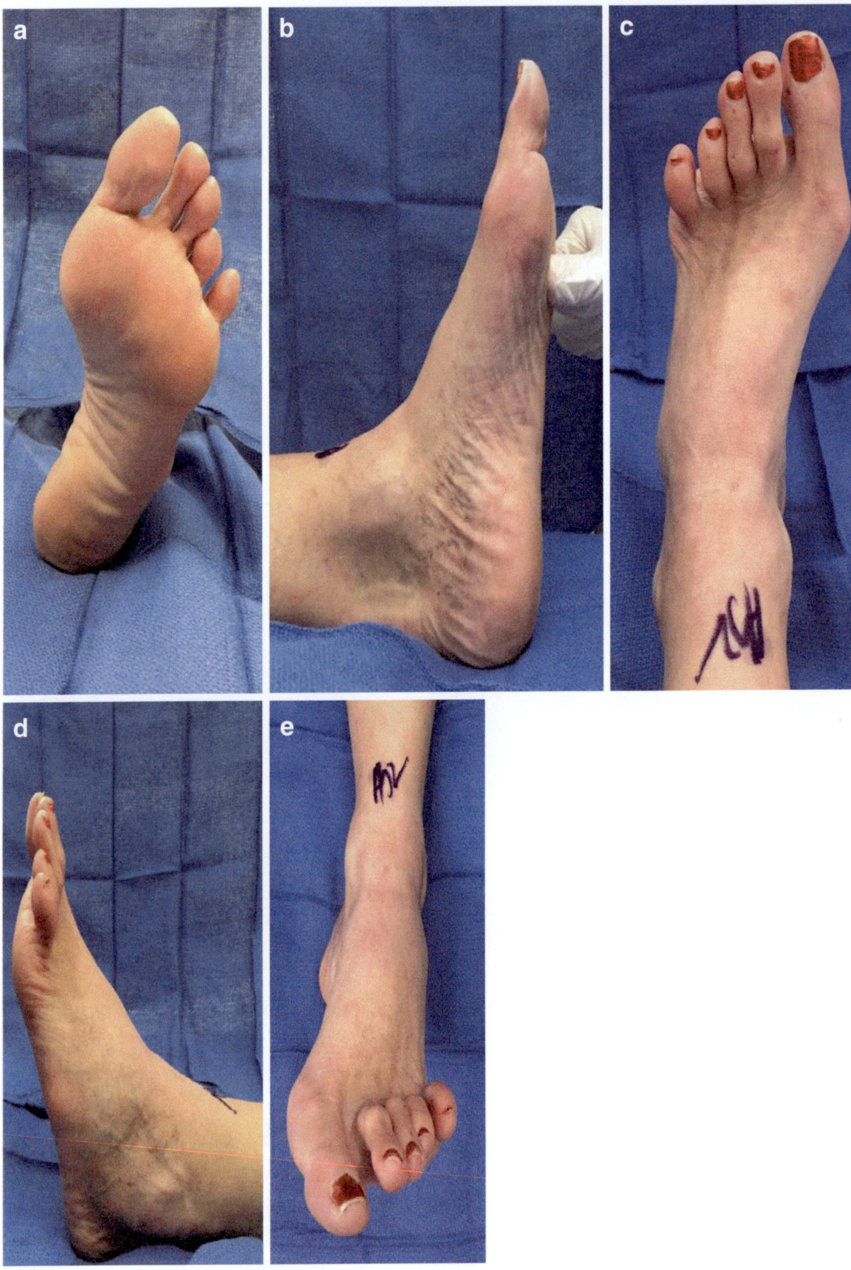

Fig. 15.1 (**a–e**) Severe flexible adductovarus foot

foot was flexible and reducible. The issue in this case was peroneal dysfunction and an associated compensatory adductovarus foot deformity with anterolateral foot and ankle instability.

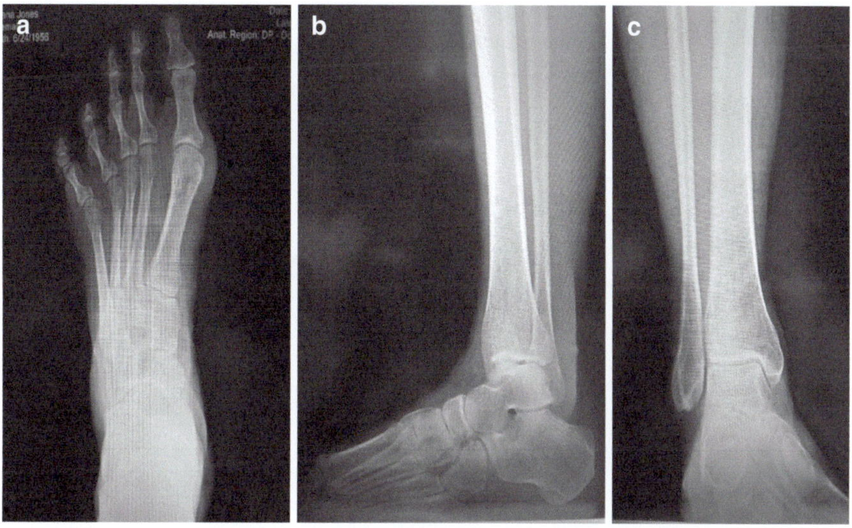

Fig. 15.2 (**a**) Talar convergence and midfoot adduction. (**b**) Bullet hole sign indicative of subtalar joint supination. (**c**) Medial position of foot to ankle anatomic axis secondary to dynamic adductovarus

Management

An initial incision was made along the course of the peroneal tendons. The peroneus brevis was extremely tendinopathic and ruptured at the peroneal tubercle (Fig. 15.3a, b). The peroneus longus was also extremely degenerated and torn in the same vicinity (Fig. 15.3c). Due to extreme tendinosis, the decision was made to excise them (Fig. 15.3d).

There was no muscle reactivity when the proximal tendon at the peroneus brevis and longus muscle interface was stretched with an Alice clamp. The distal 4 cm of the peroneus brevis was maintained for later transfer (Fig. 15.4). It had over 50% viable tendon.

A second incision was made at the navicular tuberosity. The flexor digitorum longus (FDL) tendon was then recruited near the master knot of Henry (Fig. 15.4a). The tibialis posterior tendon was resected 1 cm proximal to the navicular tuberosity (Fig. 15.4b).

The third incision was then made 9 cm above the ankle joint at the proximal medial tibia (Fig. 15.5a). The FDL tendon was then identified (Fig. 15.5b). It was then drawn through the proximal incision (Fig. 15.5c). The FDL tendon was then transferred posteriorly about the ankle [4] (Fig. 15.6a–c). The tendon was then secured to the fifth metatarsal utilizing 4 cm of the remaining peroneus brevis tendon by a Pulvertaft technique (Fig. 15.7a, b) [5]. The ankle was everted and plantarflexed, and the tendon was secured with maximal tension (Fig. 15.7c, d).

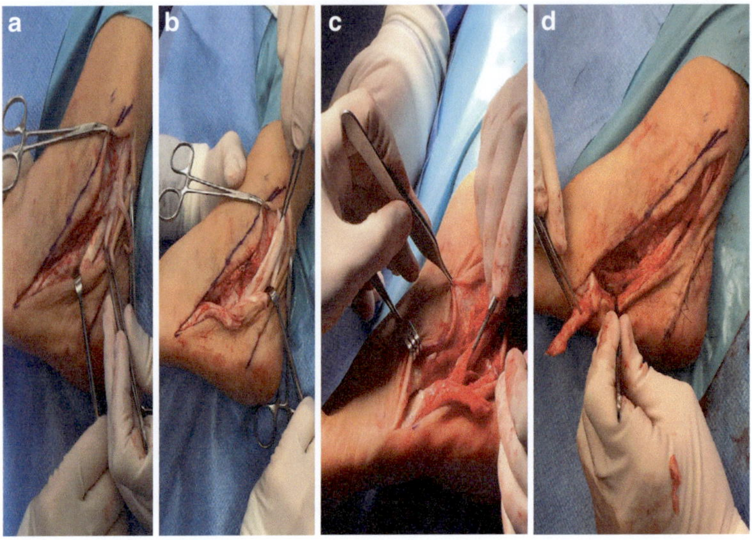

Fig. 15.3 (**a**) Peroneus brevis tendinopathic and ruptured at peroneal tubercle. (**b**) Severe tendinopathic nature of peroneus longus, with rupture. (**c**) Peroneus longus was extremely degenerated in the same vicinity (**d**) Excising both peroneal tendons maintaining distal peroneus brevis stump

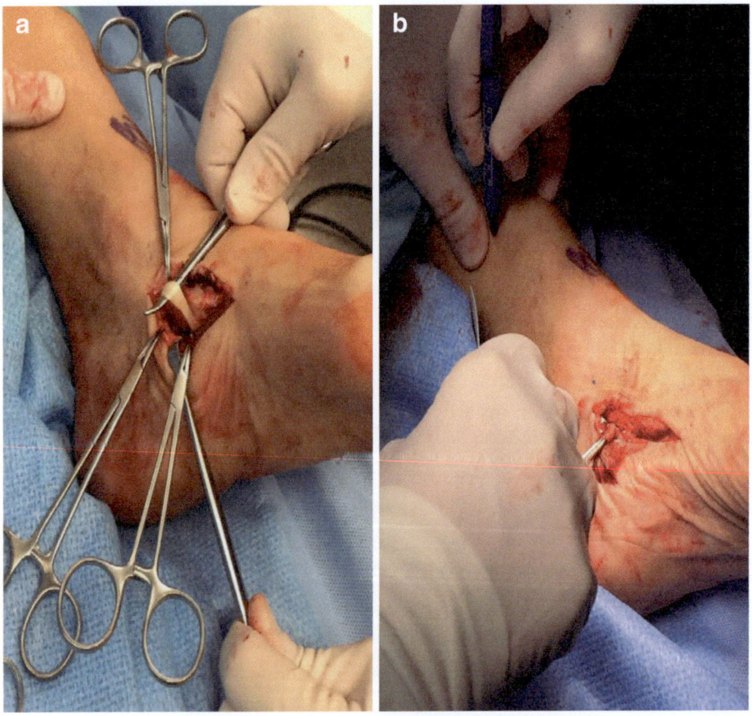

Fig. 15.4 (**a**) Recruitment of FDL tendon at navicular, master knot. (**b**) Resecting the tibialis posterior tendon

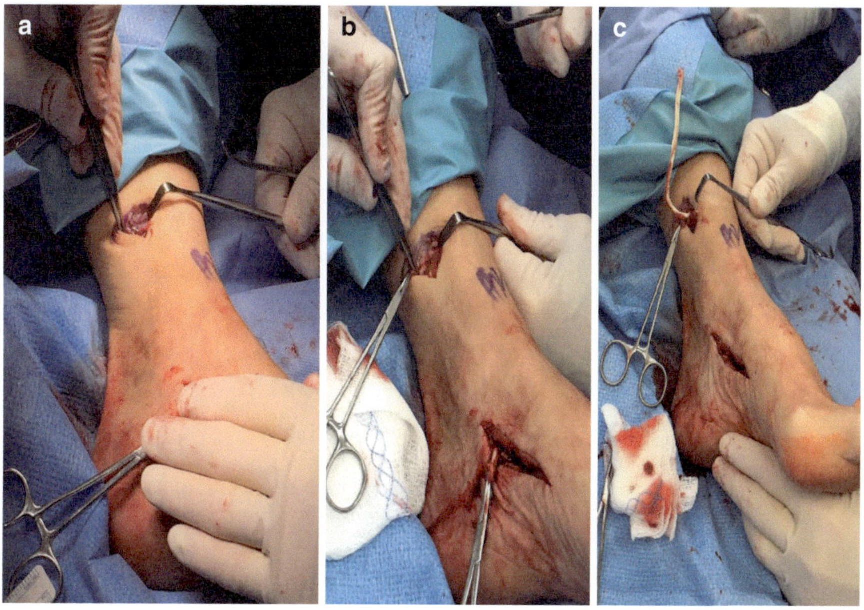

Fig. 15.5 (**a**) Incision 9 cm above the ankle joint to identify the FDL tendon. (**b**) Release of FDL tendon distally. (**c**) FDL drawn through proximal incision

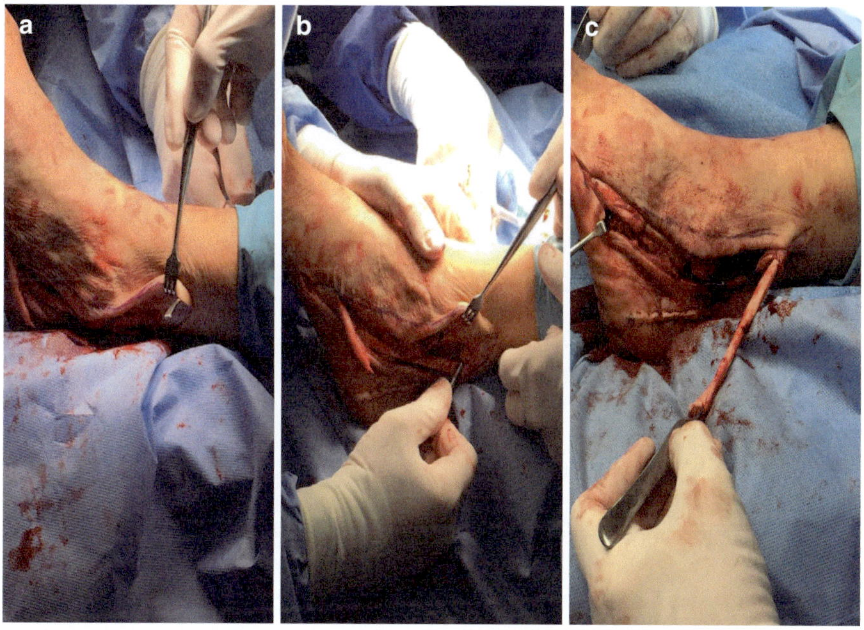

Fig. 15.6 (**a, b**) Posterior transfer of FDL around the ankle joint (**c**) FDL tendon brought into the peroneal tunnel

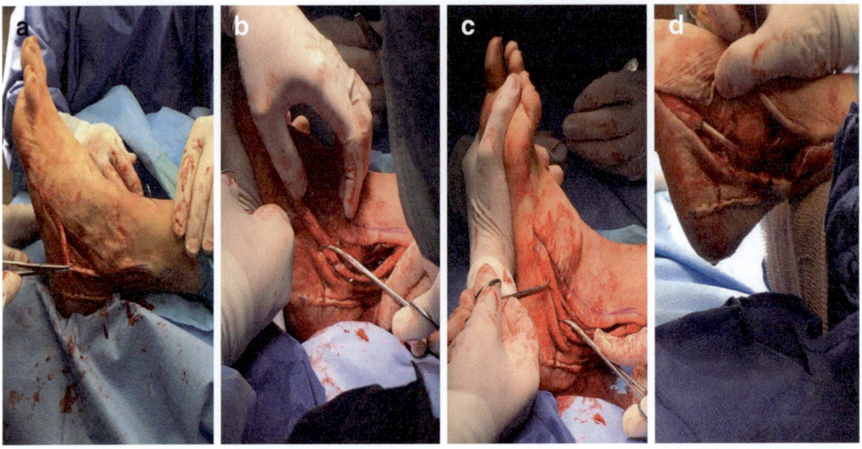

Fig. 15.7 (**a, b**) Anastomosis of FDL tendon to peroneus brevis stump. (**c, d**) Tensioning FDL to peroneus brevis via Pulvertaft technique in plantarflexion and eversion

A fourth incision was made posterior to the peroneal tendons at the calcaneal level. A Dwyer osteotomy with an appropriate 1 cm wedge with lateral translation was performed (Fig. 15.8a–f) [6]. The fifth incision included a plantar fascial release (Fig. 15.9).

Outcome

The patient was kept non-weight bearing for 4 weeks. She was then placed in a weight-bearing CAM boot. Sutures were removed at 3 weeks. Range of motion and strengthening began at 4 weeks. The patient overall had a good result but did demonstrate residual calcaneal varus. A second lateral calcaneal wedge with translation was performed 6 months later. A subtalar joint arthrodesis was recommended but the patient refused. The patient did very well with the second operation and was very happy with the outcome. No bracing was needed but she did require high-top boots for hiking.

Clinical Pearls and Pitfalls

This is a case of the patient demonstrating complete loss of peroneal function. As has been already seen, various approaches and clinical scenarios can occur. In this case, there was complete loss of peroneal muscle function. Thus, an active muscle motor must be supplied. When there is extreme flexibility, as in this case, a dynamic adductocavovarus deformity occurs [4, 7]. The degree of deformity is relevant to overall pedal fragility. In cases with more intrinsic rigidity of the subtalar joint (STJ), lesser deformities occur. A "bullet hole" sign of the canalis tarsi is seen when

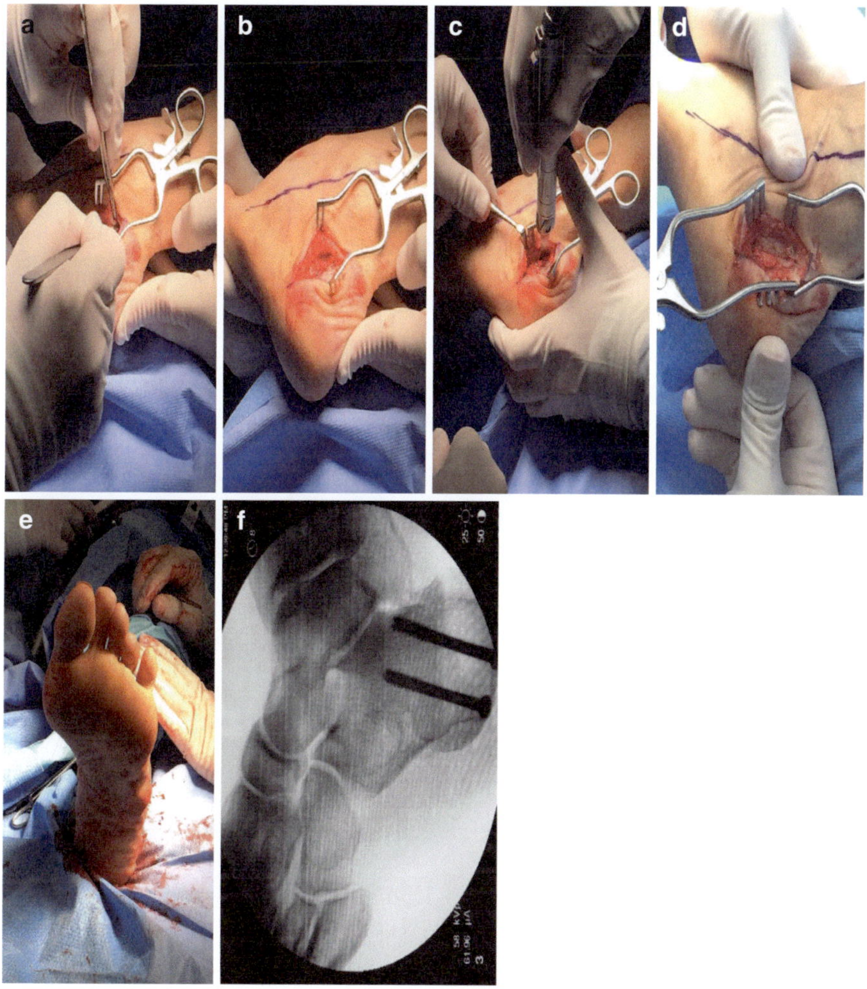

Fig. 15.8 (a–f) Dwyer calcaneal osteotomy with lateral translation and 2 screw fixation

the STJ is in maximal supination [3]. It occurs in cavus deformity with increased calcaneal inclination. The fibula is externally rotated posterior to the tibia. A foot exhibiting structural (calcaneal varus) without significant convergence of the talus will show an accentuated sinus tarsi, a circle sign [3]. The fibula is not excessively externally rotated posterior to the tibia.

Options in this case were to transfer an active motor muscle tendon. This included either the FDL or FHL muscles [4]. The FDL was chosen in this case. This represents a "phasic transfer" with loss of 1 grade of muscle strength [8]. The FDL now works as a plantarflexor and everter rather than an inverter. It is weaker than the peroneal muscles which it is to replace to produce balance [4, 9]. Its antagonist, the

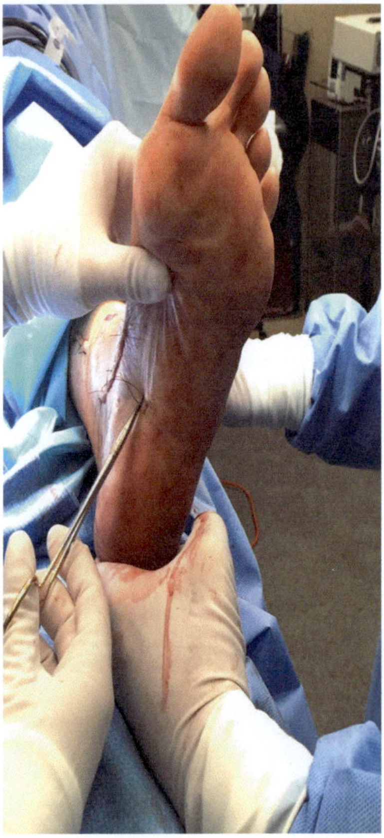

Fig. 15.9 A fifth incision included a plantar fascial release

tibialis posterior muscle, was resected at its insertion. This eliminates its function. Also, further assistance to the FDL is rendered by the valgalizing calcaneal osteotomy.

Case #15A: Tibialis Anterior Tendon Transfer Post Triple Arthrodesis for Residual Forefoot Varus with Associated Dual Loss of Peroneal Tendon and Muscle Function

Case Presentation

This represents a 56-year-old Caucasian female who had given a history of a prior triple arthrodesis. Due to her residual forefoot varus with lack of ground contact, a second procedure was performed 1 year later. It included a derotation osteotomy about the presumed talonavicular malunion. She presents here 6 months later with, again, recurrent forefoot varus (Fig. 15A.1a, b).

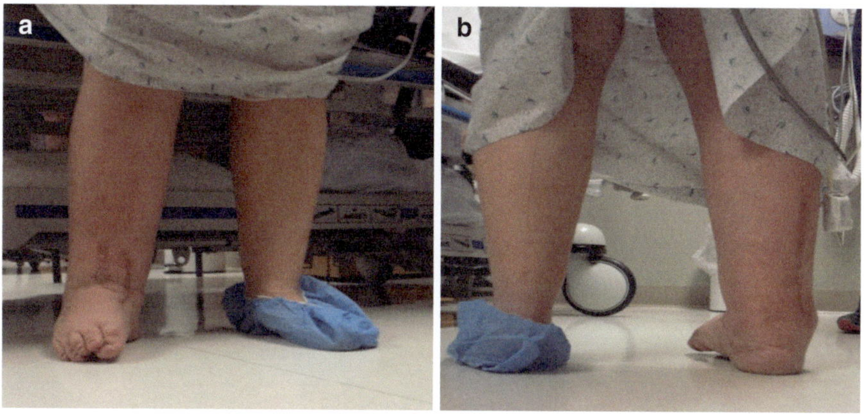

Fig. 15A.1 (**a, b**) Residual forefoot varus post triple arthrodesis, residual talon navicular malunion, right foot

Diagnosis and Assessment

On examination and attained history, the patient had documented peroneus longus and brevis ruptures. She had developed a compensatory adductocavovarus foot deformity. The surgeon, due to "lack of mobility," performed a triple arthrodesis. No attempt was made to assess or treat the peroneal ruptures.

On examination, the issue was not about the talonavicular (TN) joint but about the navicular-medial cuneiform joint (first ray). As this was mobile and reducible, the decision was to perform a transfer of the tibialis anterior to the cuboid.

Management

The tibialis anterior tendon was recruited at the insertion at the base of the first metatarsal. A second incision was made 6 cm above the ankle joint lateral to the tibia [10, 11]. The cuboid was prepared and the tibialis anterior tendon was secured with an interference screw (Fig. 15A.2). The patient was kept non-weight bearing for 4 weeks and then placed in a weight-bearing controlled ankle motion (CAM) boot for a further 4 weeks.

Outcome

The patient had complete correction of the forefoot varus deformity. She was ecstatic that after nearly 3 years, she had a functional foot (Fig. 15A.3).

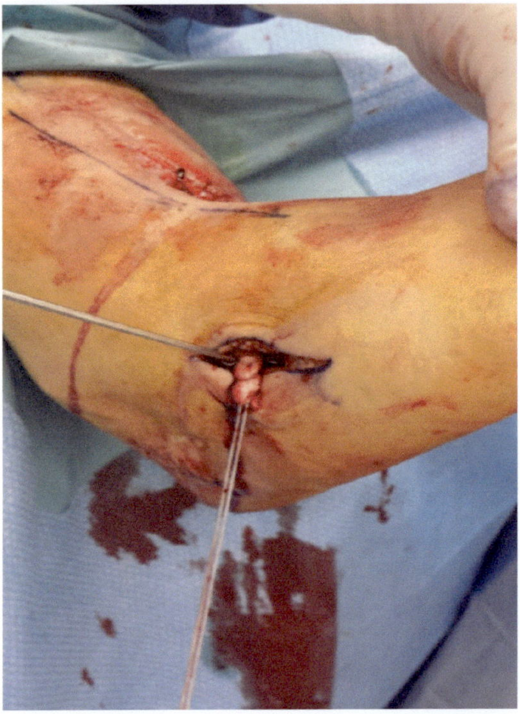

Fig. 15A.2 Transfer of tibial anterior to cuboid with interference screw, right foot. Note: incision at anterior ankle over tibial anterior tendon, 4 cm above ankle joint

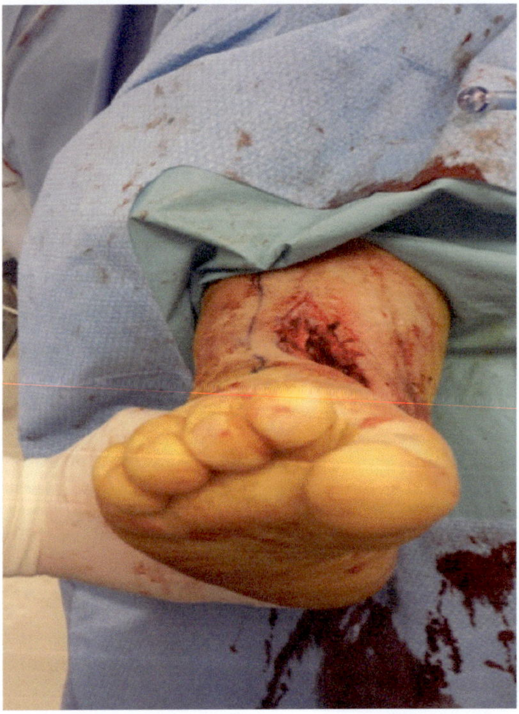

Fig. 15A.3 Reduction of forefoot varus centered at first ray (first metatarsal navicular medical cuneiform fault), right foot

Clinical Pearls and Pitfalls

The case represents the importance of neuromuscular imbalance. With the performance of a triple arthrodesis, this did neutralize the tibialis posterior in regard to loss of peroneal function. In this case, the tibialis anterior produced forefoot varus and adductus due to its distal insertion into the medial cuneiform and metatarsal bases.

In this case, the loss of peroneus longus function gave a distinct mechanical advantage to the tibialis anterior muscle [10, 12]. Unopposed, it pulled the forefoot into varus at the first ray (first metatarsal medial cuneiform-navicular joint) its insertion. The TN joint was stable by fusion. This imbalance and resulting deformity was neutralized and corrected by transfer of the neuromuscular unit.

References

1. Khoury NJ, El-Khoury GY, Saltzman CL, Kathol MH. Peroneus longus and brevis tendon tears: MR imaging evaluation. Radiology. 1996;200(3):833–41.
2. Sammarco GJ. Peroneal tendon injuries. Orthop Clin North Am. 1994;25(1):135–45.
3. Meyr AJ, Sansosti LE, Ali S. A pictorial review of reconstructive foot and ankle surgery: evaluation and intervention of the flatfoot deformity. J Radiol Case Rep. 2017;11(6):26–36.
4. Seybold JD, Campbell JT, Jeng CL, Short KW, Myerson MS. Outcome of lateral transfer of the FHL or FDL for concomitant peroneal tendon tears. Foot Ankle Int. 2016;37(6):576–81.
5. Hashimoto T, Thoreson AR, An KN, Amadio PC, Zhao C. Comparison of step-cut and Pulvertaft attachment for flexor tendon graft: a biomechanics evaluation in an in vitro canine model. J Hand Surg Eru Vol. 2012;37(9):848–54.
6. Tennant JN, Carmont M, Phisitkul P. Calcaneus osteotomy. Curr Rev Musculoskelet Med. 2014;7(4):271–6.
7. Bassett FH 3rd, Speer KP. Longitudinal rupture of the peroneal tendons. Am J Sports Med. 1993;21(3):354–7.
8. Close JR, Todd FN. The phasic activity of the muscles of the lower extremity and the effect of tendon transfer. J Bone Joint Surg Am. 1959;41-A(2):189–208.
9. Song SJ, Deland JT. Outcome following addition of peroneus brevis tendon transfer to treatment of acquired posterior Tibial tendon insufficiency. Foot Ankle Int. 2001;22(4):301–4.
10. Knutsen AR, Avoian T, Sangiorgio SN, Borkowski SL, Ebramzadeh E, Zionts LE. How do different anterior tibial tendon transfer techniques influence forefoot and hindfoot motion? Clin Orthop Relat Res. 2015;473(5):1737–43.
11. Holt JB, Westerlind B, Morcuende JA. Tibialis anterior tendon transfer for relapsing idiopathic clubfoot. JBJS Essent Surg Tech. 2015;5(3):e16.
12. Jockel JR, Brodsky JW. Single-stage flexor tendon transfer for the treatment of severe concomitant peroneus longus and brevis tendon tears. Foot Ankle Int. 2013;34(5):666–72.

Case #16: Supramalleolar Osteotomy for Ankle Varus Malunion Post Ankle and Subtalar Joint Arthrodesis

16

Case Presentation

This is a 42-year-old female Caucasian with a recent 3-year history of an ankle varus malunion involving the right foot and ankle. The patient, beginning some 7 years ago, had two attempts of attaining a tibio-talo-calcaneal (TTC) arthrodesis. They all went on to a nonunion. Her third operation performed 5 years prior did proceed to a solid TTC fusion. Unfortunately, it attained a varus position. The patient has since been ambulating in an Arizona brace with crutch assistance. Her past history is significant with obesity. Otherwise, she was in good overall health.

Diagnosis and Assessment

On clinical exam, her vascular status noted a strong +¾ dorsalis pedis (DP) pulse but nonpalpable posterior tibial (PT) pulse secondary to induration from prior surgical scarring. Arterial doppler studies showed triphasic flow patterns involving the DP, PT, and peroneal arteries. Neurologically, her sensation was intact and she was able to perceive a Semmes-Weinstein (SW) monofilament at all plantar pedal locations and above her ankle.

Her foot and ankle noted adduction of the forefoot with varus rotation and equinus (Fig. 16.1a, b). Her center of rotational axis (CORA) was at the ankle. The patient walked on the lateral side of her foot and demonstrated pain at the calcaneal cuboid (CC) joint level (Fig. 16.2a). She had a tyloma over the fifth metatarsal styloid process. The forefoot was not in contact with the ground and thus a non-plantar grade condition was present.

H. J. Visser, *Challenges in Foot and Ankle Reconstructive Surgery*,
https://doi.org/10.1007/978-3-031-07893-4_16

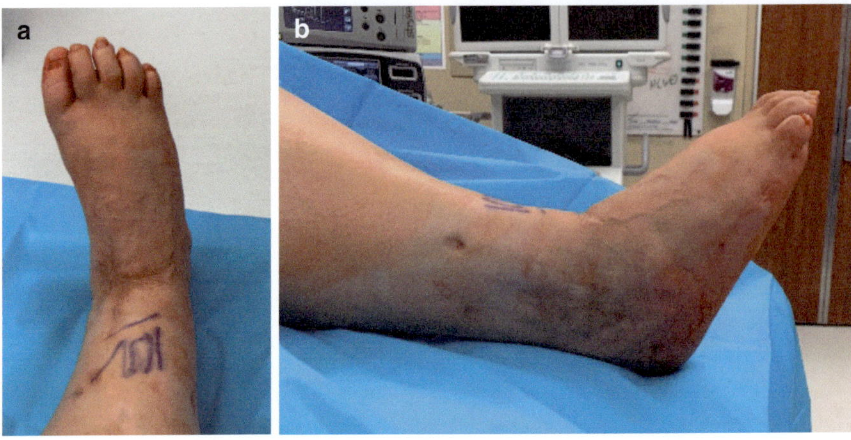

Fig. 16.1 (**a**) Residual forefoot varus and adduction post ankle arthrodesis malunion, right foot. (**b**) Residual equinus post ankle fusion malunion, right foot

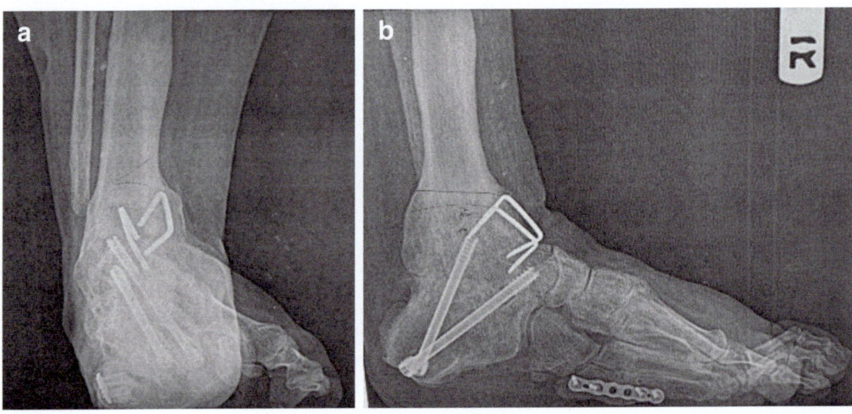

Fig. 16.2 (**a**) Forefoot varus rotation. CORA at ankle joint lateral and in line with the fifth metatarsal. (**b**) Patient developed genu recurvatum secondary to ankle and STJ arthrodesis is plantarflexed position

Radiographs showed on the lateral view her ankle and foot in 10 degrees of equinus. Recurvatum of the knee was present (Fig. 16.2b). The ankle and STJ showed complete fusion (Fig. 16.2a, b). On the AP ankle view, there was a significant increase in varus positioning involving the medial tibio talar angle. A vertical line bisecting the tibia was perpendicular to the fifth metatarsal. Compression staples were noted in the anterior ankle and 7.0 cannulated screws through the STJ (subtalar joint) (Fig. 16.2a).

Management

The decision to create a plantigrade foot involved a supramalleolar osteotomy through the arthrodesis site at the level of the ankle joint (Fig. 16.3). A lateral incision was made and the anterior, lateral, and posterior soft tissues were subperiosteally dissected from the malunion site (Fig. 16.4) [1]. The osteotomy was made utilizing fluoroscopically placed guide pins at the level of prior ankle arthrodesis (Fig. 16.5). A 4 mm wedge was then created with the apex medial and wedge lateral [1]. An osteotome was used to carefully hinge the medial cortex (Fig. 16.6a, b). With closure of the osteotomy, the varus deformity was fully corrected in the frontal plane [2]. The adduction of the forefoot was corrected simultaneously as well as the forefoot varus (Fig. 16.6c). Residual equinus was present and this was corrected by kerfing (Fig. 16.6d) the anterior cortex until a plantigrade foot was attained at 90° (Fig. 16.6e) compression staples were utilized for fixation (Fig. 16.7). Postoperative radiographs show CORA aligned on AP (Fig. 16.8a), equinus reduced, and plantigrade foot (Fig. 16.8b).

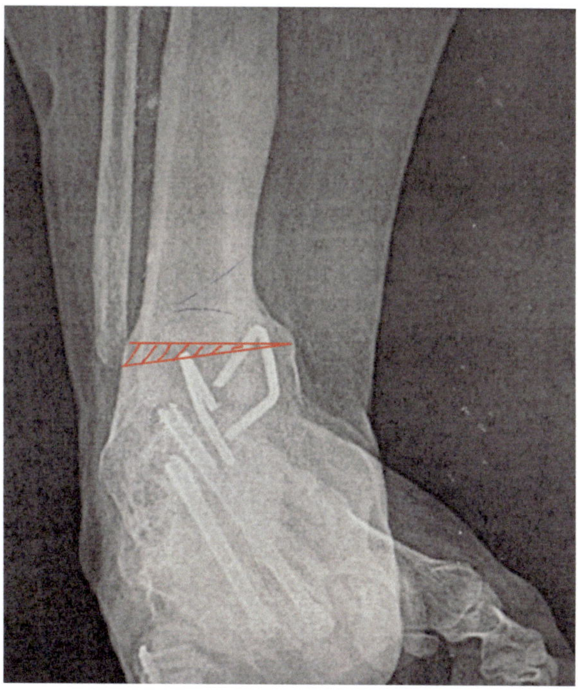

Fig. 16.3 Proposed osteotomy at malunion site

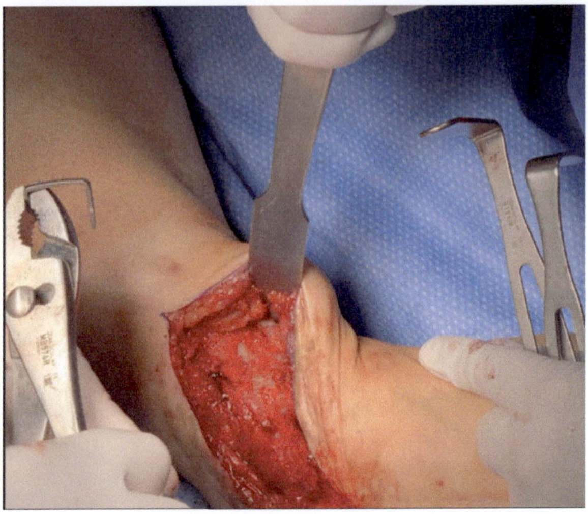

Fig. 16.4 Lateral incision, soft tissue reflection to exposure anterior, lateral and posterior ankle

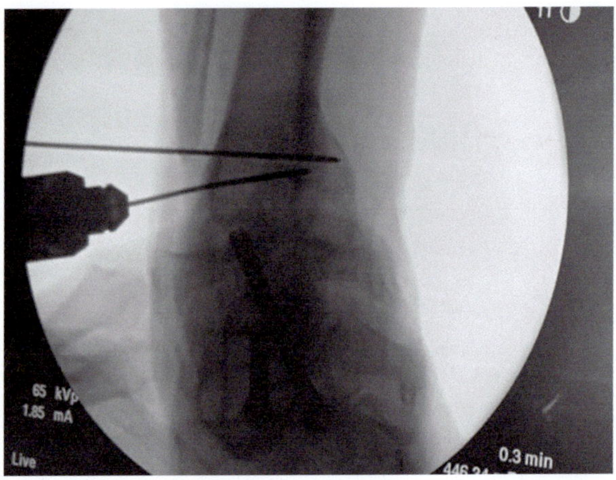

Fig. 16.5 Guide pins for proposed osteotomy, right foot

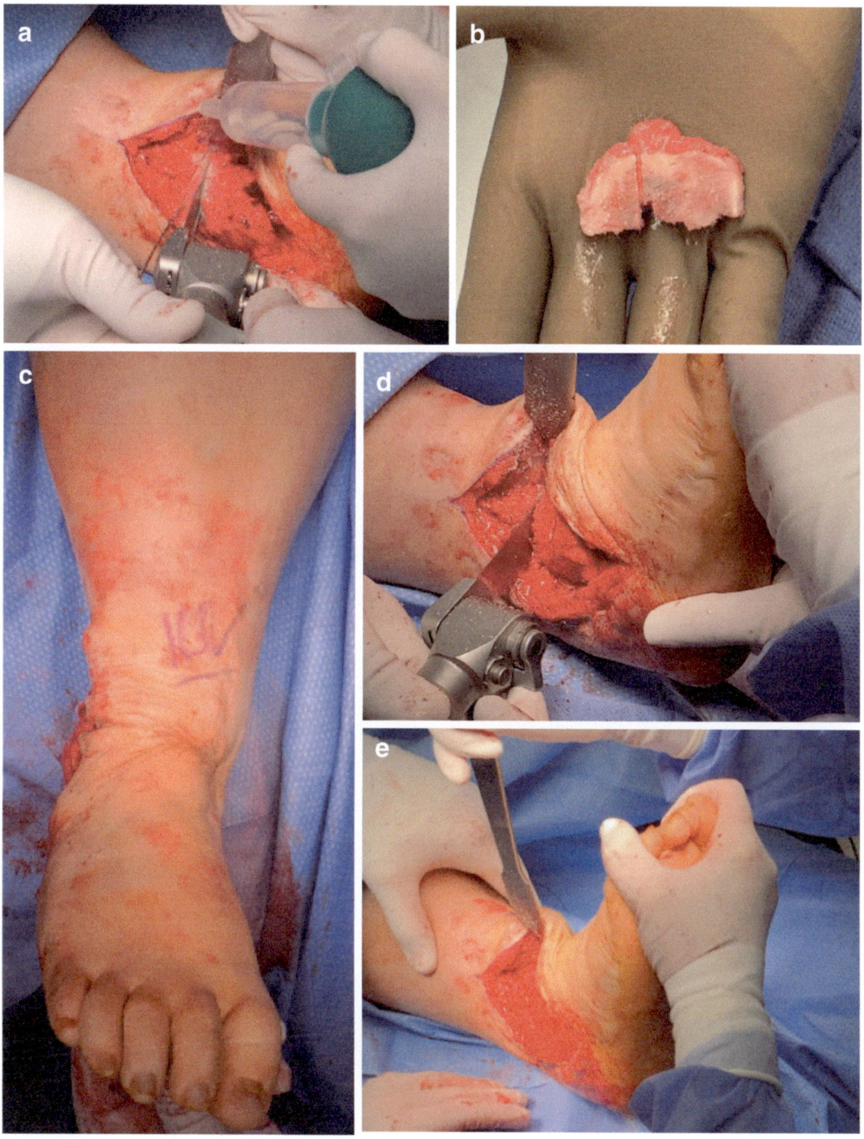

Fig. 16.6 (**a, b**) Osteotomy performed at CORA. (**c**) Simultaneous reduction of forefoot adduction and varus. (**d**) Kerfing osteotomy to reduce equinus (**e**) Final position with correction of varus and equinus

The patient was placed in a posterior splint and sutures removed at 3 weeks. Strict NWB was maintained for 9 weeks. WB began in a CAM boot for 6 more weeks. An Arizona brace (new) was then prescribed.

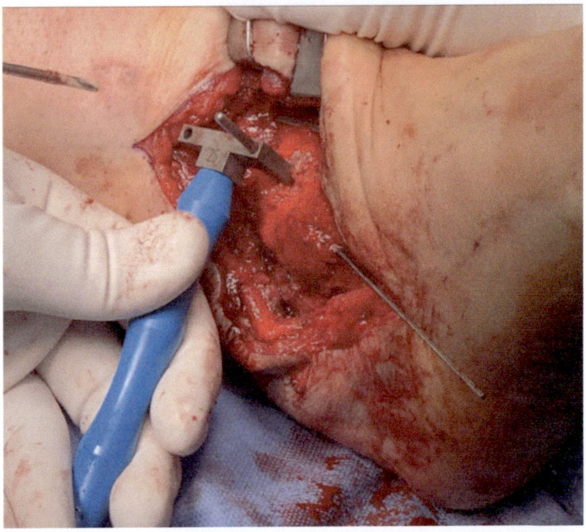

Fig. 16.7 Fixation with compression staples

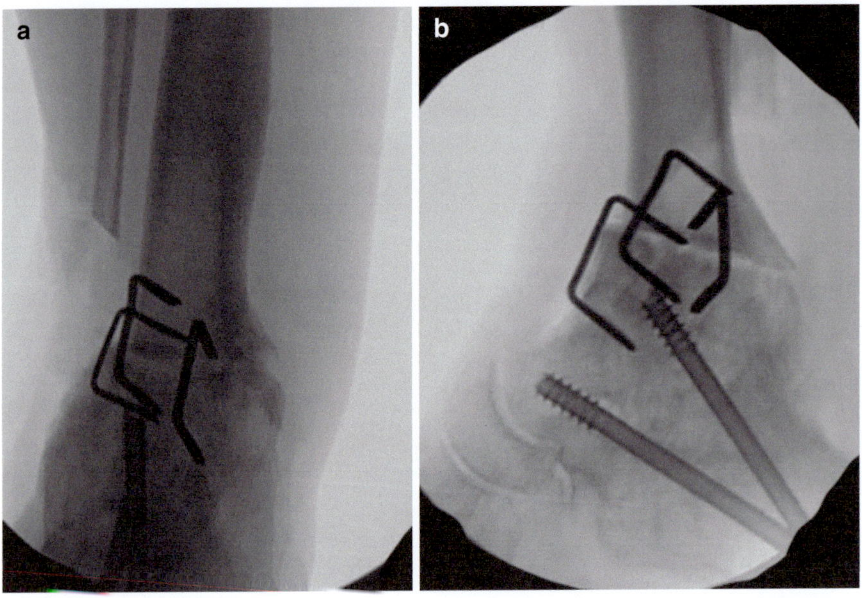

Fig. 16.8 (**a**) AP view: ankle realigned with foot. (**b**) Creating a plantigrade foot

Outcome

The patient had a prolonged post operative course. By 9 months post-op it became apparent that a non union had occurred (Fig. 16.9 a–c). The patient then underwent a further revision surgery, this included staple removal and bone grafting with insertion of an intramedullary nail (IM). The patient recovered completely and ambulates in normal shoe wear.

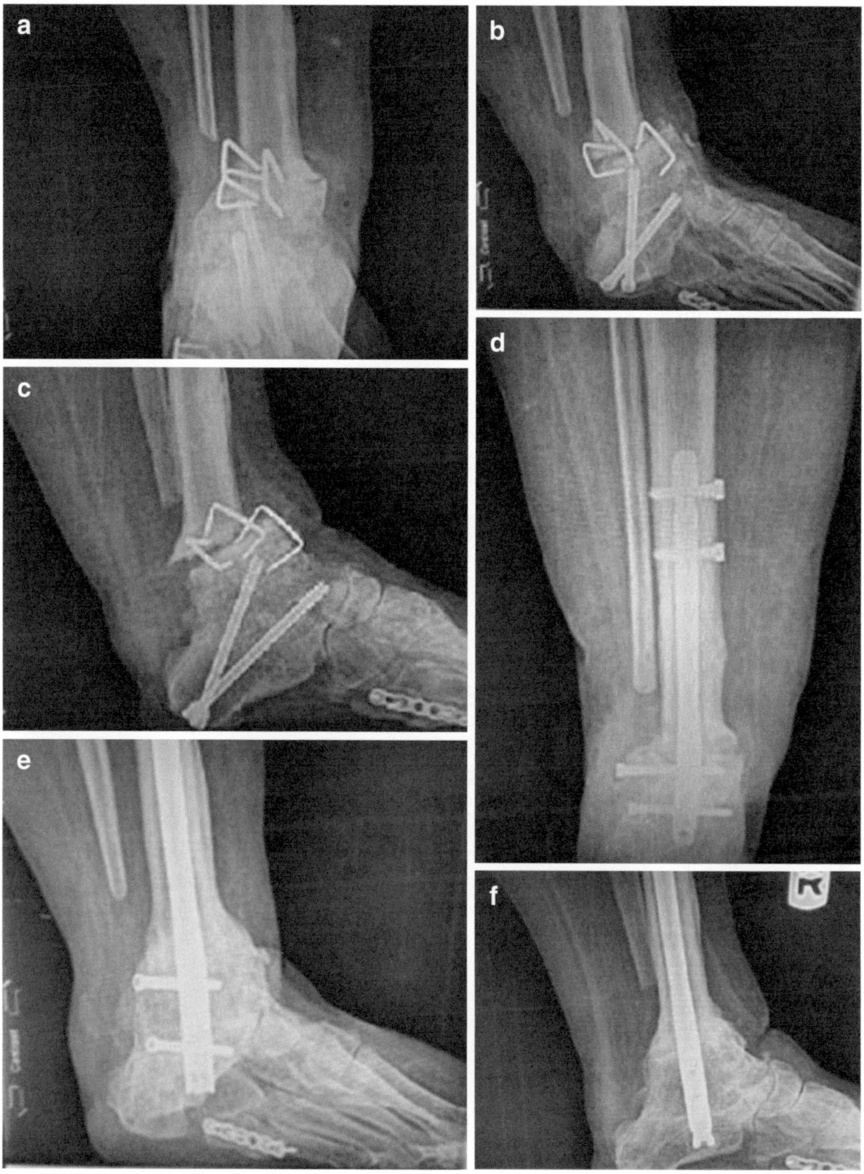

Fig. 16.9 (**a**–**c**) Failure of staple fixation and development of a non union. (**d**–**f**) Resection with bone grafting and IM nail

Clinical Pearls and Pitfall

Malunion of arthrodesis at the ankle and STJ level is a complex problem [1, 3, 4]. As the ankle goes so does the remaining foot. The STJ in this case had already undergone an arthrodesis and was in 2° (degrees) of valgus in relation to the talus. Thus, an osteotomy at the CORA (tibiotalar arthrodesis site) allowed correction of the foot inferior to this site [5, 6]. It is of utmost importance to utilize fluoroscopy and guide pins to perform an osteotomy through the malunion site centered at the CORA [7]. Osteotomes are utilized and critical for completing the osteotomy at the apex. A green stick hinge is created. If a full fracture occurs, stabilization of the hinge is needed [7]. It is obvious in this case a poor choice of fixation was utilized.

A nonunion occurred and a revision with an IM nail was performed. This choice of fixation should have most probably been utilized initially.

References

1. Graehl PM, Hersh MR, Heckman JD. Supramalleolar osteotomy for the treatment of symptomatic tibial malunion. J Orthop Trauma. 1987;1(4):281–92.
2. Harstall R, Lehmann O, Krause F, Weber M. Supramalleolar lateral closing wedge osteotomy for the treatment of varus ankle arthrosis. Foot Ankle Int. 2007 May;28(5):542–8.
3. Colin F, Gaudot F, Odri G, Judet T. Supramalleolar osteotomy: techniques, indications and outcomes in a series of 83 cases. Orthop Traumatol Surg Res. 2014;100(4):413–8.
4. Myerson MS. Reconstruction foot and ankle surgery: management of complications: Chapter 26, Osteotomy of the tibia and fibula; 2010. p. 317–30.
5. Knupp M, Stufkens SA, Bolliger L, Barg A, Hintermann B. Classification and treatment of supramalleolar deformities. Foot Ankle Int. 2011;32(11):1023–31.
6. Siddiqui NA, Herzenberg JE, Lamm BM. Supramalleolar osteotomy for realignment of the ankle joint. Clin Podiatr Med Surg. 2012 Oct;29(4):465–82.
7. Becker AS, Myerson MS. The indications and technique of supramalleolar osteotomy. Foot Ankle Clin. 2009;14(3):549–61.

Case #17: Tendon Transfer and Balancing for Combined Upper Motor Neuron and Lower Motor Neuron Equinoadductovarus Foot and Ankle Deformity

17

Case Presentation

This is a 76-year-old female Caucasian who gives a history of having lumbar spine surgery 1 year prior. She then, during the postoperative course, fell and sustained a subdural hematoma. As a result, she developed a bilateral fixed, rigid equinoadductovarus foot deformities (Fig. 17.1a, b). She was confined to a wheelchair. She was seen at a wound clinic due to the development of an ulceration over the styloid process of her fifth metatarsal (Fig. 17.1c). This occurred during transferring from her wheelchair. It affected the left extremity, but she also had a milder form of adductovarus on the right foot and ankle. The patient was referred for evaluation from the wound clinic. Radiographs (Fig. 17.2a, b) show severe adductovarus on DP view and severe equinus on lateral view.

Diagnosis and Assessment

This represents a very difficult case as it manifests characteristics of both upper motor neuron (brain) and lower motor neuron (lumbar spine) lesions. On examination, the deformity with stress could be reduced to neutral. Her deformity noted weakness of the peroneals, extensor digitorum longus (EDL), and extensor hallucis longus (EHL) muscles. This corresponded to her L5-S1 fusion. Her family noted her foot deformity before her fall. A nerve conduction velocity study (NCV) and electromyography (EMG) noted L5-S1 radiculopathy with demyelination and axonal loss. Fibrillation potentials involving the gastrocnemius and soleus, as well as, the tibialis posterior, flexor hallucis longus (FHL), and flexor digitorum longus (FDL) were present. Thus, on assessment the varus was produced by unopposed

H. J. Visser, *Challenges in Foot and Ankle Reconstructive Surgery*,
https://doi.org/10.1007/978-3-031-07893-4_17

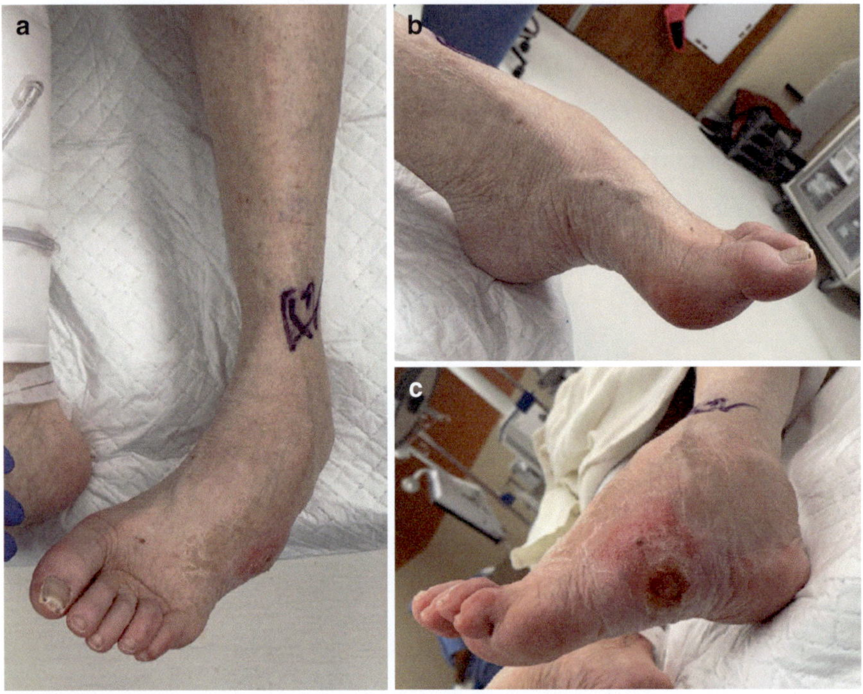

Fig. 17.1 (**a, b**) Fixed, rigid equinoadductovarus left foot deformity. (**c**) Ulceration to fifth metatarsal base, left foot, secondary to equinoadductovarus foot deformity

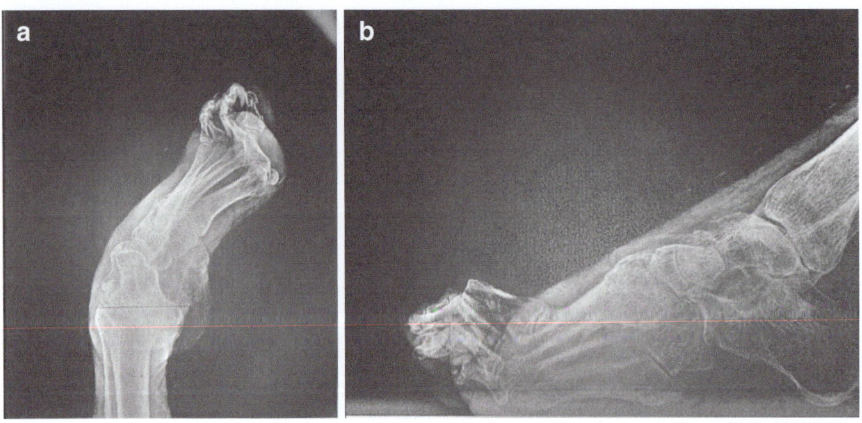

Fig. 17.2 (**a**) Severe adductovarus deformity. (**b**) Severe residual gastro-soleus equinus with cavus

tibialis anterior function (L4) and equinoadductovarus due to a spastic gastrocnemius-soleus complex and deep flexor group. This was secondary to the brain injury. Surgery was chosen due to fear of osteomyelitis associated with the deep ulceration over the fifth metatarsal. This was compounded by her loss of protective sensation about the L5-S1 dermatome. The hope was to produce a plantigrade foot in this paraplegic condition. Full ambulatory function with correction of the opposite foot was the goal.

Management

Wound care (wound care clinic) initially attempted to heal the ulceration with contact casting. The patient however was unable to tolerate the total contact cast due to her spasticity. Preoperative vascular studies were performed, and the patient was found to have adequate peripheral perfusion.

The surgical approach was first to address the Achilles contracture with an open z-plasty lengthening (Fig. 17.3). It is of note that with the popliteal nerve block and general anesthesia, the deformity failed to reduce. The ulceration over the fifth metatarsal styloid process was barriered with a Tegaderm patch. The deformity could somewhat be reduced with great stress. A tenotomy of the tibialis posterior tendon, and a talonavicular joint capsulotomy and spring ligament release were the second procedures performed (Fig. 17.4a, b). This, in conjunction with the Achilles tendon lengthening, produced great reduction of the deformity. The third procedure was to address the tibialis anterior tendon. It was transferred to the cuboid with an interference screw (Fig. 17.5a–d). Full correction of the equinoadductovarus deformity was accomplished. A 5/32" Steinmann pin was then placed across the ankle into the posterior tibia (Fig. 17.6). This positioned and splinted the plantigrade foot. A delta frame was then applied to protect the tendon balance during the healing process (Fig. 17.7a, b). The wounds were closed with 2 g of vancomycin powder over concern of potential ulcer contamination.

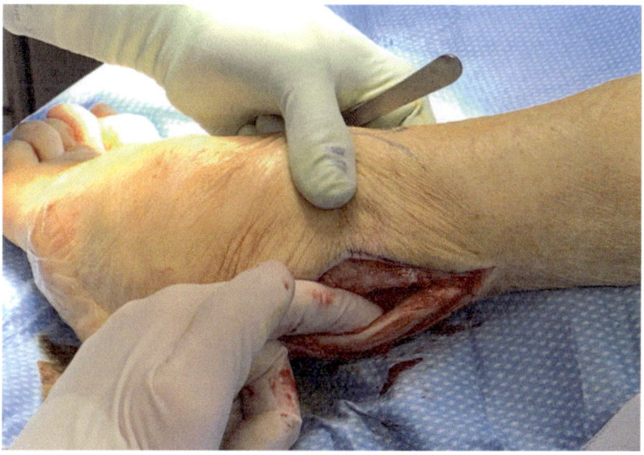

Fig. 17.3 Z-plasty lengthening of Achilles tendon, left foot

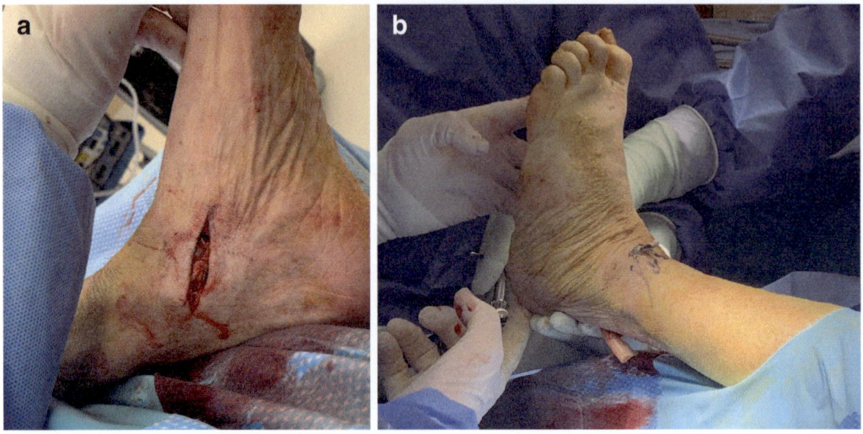

Fig. 17.4 (**a**) Tibialis posterior tenotomy, talonavicular joint capsulotomy and spring ligament release, left foot. (**b**) Foot position post tendon achilles lengthening, tibialis posterior release and TN capsulotomy

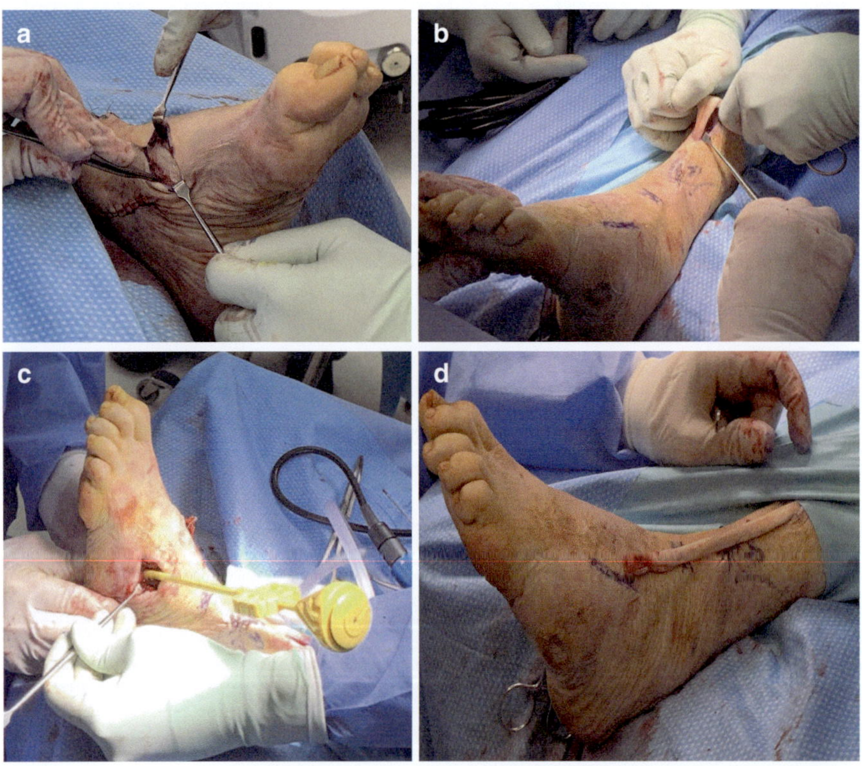

Fig. 17.5 (**a**) Recruitment of tibialis anterior tendon at insertion. (**b**) Proximal pursage of tibialis anterior tendon. (**c**) Transfer of tibialis anterior to cuboid with an interference screw. (**d**) Tibialis anterior tendon orientation for transfer

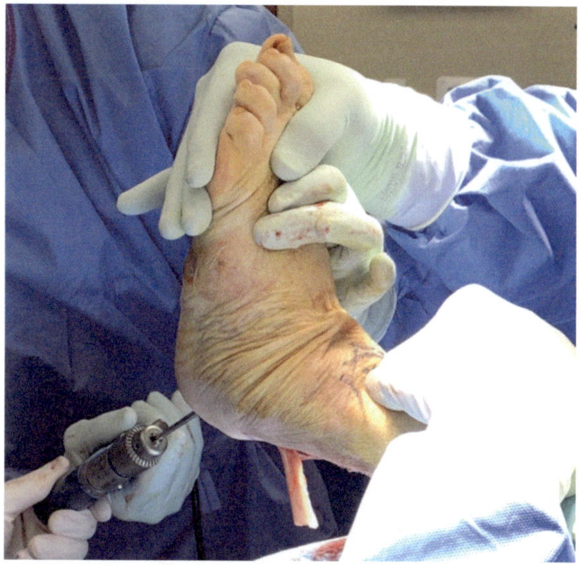

Fig. 17.6 To preserve correction, a 5/32 Steinmann pin was placed from the calcaneus into the posterior tibia

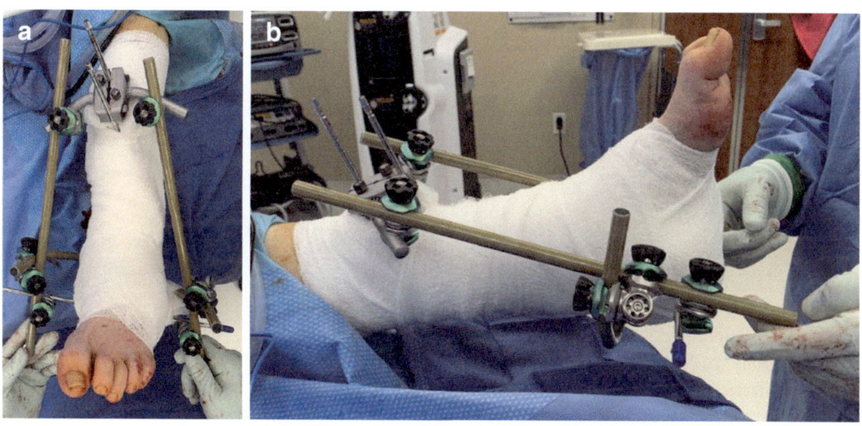

Fig. 17.7 (**a, b**) Application of delta frame

Outcome

The patient was placed in a below knee cast at the time of delta frame removal. This was 3 months post-op. The contralateral foot had the same procedure performed at the time of removal of the delta frame. The patient was prescribed an Arizona brace. She is now ambulatory with a walker for assistance.

Clinical Pearls and Pitfalls

This represents a difficult presentation of spasticity (upper motor neuron) due to her brain injury. Her forefoot supinatus was secondary to tibialis anterior muscle overactivity created by loss of function of the peroneals (S1), EHL and EDL muscles (L5). This represents lower motor neuron loss secondary to radiculopathy. [1].

Preoperative evaluation, EMG and NCV are critical to determine a surgical approach. On first viewing the patient, one would consider a more aggressive osseous approach as a need for correction. However, examination noted that the deformity could be reduced with stress. Clonus was noted when attempted reduction of the gastrocnemius-soleus complex and deep flexor group (FDL, FHL). Hyperreflexia was also present in these muscle groups.

Overpowering of the tibialis anterior secondary to L5-S1 muscle loss and equinoadductovarus from spasticity of the gastrocnemius-soleus complex and deep flexors represents combined upper motor neuron (UMN) and lower motor neuron (LMN) lesions. [2]. Transfer of the tibialis anterior to reduce forefoot varus was due to the loss of EHL, EDL, and peroneal function [3]. Weakening the spastic muscle groups involved lengthening of the triceps surae and tibialis posterior tendons. The FDL and FHL were not considered significant factors. The adduction deformity was greatly reduced by release of the supporting structures that included the talonavicular joint capsule and spring ligament. Bracing and physical therapy were also critical aspects to return her to ambulatory function.

References

1. Acosta JA, Raynor EM. Radiculopathy and motor neuron disorders. In: The clinical neurophysiology primer. Humana Press; 2007. p. 289–98.
2. Fuller DA, Keenan MAE, Esquenazi A, Whyte J, Mayer NH, Fidler-Sheppard R. The impact of instrumented gait analysis on surgical planning: treatment of spastic equinovarus deformity of the foot and ankle. Foot Ankle Int. 2002;23(8):738–43.
3. Limpaphayom N, Chantarasongsuk B, Osateerakun P, Prasongchin P. The split anterior tibialis tendon transfer procedure for spastic equinovarus foot in children with cerebral palsy: results and factors associated with a failed outcome. Int Orthop. 2015;39(8):1593–8.

18 Case #18: Tendon Lengthening Management of Rigid Equinoadductovarus Foot Deformity Post CVA

Case Presentation

This is a 43-year-old male who gives a history of having suffered a cerebrovascular accident (CVA) 2 years prior. The patient's pattern of involvement was spastic diplegia. The patient was managed with Aspirin and Plavix. Also, aggressive pharmacologic control of hypertension was done with lisinopril 20 mg and Bystolic 10 mg. His hypercholesterolemia was addressed with Lipitor and this with a higher dose at 40 mg. He underwent physical therapy but demonstrated a persistent equinoadductovarus foot deformity (Fig. 18.1a, b). He was placed in a total ankle foot orthosis (AFO). However, he was unable to tolerate the brace with ambulation. He had been given Botox injections of the involved spastic muscles (gastroc-soleus complex and tibialis posterior). This, however, failed to reduce the deformity and allow him to walk in the brace.

Diagnosis and Assessment

The patient had a presentation of an equinoadductovarus right foot secondary to spasticity from an upper motor neuron lesion secondary to a stroke (CVA).

The deformity was associated with extensive hypertonicity and clonus. With attempted reduction, spasticity could not be overcome. This presentation represents the more common of the four types of foot deformity present post CVA. The deformity was created by spasticity of the gastroc-soleus and deep flexor group. The patient also had considerable discomfort secondary to callus formation over the styloid process. This was from brace irritation.

Vascular and cutaneous nerve function were normal as CVA, in most cases, there is not a loss of protective sensation.

H. J. Visser, *Challenges in Foot and Ankle Reconstructive Surgery*,
https://doi.org/10.1007/978-3-031-07893-4_18

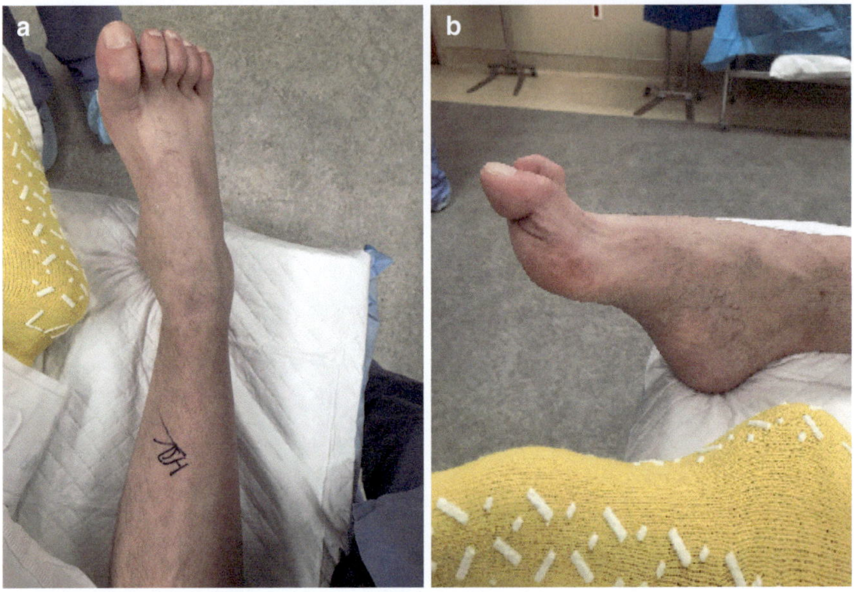

Fig. 18.1 (**a**) Post-CVA, spastic adductovarus, right foot. (**b**) Post CVA spastic equinus, right foot

Management

This first incision was to lengthen the Achilles tendon by a z-plasty (Fig. 18.2a, b). Much of the patient's deformity and residual spasticity reduced under general anesthesia. The second incision addressed the enlarged styloid process of the fifth metatarsal (Fig. 18.3a). The base was resected with care to preserve the insertion of the peroneus brevis tendon (Fig. 18.3b). The third incision involved the performance of a plantar fasciotomy (Fig. 18.4a, b). It would assist in reducing some of the arch height. The fourth incision was to lengthen the deep flexor group that included the tibialis posterior, flexor digitorum longus (FDL), and flexor hallucis longus (FHL) (Fig. 18.5). This assisted in reducing the influence of the musculotendinous structures that produced the dynamic adductovarus foot deformity [1]. This was created by a weight-bearing challenge.

Outcome

The procedure was able to create a plantigrade foot (Fig. 18.6a–c). This allowed him to comfortably ambulate in an AFO brace. He, with physical therapy, is able to ambulate at home without bracing.

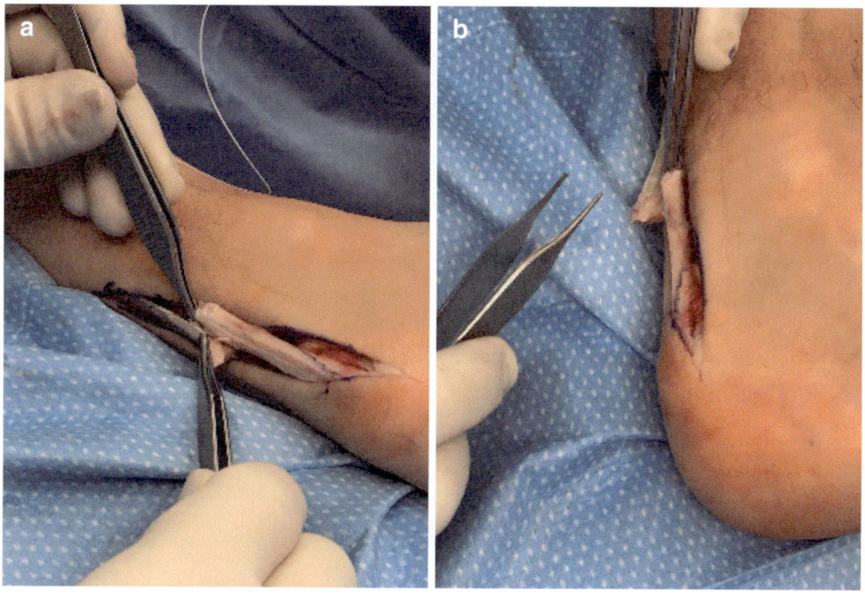

Fig. 18.2 (**a, b**) Z-plasty of Achilles tendon, right foot

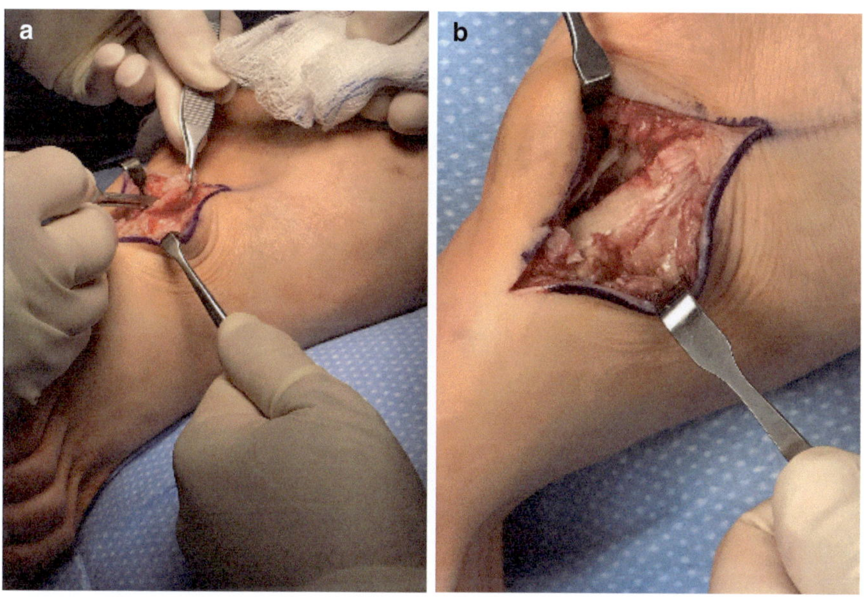

Fig. 18.3 (**a**) Enlarged styloid process, resection of the base of fifth metatarsal. (**b**) Preservation of peroneus brevis insertion

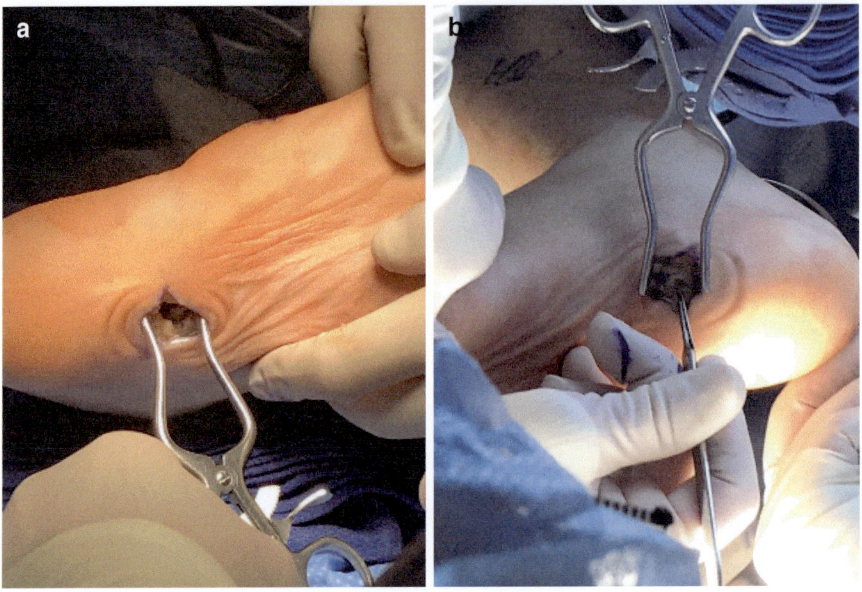

Fig. 18.4 (**a, b**) Plantar fasciotomy

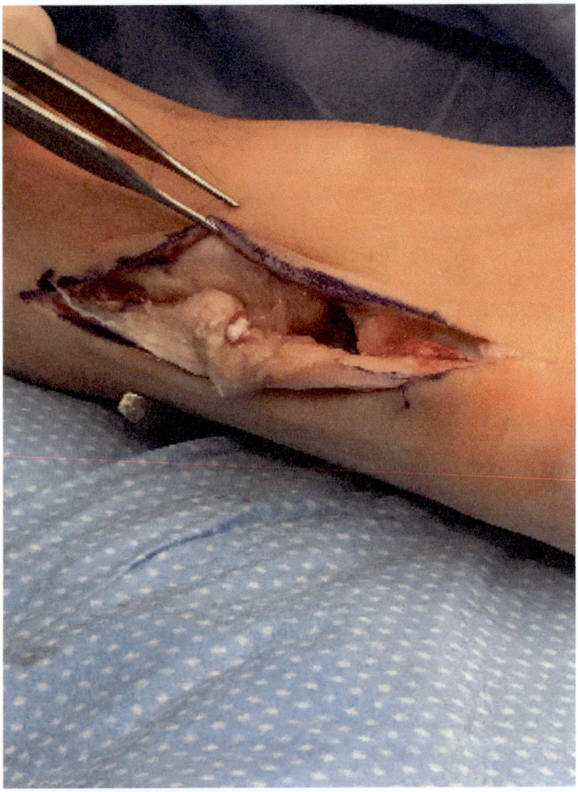

Fig. 18.5 Z-lengthening of FHL, FDL and tibialis posterior

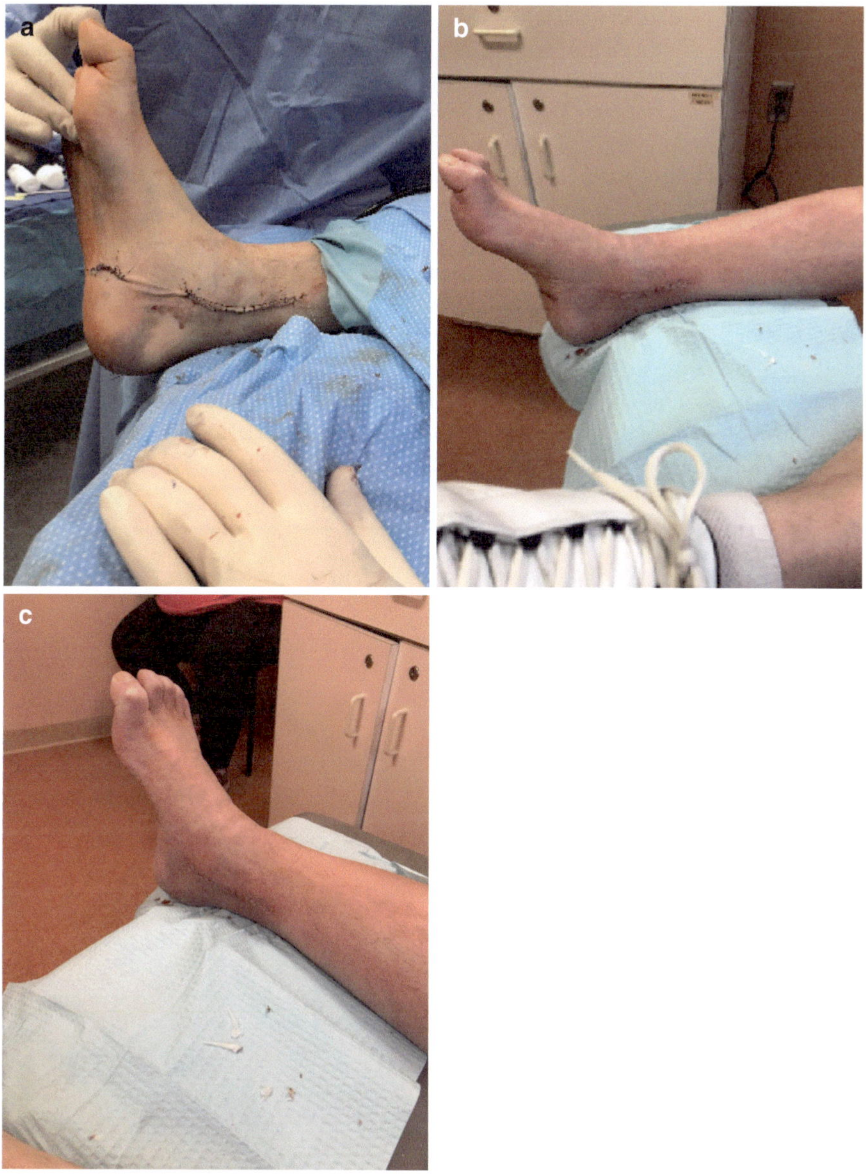

Fig. 18.6 (**a–c**) Post-operative correction of equinus and adduction deformities

Clinical Pearls and Pitfalls

The spastic equinovarus foot deformity is one of the four manifestations of spastic foot deformities post CVA. They are (1) equinus, (2) varus, (3) equinovarus, and (4) striated toe. The plan in this case was to establish a pain-free, plantigrade foot that could be accommodated by bracing. First attempts should be time and physical therapy. CVA patients should be allowed at least 9 months for recovery. Also the use of botulinum toxin or phenol has proven to be helpful to reduce spasticity created by such brain lesions [2]. While these can be useful during the long healing process, in this case it did not allow a plantigrade foot and bracing proved to be unhelpful. In essence, the patient could not ambulate. The brace was an irritant due to activated weight-bearing tone (spasticity). The spastic equinovarus is addressed with weakening by tendon lengthening. One must always be concerned when addressing spasticity about antagonist muscle groups. Use of tendon transfer can produce a reversal of existing deformity [3]. Transfer in cases of spasticity is normally ill advised. It can give a very distinct advantage to the antagonist group. Anterior transposition as described by Baker and Hill [4] of the tibialis posterior weakens and reduces spasticity by eliminating its fulcrum at the retromalleolar groove. This serves as another method of weakening the spastic muscle tendon. It will then allow balancing of its antagonist. Also, the use of split transfers can be another useful adjunct in the toolbox of addressing spasticity involving musculotendinous disorders.

References

1. Rutz E, Baker R, Tirosh O, Romkes J, Haase C, Brunner R. Tibialis anterior tendon shortening in combination with Achilles tendon lengthening in spastic equinus in cerebral palsy. Gait Posture. 2011;33(2):152–7.
2. Kuo CL, Hu GC. Post-stroke spasticity: a review of epidemiology, pathophysiology, and treatments. Int J Gerontol. 2018;12(4):280–4.
3. Medina PA, Karpman RR, Yeung AT. Split posterior tibial tendon transfer for spastic equinovarus foot deformity. Foot Ankle. 1989;10(2):65–7.
4. Baker LD, Hill LM. Foot alignment in the cerebral palsy patient. JBJS. 1964;46(1):1–15.

Case #19: Management of Avascular Necrosis of the Navicular Secondary to Mueller-Weiss Disease by Midtarsal Joint Arthrodesis

19

Case Presentation

This is a 51-year-old female with a medical history of generalized osteoarthritis and fibromyalgia. The patient gave a history of left foot pain and low-grade edema involving the midfoot. The patient, over the ensuing 1.5 years, was managed by corticosteroid injections (multiple) and two procedures that involved removal of bone spurs, in the vicinity of the navicular, from the dorsum of her left foot. She also felt that her foot had changed. She was walking more to the outside of her foot and felt unstable.

Diagnosis and Assessment

Evaluation of her left foot noted a varus heel position (Fig. 19.1a, b). Motion restriction involved both the subtalar joint and midtarsal joint motion. There was palpable pain across the midfoot with attempted range of motion. The patient demonstrated ample ankle dorsiflexion when performing the Silfverskiold test.

Radiographs were taken. On the dorsal-plantar view, abduction or convergence of the talus was noted. There was also loss of volume, (crescent sign) of the navicular, involving its central and lateral pole (Fig. 19.2a). The lateral view noted dorsal bony fragmentation involving the navicular. There was complete loss of the talonavicular joint space. There was plantarflexion of the talus and a decrease in calcaneal inclination (Fig. 19.2b). The impression was that the patient demonstrated Mueller-Weiss disease or spontaneous osteonecrosis of the navicular.

H. J. Visser, *Challenges in Foot and Ankle Reconstructive Surgery*,
https://doi.org/10.1007/978-3-031-07893-4_19

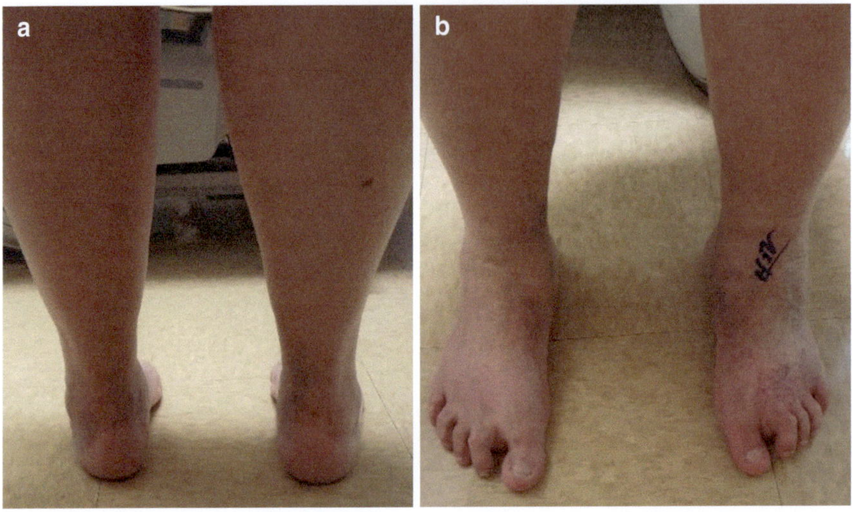

Fig. 19.1 (**a**) varus heel position, posterior view, left foot (**b**) varus heel position, anterior view, left foot

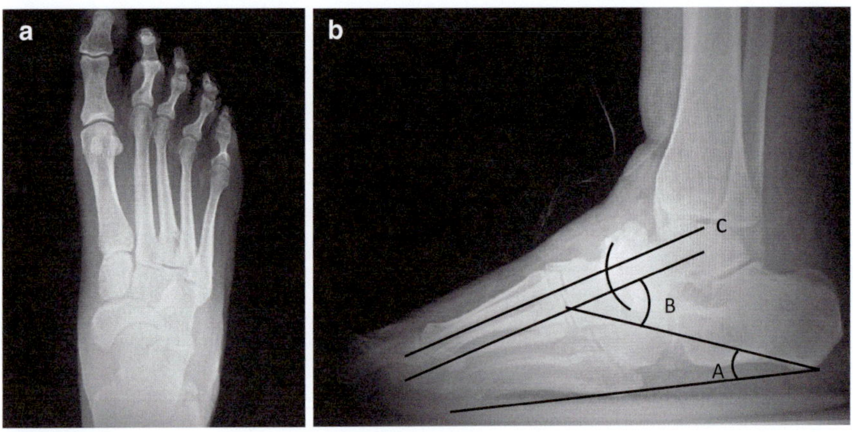

Fig. 19.2 (**a**) Convergence of talus with decreased talocalcaneal angle. (**b**) Fragmentation of navicular, talonavicular joint space loss, plantarflexed talus with decreased calcaneal inclination

Management

The approach was to perform a midtarsal arthrodesis. The central and lateral pole of the navicular body was osteonecrotic. It was thus felt that a significant portion of the navicular tuberosity and medial navicular body were viable for available arthrodesis.

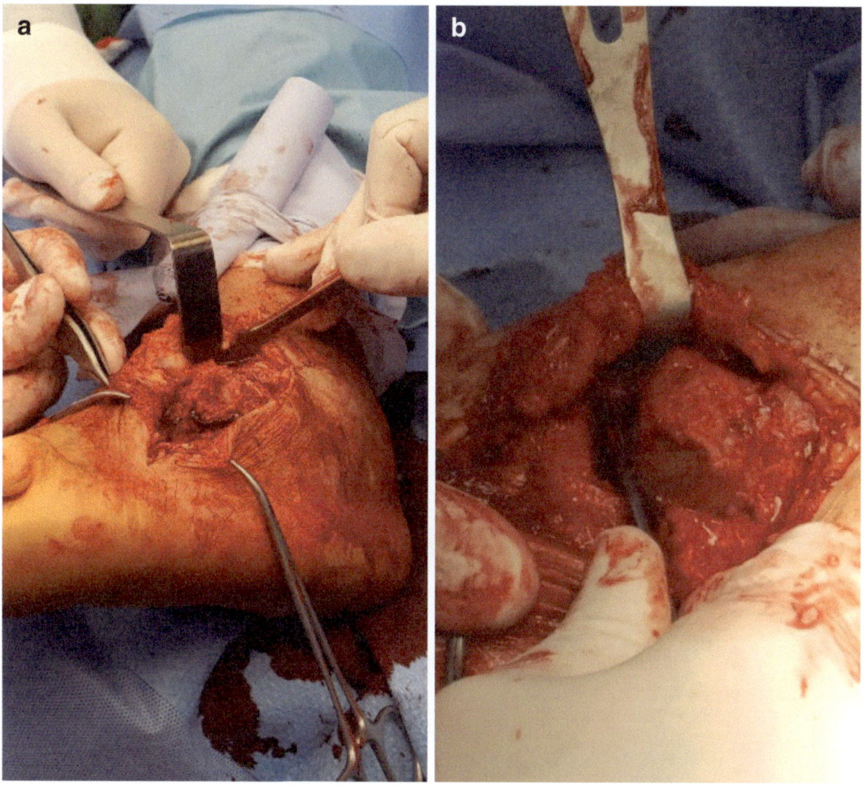

Fig. 19.3 (**a**) lateral incision over calcaneal cuboid joint. (**b**) Visualization of talar head through lateral incision

As can be seen with the lateral incision over the calcaneocuboid joint, the talar head was fully visible in line with the cuboid (Fig. 19.3a, b). This same lateral incision was also utilized to remove necrotic bone involving the central and lateral pole of the navicular body.

Through a medial incision, the remaining navicular medial body and convex tuberosity were flattened with a sagittal saw (Fig. 19.4a). A large bone hook was then used to capture the lateral neck of the talus and pull it in line with the remaining navicular tuberosity and body (Fig. 19.4b, c). This maneuver produced closed kinetic chain pronation and positioned the heel within 2 degrees of valgus. Had reduction not occurred, a subtalar joint arthrodesis or calcaneal osteotomy (valgalizing) would have been utilized. Screw fixation was accomplished with two 5.0 mm headless screws through the talonavicular joint. One 5.0 mm headless screw was then placed across the calcaneocuboid joint (Fig. 19.4d).

As can be seen by the postoperative views, talar positioning and calcaneal height were restored. The midfoot was properly aligned in all three planes.

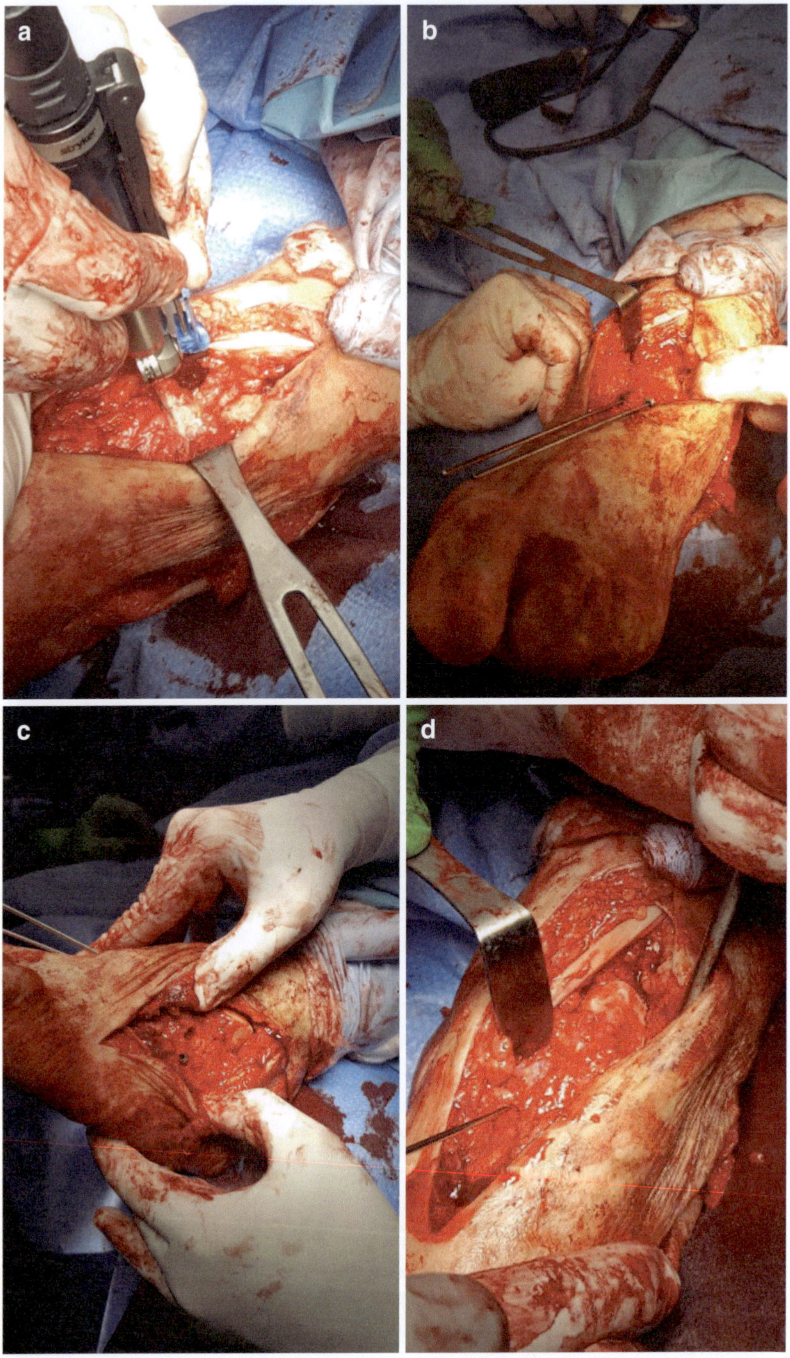

Fig. 19.4 (**a**) Preparation of talonavicular joint. (**b**) Positioning talar head in medial incision at talonavicular joint. (**c**) Repositioned talus as visualized through the lateral incision. (**d**) Fixation of talonavicular joint with 5.0 headless screws

Outcome

The patient was kept non-weight bearing for 6 weeks and then began weight bearing in a CAM boot for a further 6 weeks. A solid arthrodesis was noted and she was ambulating well by 6 months. As she had only unilateral involvement and was not highly mobile, she was pleased with her postoperative result.

Clinical Pearls and Pitfalls

This case demonstrates another condition that can produce an adult acquired flatfoot deformity. In this case, Mueller-Weiss disease is often seen in middle aged women during their 40s and 50s [1]. This age range is similar to tibialis posterior dysfunction, the most common cause of adult acquired flatfoot.

Mueller-Weiss disease produces a condition that can be termed a "paradoxical pes planovarus foot." When viewing the dorsoplantar view, convergence (talar abduction) occurs here due to volume loss of the lateral navicular body. This produces closed kinetic chain supination [2]. The result is the subtalar joint supinates and calcaneus tilts into varus in the frontal plane (Fig. 19.5).

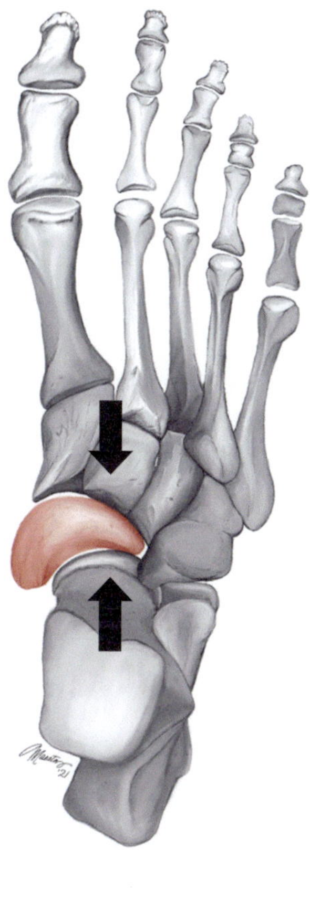

Fig. 19.5 AVN of the central and lateral pole at the navicular. With loss of buttressing supporting the talus positions in abduction which then creates closed kinetic chain supination of the subtalar joint

The "pes plano" portion occurs where there is no further support for the talar head with loss of the central navicular body (Fig. 19.2b) [3]. The talus tilts plantarly into the created defect. This places force on the anterior calcaneal body (anterior subtalar joint). Thus, it forces the calcaneus into plantarflexion and "lowers the arch." The result is complete loss of talonavicular motion. The subtalar joint also becomes locked. The foot is, thus, fixed and rigid.

Other approaches to addressing the avascular portion of the navicular can include the following: First, grafting the excised central or lateral pole and using structural autograft or allograft [4]. Second, excising the complete navicular and replacing it with a carved autograft. Both require extended periods of non-weight bearing and, thus, carry a much higher risk of nonunion. Third is performing a Naughton-Dunn type of triple arthrodesis [5]. This involves removing the navicular and then the talus is fused to the three cuneiforms. The calcaneocuboid joint is shortened to accommodate medial column shortening. It is preferable, as in this case, that if enough remaining tuberosity and medial body are available, that a primary talonavicular arthrodesis can be performed.

References

1. Doyle T, Napier RJ, Wong-Chung J. Recognition and management of Müller-Weiss disease. Foot Ankle Int. 2012;33(4):275–81.
2. Rivera JE. Open versus closed kinetic chain rehabilitation of the lower extremity: a functional and biomechanical analysis. J Sport Rehabil. 1994;3(2):154–67.
3. Woodburn J, Cornwall MW, Soames RW, Helliwell PS. Selectively attenuating soft tissues close to sites of inflammation in the peritalar region of patients with rheumatoid arthritis leads to development of pes planovalgus. J Rheumatol. 2005;32(2):268–74.
4. Mayich DJ. The treatment of Mueller-Weiss disease: a systematic approach. Techniq Foot Ankle Surg. 2016;15(2):59–73.
5. Dunn N. Stabilizing operations in the treatment of paralytic deformities of the foot. Proc R Soc Med. 1922;15(Surg Sect):15–22.

Case #20: Management of Adductocavovarus Foot Deformity Secondary to Post Talar Neck Fracture Malunion

20

Case Presentation

This is a 52-year-old female who fell into a deep hole and twisted her right foot. She was seen in the ER with increased edema and pain. Original X-rays were negative. The conclusion was that a Lisfranc ligament disruption was not present.

She then followed up with her primary care physician (PCP) who managed her with rest, ice, compression, and elevation (RICE), nonsteroidal anti-inflammatory drugs (NSAIDs), and a controlled ankle motion (CAM) boot. She states she could not really put weight on her foot for 3 weeks. Repeat X-rays were taken and she was told there were no signs of fracture. As the edema reduced, she was sent for physical therapy (PT). She states she could not tolerate it. Now at 3 months post injury, she was still experiencing pain and could not get back into shoe wear. This led to her PCP to order a magnetic resonance imaging (MRI). The MRI related a mildly displaced (Hawkins type II) talar neck fracture with medial comminution. She then underwent open reduction internal fixation (ORIF) with two headless screws through "percutaneous" incision.

Over the next 2 years, she described her pain as tolerable. But was still having problems with increased activity. She also noted her foot felt "stiff." She also stated that she was walking on the outside and felt unstable.

Diagnosis and Assessment

When she was initially evaluated, the patient was noted to have restricted range of motion (ROM) of both the subtalar (STJ) and midtarsal (MTJ) joints, right foot. There was some available motion but with a maximal pronation force the calcaneus

H. J. Visser, *Challenges in Foot and Ankle Reconstructive Surgery*,
https://doi.org/10.1007/978-3-031-07893-4_20

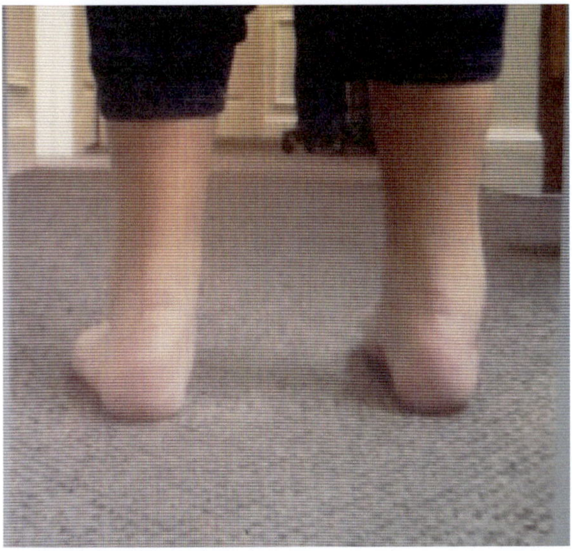

Fig. 20.1 Calcaneal varus, right foot

was in varus. On relaxed calcaneal stance position (RSCP), she had 6° (degrees) of calcaneal varus and residual midfoot adduction. Her contralateral foot noted a mildly pronated foot with some left heel valgus (Fig. 20.1).

The dorsal-plantar (DP) radiograph noted a healed neck fracture of the talus. There was increased talar convergence (talar abduction). The talo-navicular joint (TNJ) looked preserved, and there were no signs of avascular (AVN). Forefoot (FF) adduction was noted at the MTJ (Fig. 20.2a). The lateral view noted a healed talar neck fracture with a preserved STJ. Her Meary's angle however was increased. Overall, arch elevation secondary to STJ supination was noted (Fig. 20.2b).

The calcaneal long leg axial view was telling with the presence of an STJ varus. The calcaneus was in approximately 6° of varus (Fig. 20.3a, b).

The assessment was a healed talar neck fracture without AVN. However, during the healing process shortening of the talar neck occurred producing an adductocavovarus foot deformity. Thus, the patient demonstrated a talar neck malunion.

Management

The surgical approach was to perform an opening wedge osteotomy of the talar neck (Fig. 20.4a). The osteotomy was created just anterior to the medial talar tubercle. The more proximal cut would allow greater lengthening of the talar neck (collum tali). A saw was utilized to create the osteotomy ¾ of the way. It was completed with an osteotome to greenstick the lateral neck (Fig. 20.4b). A Hintermann retractor was then used for distraction to produce lengthening of the neck (Fig. 20.4c, d). This allowed closed kinetic chain pronation of the STJ (Fig. 20.5a, b). This

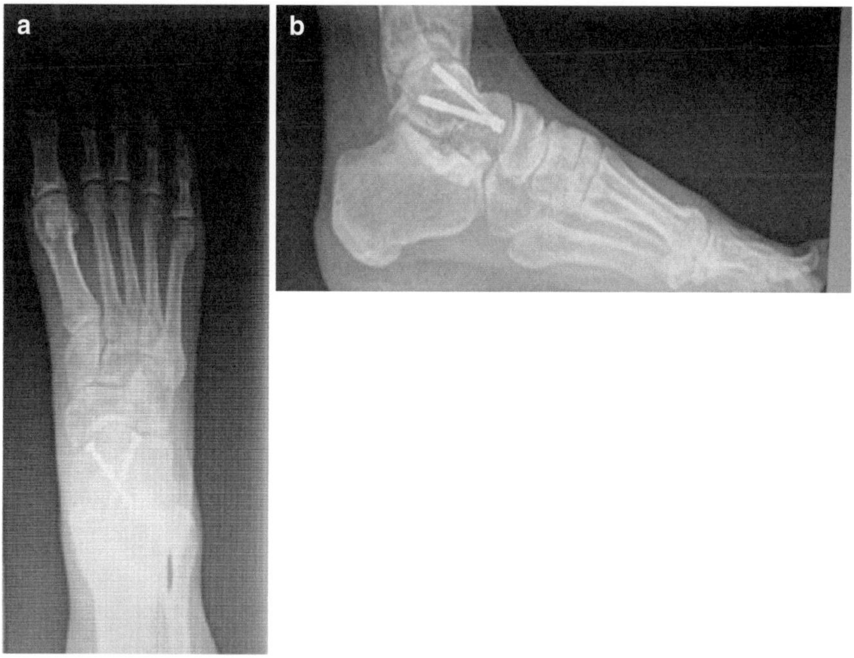

Fig. 20.2 (**a**) Increased talar abduction without signs of avascular necrosis. Forefoot adduction noted at the midtarsal joint level. (**b**) Healed talar neck fracture with preserved subtalar joint. Subtalar joint is supinated as noted by the increased arch height

produced correction of the heel varus deformity (see on the axial). A tricortical iliac autograft, secured from the ipsilateral hip, was utilized and two points of fixation were performed (Fig. 20.6). This was due to the created greenstick fracture of the lateral neck.

Outcome

The patient was kept at non-weight bearing (NWB) for nearly 3 months. The concern was graft healing and potential AVN [1]. She did heal the graft and did not develop AVN. Overall correction was good but her STJ and MTJ motion remained restricted. She had a plantigrade foot with the heel in 3° of valgus. As she was not highly active, this has sustained her. A triple arthrodesis may be in the future.

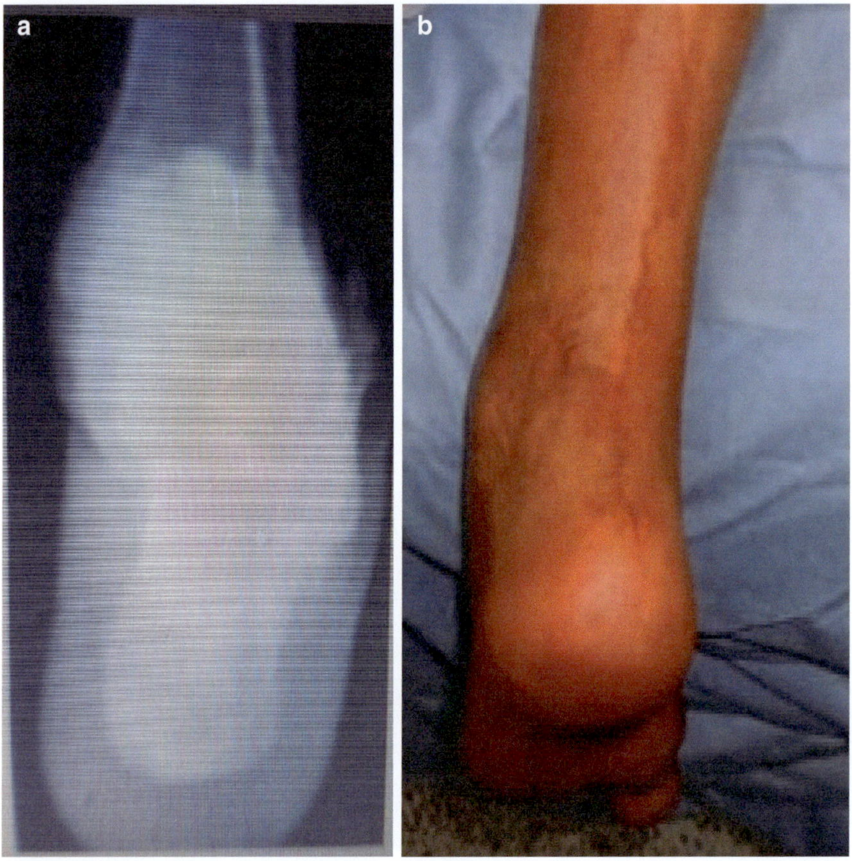

Fig. 20.3 (**a, b**) STJ varus evident both radiographically and clinically

Clinical Pearls and Pitfalls

Talar neck malunion presents intricate conditions for revision [2]. It is important that with the initial surgery, restoration of length on the medial talar neck is re-established. Traditionally, a 2-incision approach is utilized. The lateral neck is anatomically aligned first, in most cases fracture mechanisms create comminution medially [3]. Once the lateral side is aligned, fixation medially with screws or mini plates is performed.

Malunion of the talar neck creates "shortening" of the medial column. This produces a closed kinetic chain (CKC) supinatory effect leading to STJ varus, forefoot supination, and an anterior cavus. This then locks the STJ in a fixed supinated position. The midtarsal joint gets fixed in an adducted and varus state [4]. The result is loss of STJ and MTJ motion with lateral foot overload.

Management of talar neck osteotomy requires care to preserve the talar neck blood supply. A medial incision is utilized and dissection is carried to the proximal

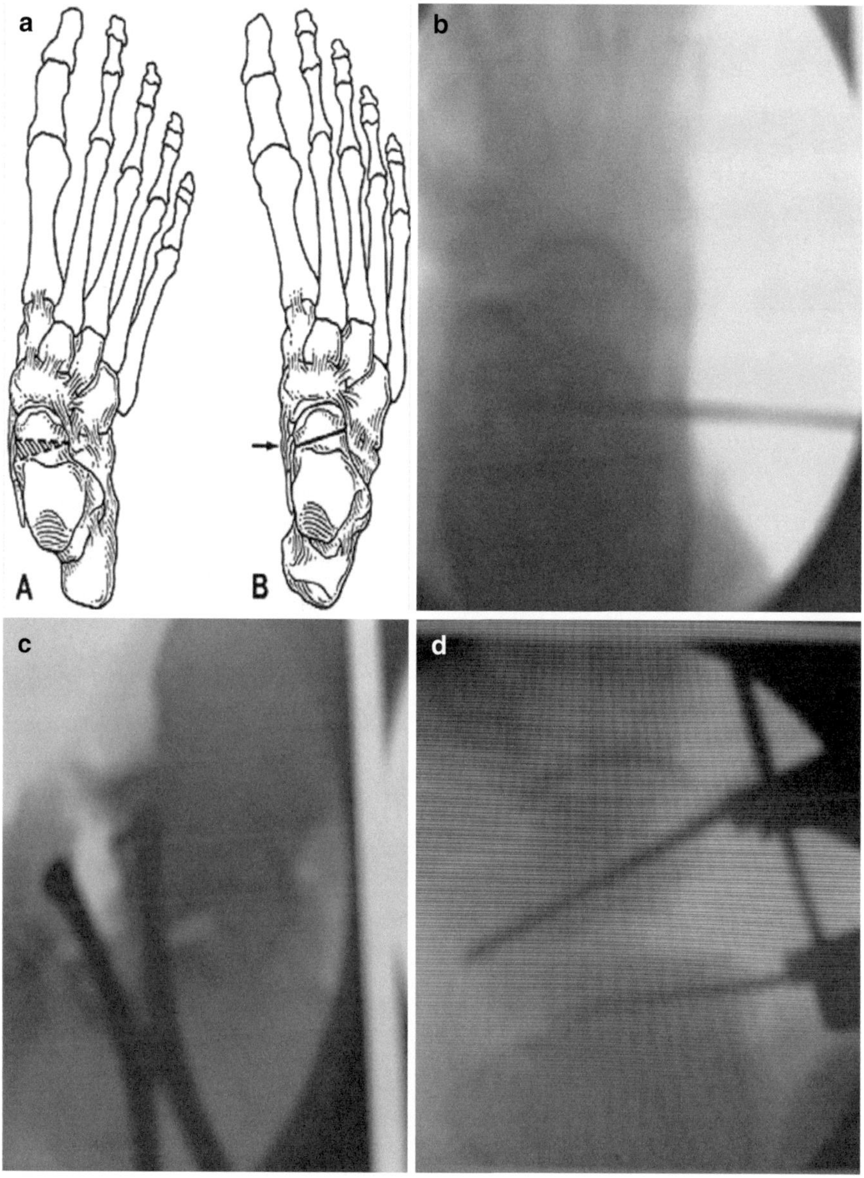

Fig. 20.4 (**a**) Opening wedge osteotomy completed just anterior to the medial talar tubercle. (**b**) An osteotome is utilized to complete the osteotomy to greenstick the lateral neck of the talus. (**c, d**) The osteotomy is distracted with a Hintermann retractor to effectively lengthen the talar neck

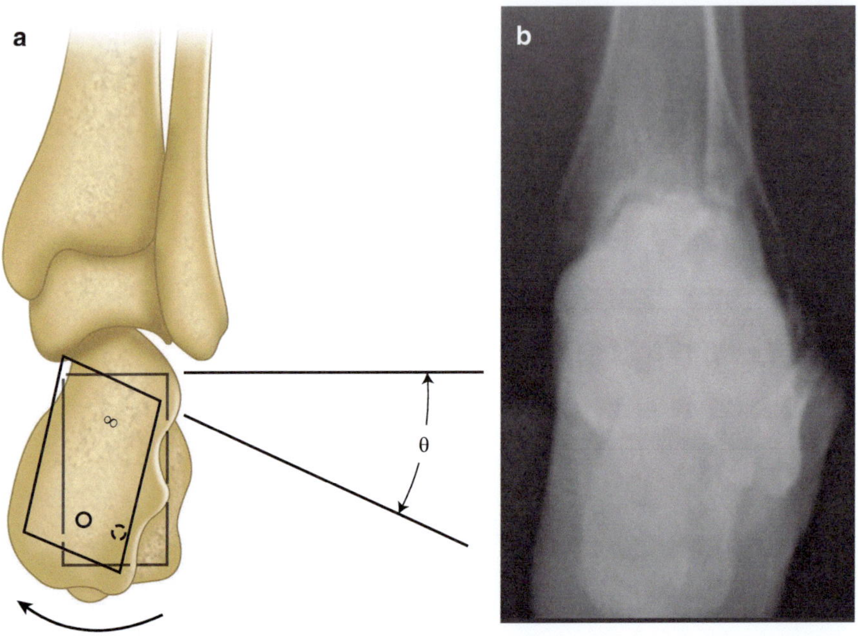

Fig. 20.5 (**a**, **b**) Lengthening of the talar neck produces closed kinetic chain pronation of the STJ resulting in correction of the heel varus deformity

Fig. 20.6 Two screws are placed to fixate a tricortical autograft in the osteotomy site

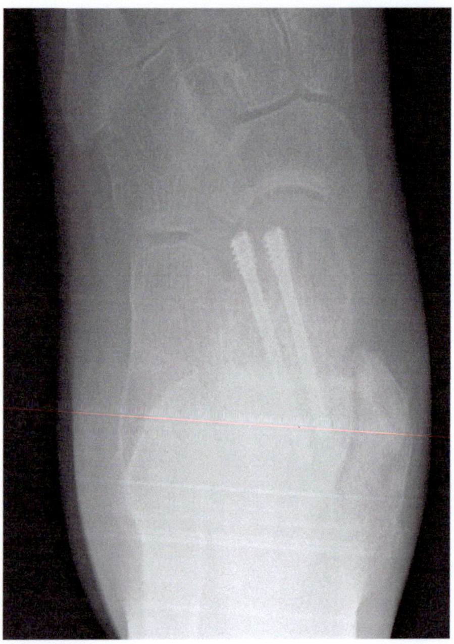

neck to avoid the nutrient artery that travels to the distal neck. Also, care is taken not to damage the anterior STJ with the osteotomy. Graft size is dependent on restoration of the STJ and MTJ position. This is determined by distraction with a Hintermann retractor. If the STJ is not "repositioned" or the midtarsal joint not reduced, a triple arthrodesis or valgalizing osteotomy may be required [5].

References

1. Huber H, Galantay R, Dutoit M. Avascular necrosis after osteotomy of the talar neck to correct residual club-foot deformity in children: a long-term review. J Bone Joint Surg Br. 2002;84(3):426–30.
2. Halvorson JJ, Winter SB, Teasdall RD, Scott AT. Talar neck fractures: a systematic review of the literature. J Foot Ankle Surg. 2013;52(1):56–61.
3. Monroe MT, Manoli A. Osteotomy for malunion of a talar neck fracture: a case report. Foot Ankle Int. 1999;20(3):192–5.
4. Daniels TR, Smith JW, Ross TI. Varus malalignment of the talar neck. Its effect on the position of the foot and on subtalar motion. JBJS. 1996;78(10):1559–67.
5. Suter T, Barg A, Knupp M, Henninger H, Hintermann B. Surgical technique: talar neck osteotomy to lengthen the medial column after a malunited talar neck fracture. Clin Orthop Relat Res. 2013;471(4):1356–64.

Case #21: Revision of the STAR Total Ankle Replacement with Iliac Autograft

21

Case Presentation

This is a 57-year-old white female who gives a history of long-term bilateral ankle pain after suffering injuries to both extremities in a motor vehicle accident (MVA) some 12 years prior. She began to develop symptoms of ankle pain some 4 years prior to evaluation. She underwent extensive conservative care for her post-traumatic ankle arthritis. Ultimately, she was referred for surgical care.

The patient was healthy and no major health issues listed. She had normal vitamin D levels and was maintained on oral D3. Vascular perfusion was normal and neurologically there were no noted deficits. The patient exhibited a very antalgic gait with associated external limb rotation. She had an initial Scandinavian Total Ankle Replacement (STAR) on the left ankle in March and did very well. The right ankle was then performed in July of the same year. She made good progress for approximately 16 months but then came for evaluation when she developed insertional Achilles tendinitis. She also related that her ankle felt unstable.

Diagnosis and Assessment

Clinically, the patient on weight bearing (WB) demonstrated calcaneal varus angulation. She had exquisite pain over the insertion of her right Achilles tendon. Radiographs were taken and the telling story was noted on the lateral view. The talar component was noted to have shifted posterior and appeared level with the posterior facet of the subtalar joint (STJ). Lateral translation of the talar implant was noted on the ankle anterior posterior view with encroachment of the lateral gutter (Fig. 21.1a, b).

H. J. Visser, *Challenges in Foot and Ankle Reconstructive Surgery*,
https://doi.org/10.1007/978-3-031-07893-4_21

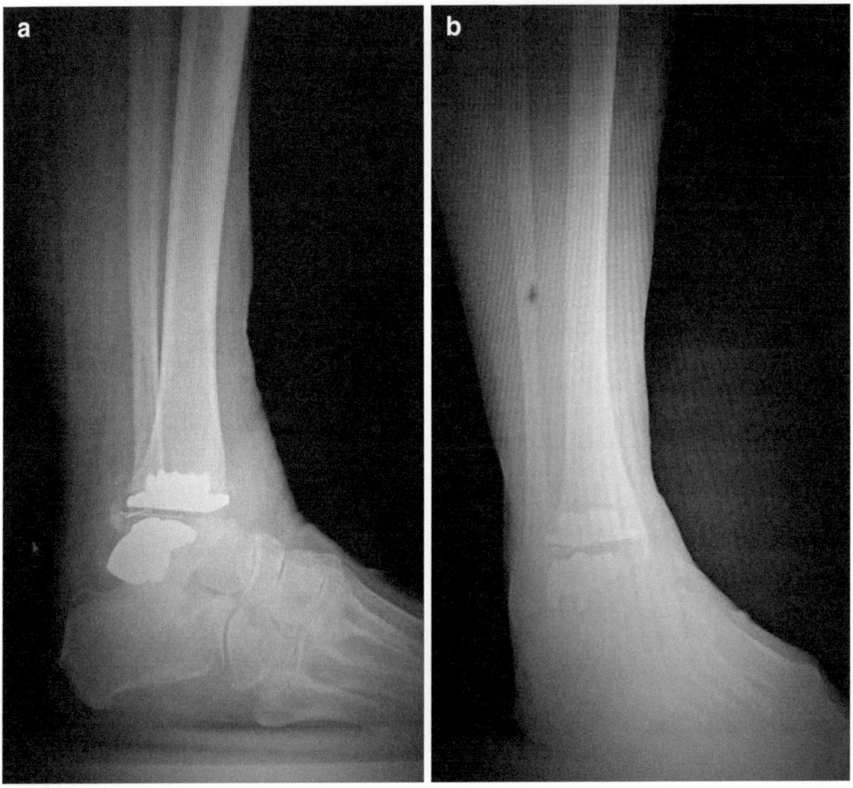

Fig. 21.1 (**a, b**) Talar subsidence with lateral and posterior translation of talar implant encroaching into lateral gutter

The obvious concern was collapse of the talar implant and thus the remaining integrity of the talar body. Computed tomography (CT) scans showed talar body subsidence. The STJ itself remained preserved.

Management

The surgical approach was through the prior anterior incision. The polyethylene spacer and talar prosthetic component were removed (Fig. 21.2a, b). The hope was to possibly reposition the implant with bone grafting. On viewing the lateral view, a significant loss of the talar body was noted (Fig. 21.2c).

Thus, the choice was then to perform an arthrodesis of the right ankle with a tricortical iliac autograft. A 7.0 mm cannulated posterior positioning screw was placed through the graft (Fig. 21.3a). A long anatomically contoured locking plate was then placed anteriorly to act as buttress, as well as neutralization. The fixation secured a plantigrade position (Fig. 21.4a–c).

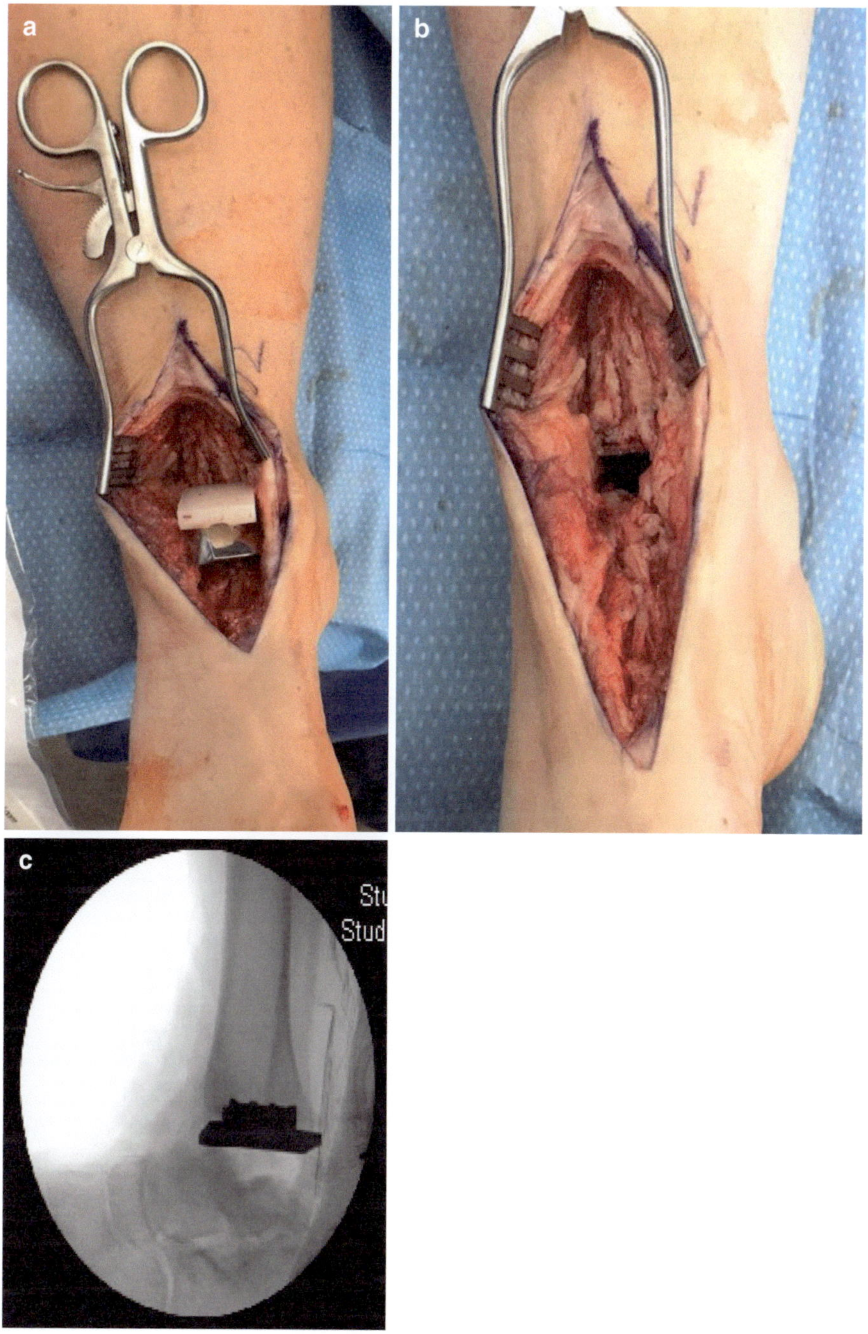

Fig. 21.2 (**a**–**c**) Removal of the poly and talar resurfacing implant revealed posterior lateral collapse of the talus

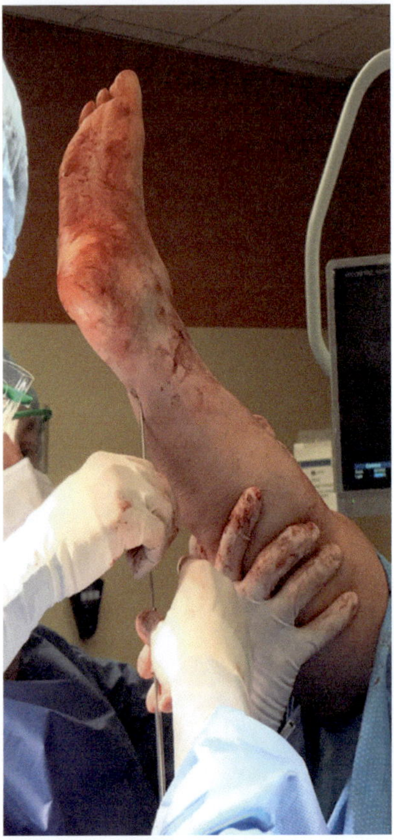

Fig. 21.3 (**a**) A cannulated posterior positioning screw was inserted through the cortical iliac graft

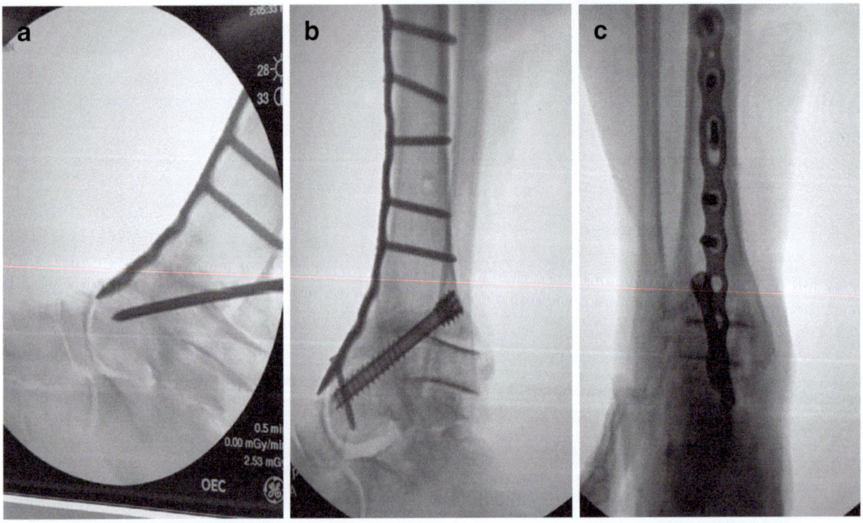

Fig. 21.4 (**a–c**) With the foot in a plantigrade position, a long anatomically contoured locking plate was placed anteriorly to act as buttress, as well as neutralization

The patient was kept at non-weight bearing (NWB) for 12 weeks. She was further protected during WB in a controlled ankle motion (CAM) boot, for a further 12 weeks. An Arizona brace was then constructed.

Outcome

The patient showed persistent signs of a delayed union. She was kept further NWB for six more weeks utilizing a capacitance coupling bone stimulator. She ultimately broke the anterior plate and went on to a nonunion. Fortunately, an arthrofibrosis occurred. Despite being sensate, she had little pain. She did exhibit motion at this site. She notes much better function on the successful left total ankle replacement (TAR) site.

Clinical Pearls and Pitfalls

Performance of bilateral TARs can establish much improved function in a patient demonstrating bilateral ankle joint osteoarthritis (OA). The issue in this case where AVN of talus occurred, it required removal of the implant with insertion of a bone graft to attain arthrodesis. Unfortunately, it went on to nonunion on the right lower extremity. It may have been prudent to have had a longer window of recovery between cases. There is, however, no substantial evidence in the literature concerning bilateral TAR's recovery and associated timing [1, 2].

When performing a revision of this nature, it makes a difficult situation. A large defect exhibited with filling of bone graft and maintaining anatomic position is difficult. Failure in this case probably was due to the large graft size and also the presence of residual talar avascular changes on the remaining posterior talar surface [3–5].

When utilizing a large bone graft in a situation like this, placement of a strut 7.0 mm screw without compression is preferred. Compression of the graft with screw fixation can lead to bone graft accretion [6]. As a compression screw was used in this case, it could have contributed to graft collaspe. A long locking plate was utilized to dissipate bending, shearing, and torsional forces.

References

1. Barg A, Henninger HB, Knupp M, Hintermann B. Simultaneous bilateral total ankle replacement using a 3-component prosthesis: outcome in 26 patients followed for 2–10 years. Acta Orthop. 2011;82(6):704–10.
2. Barg A, Knupp M, Hintermann B. Simultaneous bilateral versus unilateral total ankle replacement: a patient-based comparison of pain relief, quality of life and functional outcome. J Bone Joint Surg. 2010;92(12):1659–63.
3. Berkowitz MJ, Sanders RW, Walling AK. Salvage arthrodesis after failed ankle replacement: surgical decision making. Foot Ankle Clin. 2012;17(4):725–40.

4. Deleu PA, Devos Bevernage B, Maldague P, Gombault V, Leemrijse T. Arthrodesis after failed total ankle replacement. Foot Ankle Int. 2014;35(6):549–57.
5. Horisberger M, Henninger HB, Valderrabano V, Barg A. Bone augmentation for revision total ankle arthroplasty with large bone defects: a technical note on 10 cases. Acta Orthop. 2015;86(4):412–4.
6. Berkowitz MJ, Clare MP, Walling AK, Sanders R. Salvage of failed total ankle arthroplasty with fusion using structural allograft and internal fixation. Foot Ankle Int. 2011;32(5):493–502.

Part III

The Valgus Foot and Ankle

Case #22: Reconstruction of Adult-Acquired Flatfoot Deformity with Ruptured Tibialis Posterior Tendon and Spring Ligament

22

Case Presentation

This is a 51-year-old Caucasian male who presents with a unilateral flatfoot deformity of long-term duration. He was told 3 years prior after magnetic resonance imaging (MRI) was performed that he had a completely ruptured tibialis posterior (PT) tendon involving his right foot and ankle. The patient clinically demonstrated a unilateral peritalar subluxation (flatfoot) and associated antalgic gait of right foot. The deformity was flexible and reducible. It did require plantarflexion of the ankle however to attain reduction of subtalar joint (STJ) and midtarsal joint (MTJ) position.

Diagnosis and Assessment

Radiographs were performed showing on the dorsal plantar (DP) view about 35% uncoverage of the talus (Fig. 22.1a). The cuboid abduction angle was increased. The lateral view showed an uncharacteristic talonavicular (TN) fault on right foot (Fig. 22.1b). The talus was stepped off in reference to the navicular by about 3 mm. The remaining medial column was well aligned. There were no associated signs of degenerative joint disease (DJD). An AP of an ankle revealed no deltoid insufficieny.

The MRI indicated a complete rupture of the PT tendon with retraction. Also a tear of the spring ligament was present.

Since the deformity centered completely about the talus, a double calcaneal osteotomy and soft tissue tendon balancing procedures were chosen.

H. J. Visser, *Challenges in Foot and Ankle Reconstructive Surgery*,
https://doi.org/10.1007/978-3-031-07893-4_22

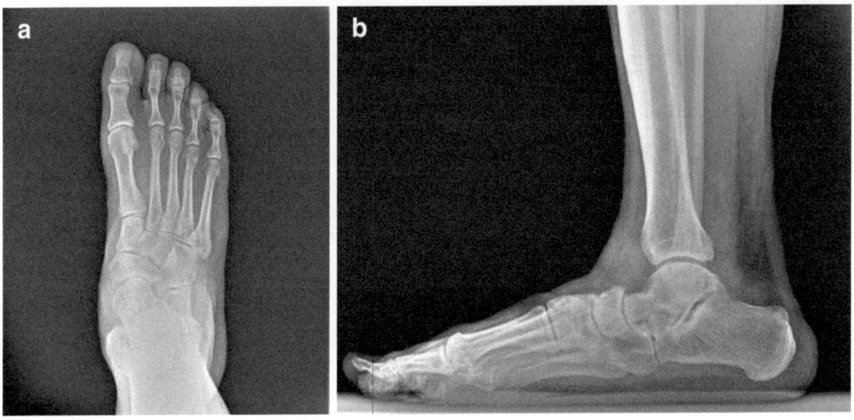

Fig. 22.1 (**a**) Dorsoplantar view radiograph demonstrates 35% talonavicular uncoverage. (**b**) Lateral radiograph shoes an uncharacteristic TN fault, indicating a possible spring ligament tear

Management

The initial double calcaneal osteotomy was performed through two separate incisions. A posterior (koutsogiannis-first incision) calcaneal osteotomy was performed and fixed with two (5.0 mm) cannulated screws to reduce the valgus heel position (Fig. 22.2a, b). An anterior (Evans-second incision) calcaneal osteotomy was performed to create closed kinetic chain supination of the STJ by lengthening the lateral column (Figs. 22.3a, b and 22.4a–c). A cancellous titanium wedge of 8 mm was utilized. This acted to reposition the talus and restore its normal coverage with navicular. Longitudinal arch height was re-established by tensioning the plantar fascia and restoring the function of the peroneus longus tendon (Fig. 22.5a, b).

A peroneus brevis to longus transfer was performed above the retromalleolar groove posterior to the fibula through the third incision (Fig. 22.5a). The fourth incision included a Baumann type gastrocnemius recession for the gastrocnemius equinus which was determined by the Silfverskiold test (Fig. 22.6a–f).

A fifth incision was performed medially to transfer the flexor digitorum longus (FDL) tendon to the navicular. The remaining ruptured tibialis posterior tendon stump was found at the retro malleolar groove. It was excised. The spring ligament was repaired via an internal bracing system. Two interference screws were placed. One at the sustentaculum tali and then the distal end of the tape completing the spring ligament tear repair was then placed through a 5.0 mm drill hole in the navicular. The FDL tendon was run through the same drill hole inferior to superior. The FDL tendon was then tensioned with the foot in a fully adducted, plantarflexed, and inverted position about the TN joint. A 7.0 mm interference screw was utilized. The patient was kept NWB for 4 weeks in a posterior splint. He was then converted to a WB CAM boot for a further 4 weeks. He was then sent to physical therapy (PT) for approximately 6 weeks.

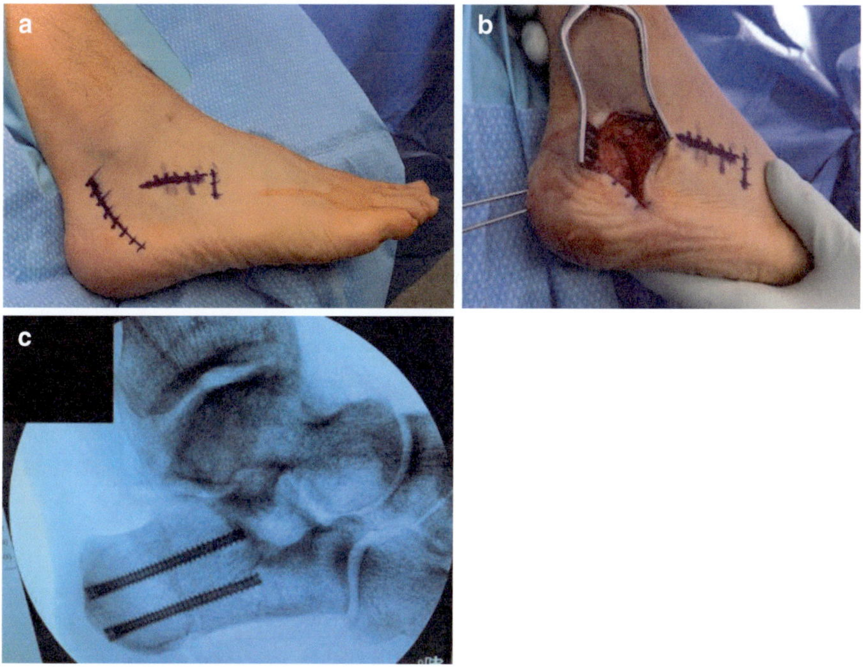

Fig. 22.2 (**a–c**) Lateral incision for medializing calcaneal osteotomy. Fixated with two 5.0 mm screws

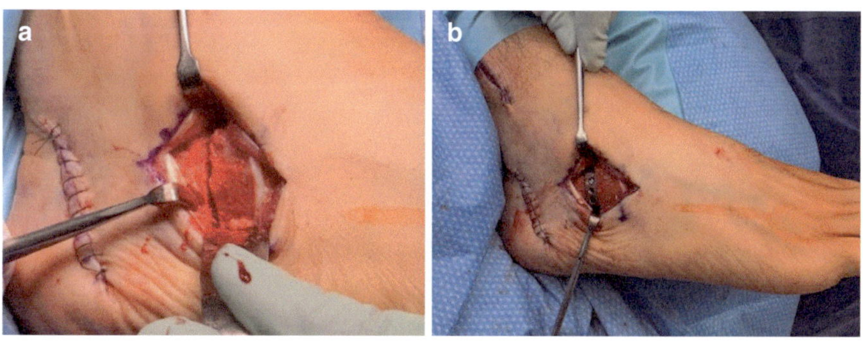

Fig. 22.3 (**a, b**) Lateral column lengthening made through an anterior lateral calcaneal incision with placement of 8 mm cancellous titanium wedge

Outcome

The patient did extremely well and benefited greatly from PT. He was able to resume full activity at 6 months. Deformity correction was maintained. He was then placed in a rigid orthotic device to help maintain the corrected position.

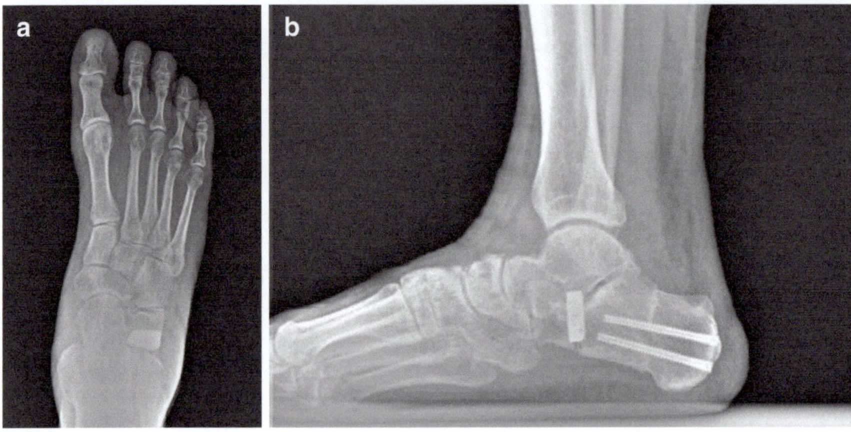

Fig. 22.4 (**a, b**) Lateral column lengthening repositioned the talus to restore normal coverage with the navicular. Longitudinal arch height is re-established, allowing restoration of peroneus longus tendon function

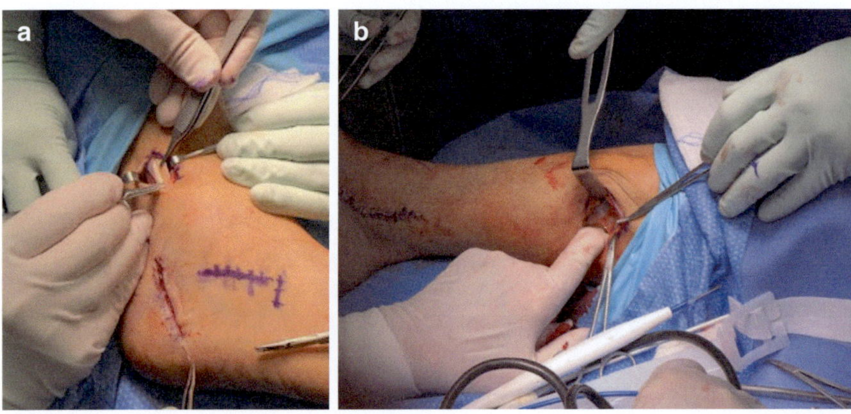

Fig. 22.5 (**a**) Peroneus brevis to longus transfer was performed above the fibular retromalleolar groove. (**b**) Baumann type gastrocnemius recession

Clinical Pearls and Pitfalls

Patients with tibialis posterior dysfunction can be staged as originally described by Johnson and Strom. This is a case of a stage 2 deformity which indicated reducibility and flexibility of the foot deformity [1]. A long-term tibialis posterior tendon rupture and an associated spring ligament rupture served to destabilize the talus [2]. The 3 mm step off of the talus that was viewed on the lateral radiograph can be indicative of spring ligament rupture [3, 4]. In most cases, stage 2 tibialis posterior dysfunction (PTT) and associated N-C fault is present. This is secondary to equinus

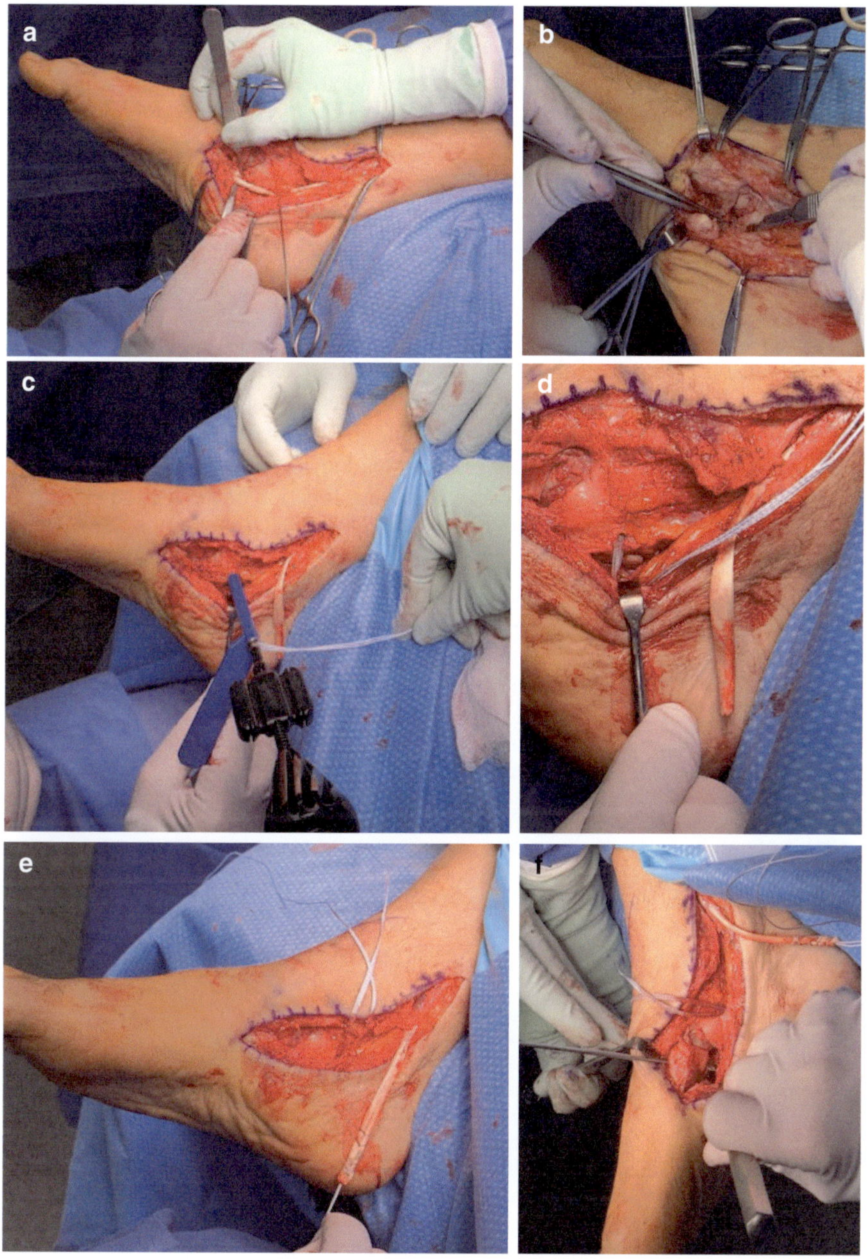

Fig. 22.6 (**a**) Identification of the FDL tendon. (**b**) Ruptured spring ligament. (**c, d**) Proximal limb of internal brace placed into the sustentaculum tali. (**e**) FDL tendon whip stitch. (**f**) Drill hole made to transfer both the FDL and fiber tape of internal brace through the navicular and secure with interference screw

and heel valgus. With loss of the spring ligament, the talus falls out of the mortise medial and inferior position thus leading to the TN "step off." In this case, restoring the talus to its anatomic position was accomplished by a double calcaneal osteotomy [5]. Certainly, an arthrodesis involving either the TNJ and combination posterior calcaneal osteotomy or double or triple arthrodesis could be considered [6, 7]. To offset the loss of tibialis posterior muscle strength, an FDL transfer was performed [8]. As this muscle provides only 40% of tibialis posterior muscle strength, the peroneus brevis was transferred to the peroneal longus to help restore the balance about the STJ and MTJ [9, 10]. As there was no associated fault of the medial column noted distal to the TNJ, there was no need for further medial column correction.

Decision for excision of the tibialis posterior tendon depends on its remaining condition. It must be assessed as its damaged state can serve as a source of pain. Severe degeneration with tendinosis involving greater than 50% of the tendon is best served with excision [11]. A more intact tendon can be debulked and repaired. Also consideration should be given to the gliding function of the tendon sheath. If this is damaged and can't be restored, excision of the tendon should be contemplated.

References

1. Giza E, Cush G, Schon LC. The flexible flatfoot in the adult. Foot Ankle Clin. 2007;12(2):251–71.
2. Mosier-Laclair S, Pomeroy G, Manoli A. Operative treatment of the difficult stage 2 adult acquired flatfoot deformity. Foot Ankle Clin. 2001;6(1):95–119.
3. Orr JD, Nunley JA. Isolated spring ligament failure as a cause of adult-acquired flatfoot deformity. Foot Ankle Int. 2013;34(6):818–23.
4. Patel MS, Barbosa MP, Kadakia AR. Role of spring and deltoid ligament reconstruction for adult acquired flatfoot deformity. Tech Foot Ankle Surg. 2017;16(3):124–35.
5. Anderson JG, Bohay DR. Lateral column lengthening in the adult acquired flatfoot. Tech Foot Ankle Surg. 2003;2(2):91–100.
6. Henry JK, Shakked R, Ellis SJ. Adult-acquired flatfoot deformity. Foot Ankle Orthopaedics. 2019;4(1):2473011418820847.
7. Conti MS, Deland JT, Ellis SJ. Stage IIB flatfoot reconstruction using literature-based equations for heel slide and lateral column lengthening. Tech Foot Ankle Surg. 2017;16(4):153–66.
8. Manoli A II. The treatment of posterior tibial tendon insufficiency using the double heel osteotomy and soft tissue reconstruction: the "all-American procedure". Fuß Sprunggelenk. 2020;18(1):37–48.
9. Peng Y, Wang Y, Wong DWC, Chen TLW, Zhang G, Tan Q, Zhang M. Extrinsic foot muscle forces and joint contact forces in flexible flatfoot adult with foot orthosis: a parametric study of tibialis posterior muscle weakness. Gait Posture. 2021;88:54–9.
10. Cifuentes-De la Portilla C, Pasapula C, Gutiérrez-Narvarte B, Larrainzar-Garijo R, Bayod J. Peroneus longus overload caused by soft tissue deficiencies associated with early adult acquired flatfoot: a finite element analysis. Clin Biomech. 2021;86:105383.
11. Dominick DR, Catanzariti AR. Posterior tibial tendon allograft reconstruction for stage II adult acquired flatfoot: a case series. J Foot Ankle Surg. 2020;59(4):821–5.

Case #23: Reconstruction of Long-Standing Adult Flatfoot Deformity and Associated Peroneal Muscle Tendon Contractures

23

Case Presentation

This is a 34-year-old male who presents with a long-standing flatfoot deformity of several years duration. He had previous treatment involving orthotic management and physical therapy. He states he could hardly wear the orthotics and they produced pain. He states they were rigid. Of note, he was obese weighing 400 lbs. He was also 6′1″ tall. His BMI was 36.

He was not diabetic and had no history of cardiovascular disease. His lower extremity vascular perfusion was excellent. He had no neurologic deficits present. Neuromuscular exam will be noted in the assessment. He had a large tyloma over the medial cuneiform and navicular at the naviculocuneiform joint. It was extremely painful with weight bearing.

Diagnosis and Assessment

When examining the reducibility of the rear foot and midfoot, it was found to be reducible. However, it required stress to attain a biomechanically reduced rectus position (Fig. 23.1b). He exhibited an extreme amount of pedal abduction (Fig. 23.1a). The Silfverskiold test noted a gastrocnemius soleus equinus of −10 degrees of ankle dorsiflexion. It was not affected by knee position (Fig. 23.2c). Tylomas with nucleation were noted separately at the plantar navicular and medial cuneiform, as well as, under the first metatarsal head (Fig. 23.1c).

Weight-bearing radiographs of the left foot on the dorsoplantar view (Fig. 23.2a) note increased talar adduction and uncoverage. The calcaneocuboid joint is well aligned with mild degenerative joint disease laterally. On the lateral view (Fig. 23.2b), there was presence of a navicular, medial cuneiform fault. Increased talar declination and a decrease in calcaneal inclination were also present.

H. J. Visser, *Challenges in Foot and Ankle Reconstructive Surgery*,
https://doi.org/10.1007/978-3-031-07893-4_23

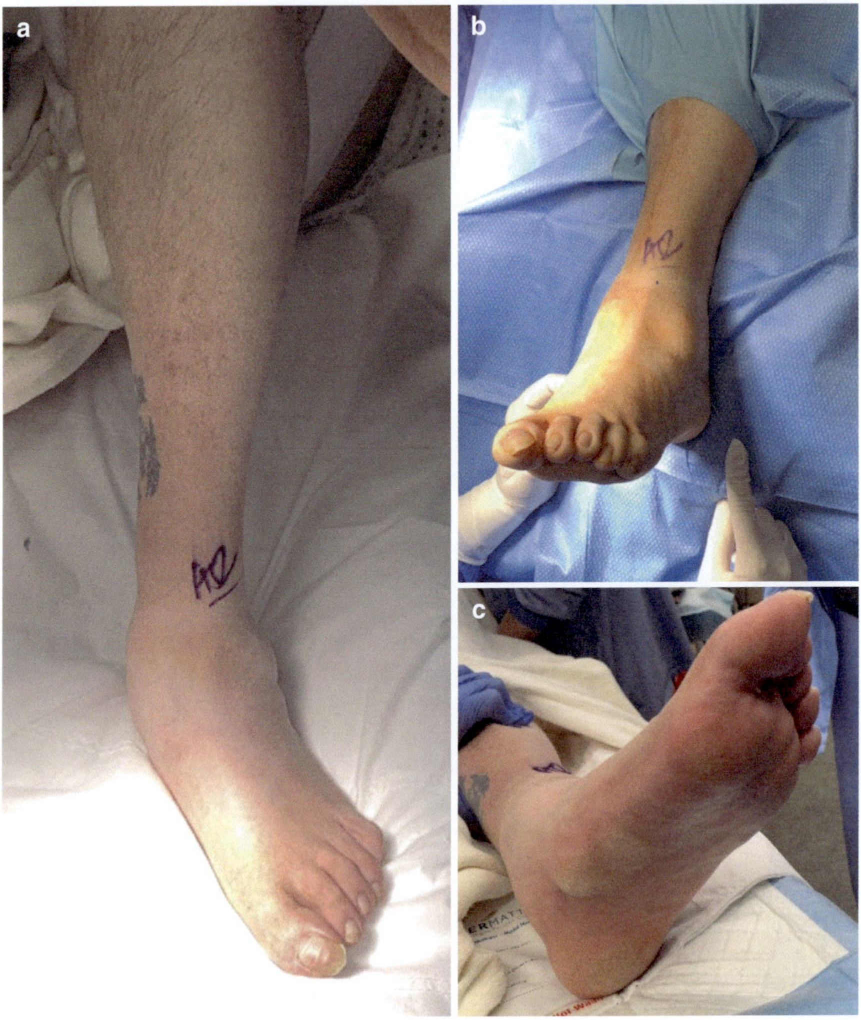

Fig. 23.1 (**a**) Extreme abduction of left foot and leg. (**b**) Reducibility with stress. (**c**) Tyloma over navicular, medial cuneiform and first metatarsal head, left foot

The diagnosis was a congenital, adult flatfoot deformity. There was significant medial column overload created by equinus, peroneal contracture, heel valgus, and obesity. This corresponded to significant nucleation of the plantar lesions under the navicular and medial cuneiform and first metatarsal head.

Management

The approach to deformity correction was to first address the soft tissue tendon contractures. The clinical presence of significant foot abduction did not seem to correlate with the weight-bearing radiographs.

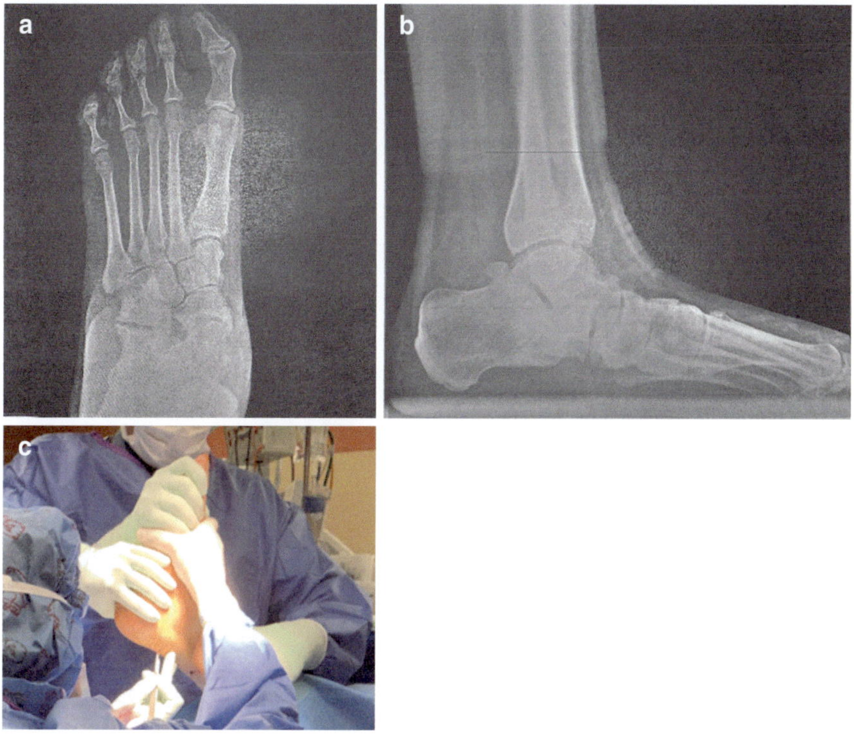

Fig. 23.2 (**a**) Increased talar adduction and uncoverage. Well aligned calcaneocuboid joint with mild degenerative joint disease. (**b**) Navicular medial cuneiform fault. Increased talar declination and decreased calcaneal inclination angles. (**c**) Silfverskiöld test

A stepwise approach was done. First performing a Hoke triple hemisection lengthening of the Achilles tendon was performed. Second, both the peroneus longus and brevis were also lengthened (Fig. 23.3a). Upon completion of these two maneuvers, the foot became completely rectus. The medial column was then addressed with a third incision carried dorsally between the tibialis anterior and extensor hallucis longus tendons and carried to the naviculocuneiform joint (Fig. 23.4a, b). A talonavicular fusion was chosen to stabilize the subtalar and midtarsal joint complex due to the patient's size. A cotton medial cuneiform opening wedge with a cancellous titanium implant wedge was chosen to address the naviculocuneiform joint fault (Fig. 23.5a, b). With the re-established medial column, the plantar callosities were no longer weight bearing (Fig. 23.6a, b).

Outcome

The patient was kept non-weight bearing for 6 weeks. He was then allowed to bear weight fully in a CAM boot. At 12 weeks, he was sent to physical therapy and a rigid orthotic device was designed. He had an excellent outcome and was very

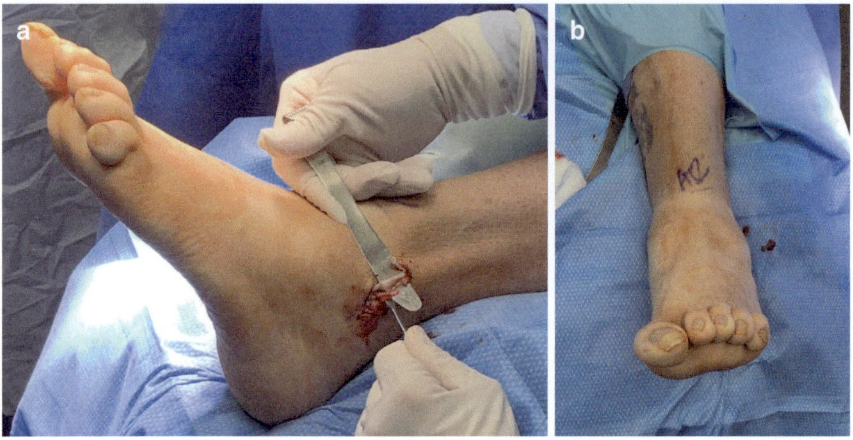

Fig. 23.3 (**a**) Lengthening the peroneus longus to the peroneus brevis, (**b**) reduced foot position post-TAL and peroneal lengthening

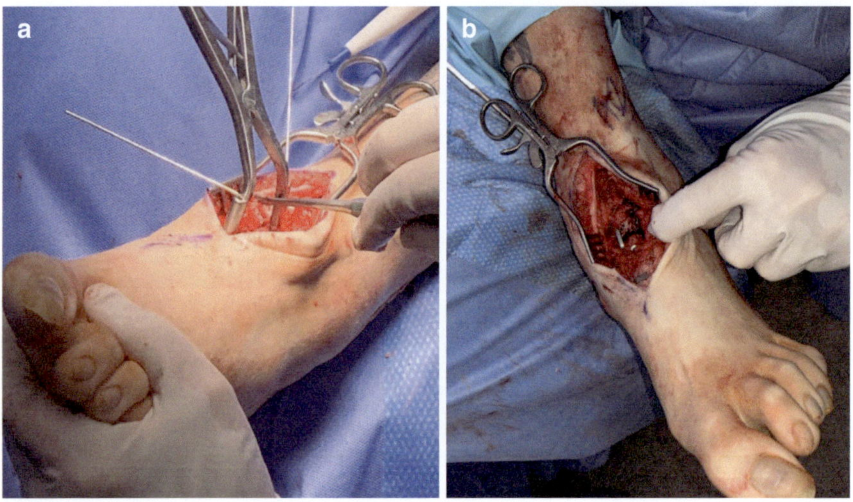

Fig. 23.4 (**a**) Incision for TN joint arthrodesis, Cotton, medial cuneiform with cancellous wedge. (**b**) Incision between the tibialis anterior and EHL

satisfied with the result. His contralateral foot was not as severe and has been controlled biomechanically with orthotics.

Clinical Pearls and Pitfalls

This case represents the importance of the clinical examination as the deformity did not match the radiographs. The patient preoperatively has extreme abduction. While the foot could be reduced it required stress to allow it. It also required plantarflexion

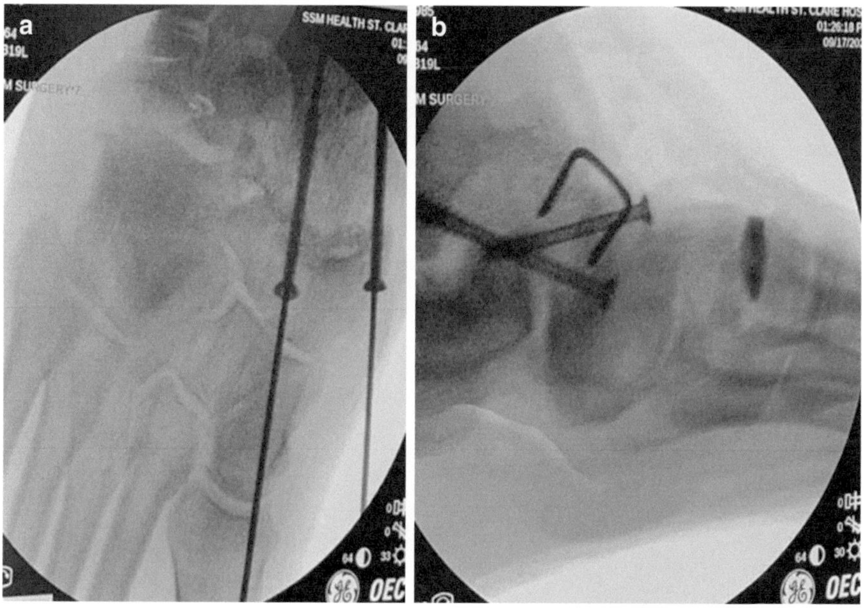

Fig. 23.5 (**a**) TN joint arthrodesis fixated with two cannulated partially threaded screws. (**b**) Navicular cuneiform fault addressed by performing a cotton medial cuneiform opening wedge with a cancellous titanium implant wedge

at the ankle indicating equinus contracture. The radiographs demonstrate a peritalar subluxation but no signs of significant midtarsal abduction.

In this case, when the equinus contracture was released and both peroneals lengthened [1–3], it showed full reduction of the deformity. The remaining medial column surgery was to stabilize the foot and resist weight-bearing forces associated with the patient's high BMI. Of interest too was the lesion pattern. The patient had three distinct lesions. The navicular and medial cuneiform plantarly as well as the first metatarsal head. This was generated by his significant equinus, peroneal contracture, heel valgus forces, and high BMI. This forced pressure directly at the fault of the naviculocuneiform joint [4, 5]. The sub first metatarsal head lesion appears to be a paradox with this form of extreme flatfoot. The lateral view does not show a plantarflexed metatarsal. This lesion can be explained by the increased tension placed on the peroneus longus created by the abducted foot position [6]. It was compounded by the equinus and also exhibited hyperactivity with associated significant forefoot abduction. Once lengthening occurred, the foot realigned and the lesion's presence was eliminated. The remaining naviculocuneiform joint fault still needed to be addressed at this juncture. A talonavicular joint arthrodesis was used to support the medial cuneiform cotton wedge [7, 8].

This case predominantly exhibits the contribution of soft tissue tendon contracture in an architectural flatfoot deformity.

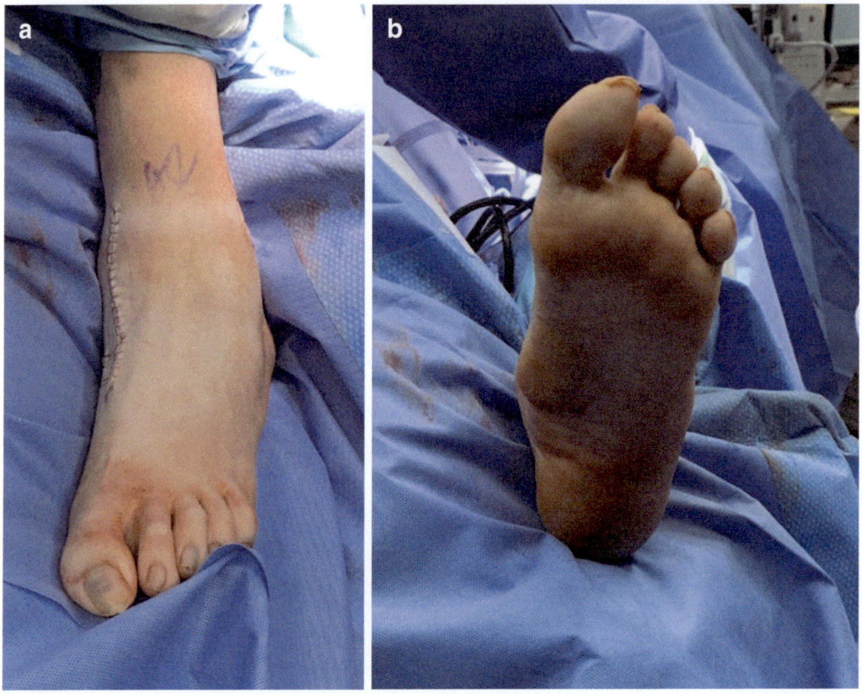

Fig. 23.6 (**a, b**) Realignment of foot and reestablishment of medial column

References

1. Harris RI, Beath T. Etiology of peroneal spastic flat foot. J Bone Joint Surg. 1948;30(4):624–34.
2. Blair J, Perdios A, Reilly CW. Peroneal spastic flatfoot caused by a talar osteochondral lesion: a case report. Foot Ankle Int. 2007;28(6):724–6.
3. Niki H, Aoki H, Hirano T, Akiyama Y, Fujiya H. Peroneal spastic flatfoot in adolescents with accessory talar facet impingement: a preliminary report. J Pediatr Orthop B. 2015;24(4):354–61.
4. Metzl JA. Naviculocuneiform sag in the acquired flatfoot: what to do. Foot Ankle Clin. 2017;22(3):529–44.
5. Gerrity M, Williams M. Naviculocuneiform arthrodesis in adult flatfoot: a case series. J Foot Ankle Surg. 2019;58(2):352–6.
6. Ellis SJ, Yu JC, Williams BR, Lee C, Chiu YL, Deland JT. New radiographic parameters assessing forefoot abduction in the adult acquired flatfoot deformity. Foot Ankle Int. 2009;30(12):1168–76.
7. Boffeli TJ, Schnell KR. Cotton osteotomy in flatfoot reconstruction: a review of consecutive cases. J Foot Ankle Surg. 2017;56(5):990–5.
8. Aiyer A, Dall GF, Shub J, Myerson MS. Radiographic correction following reconstruction of adult acquired flat foot deformity using the cotton medial cuneiform osteotomy. Foot Ankle Int. 2016;37(5):508–13.

24 Case #24: Management of a Spontaneous Peritalar Dislocation with Talocalcaneal Arthrodesis Utilizing an Intramedullary Nail

Case Presentation

This is a 51-year-old Caucasian female that had presented with a long-standing history of flat foot deformity of both pedal structures. She, however, noticed increasing pain involving the right foot over the past year. She stated that her orthotics were now painful and she noticed her foot turned out more. She felt the change in her foot structure was gradual.

Medically, she had a history of long-standing obesity. She states that she was overweight in childhood. She was not diabetic and her hypertension was controlled. She was also on Lovastatin for lipid management. Her vascular perfusion was normal and neurologically there were no deficits noted.

Diagnosis and Assessment

On biomechanical evaluation, there was the presence of a rigid flatfoot deformity. There was no ability to reduce the position of the rearfoot or midfoot. It was a fixed and rigid deformity. There was the presence of a Falstaff type of lower extremity obscuring anatomic landmarks. There was no history of ulceration. She demonstrated significant pain with weight bearing and was greatly limited in her ambulatory function. Most of her pain was lateral and severe impingement of the fibula was present.

Radiographs noted that a near vertical talus was present. A significant talonavicular (TN) break was noted on the lateral view. Also significant forefoot supinatus was present (Fig. 24.1a). Panicular undulations were noted at the ankle and increased calf girth on soft tissue evaluation. The dorsoplantar view showed a complete dislocation of the TN joint. There was an increase in cuboid abduction. Arthrosis was

H. J. Visser, *Challenges in Foot and Ankle Reconstructive Surgery*,
https://doi.org/10.1007/978-3-031-07893-4_24

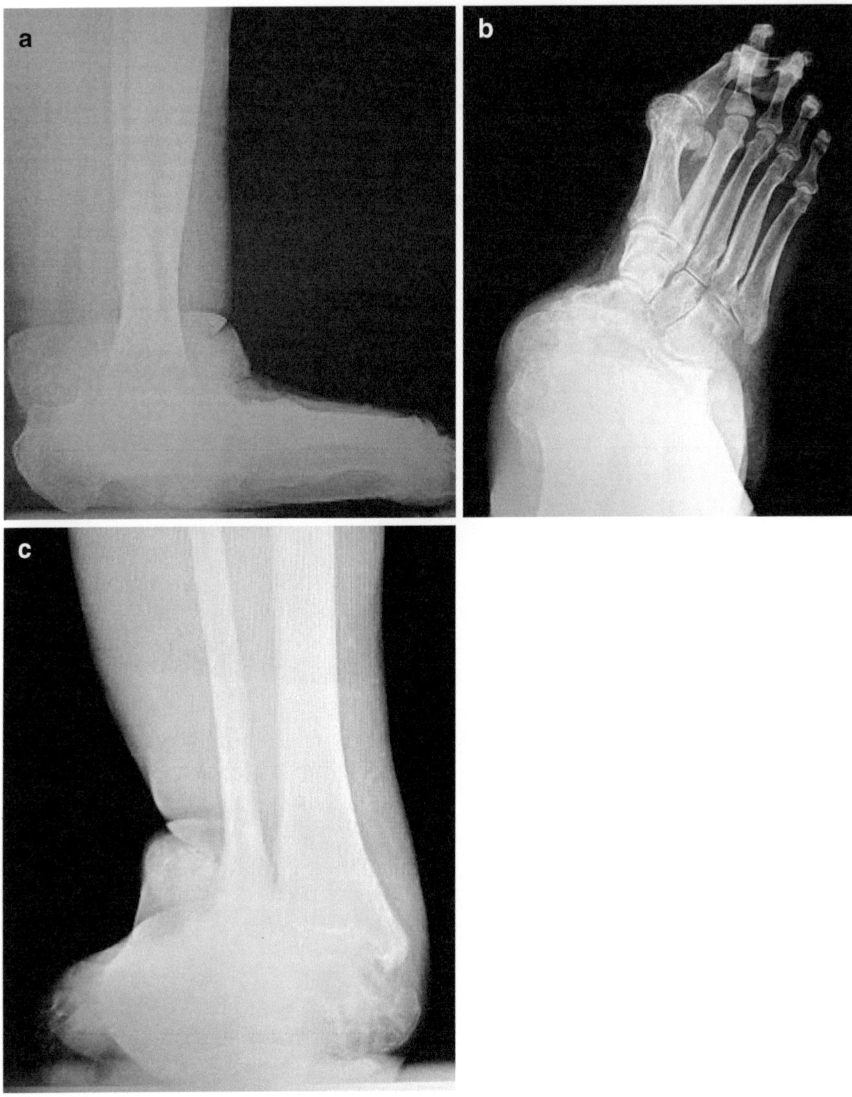

Fig. 24.1 (a–c) A near vertical talus deformity is present along with forefoot supinatus and an increased cuboid abduction angle. The forefoot is markedly abducted to the ankle joint and the talonavicular joint is completely dislocated. There is a sidecar deformity as noted by the lateral dislocation of the subtalar joint. A severe hallux valgus deformity is noted

present at the TN joint. The remaining midfoot and forefoot were relatively free of degenerative changes. There was a significant hallux abductovalgus deformity present (Fig. 24.1b). The anteroposterior view of the ankle related that the talus was still intact within the mortise. No talar tilt was present. There was severe impingement of the fibula at the calcaneal level. The foot was markedly abducted in reference to the ankle joint (Fig. 24.1c). A preoperative MRI noted a completely intact tibialis posterior tendon.

Her diagnosis was a spontaneous peritalar dislocation involving complete dislocation of the TN joint. This has also been described as a "sidecar" deformity which represents a chronic, lateral dislocation of the subtalar joint. There was severe passive valgus of the subtalar joint (subluxato tali valgo totalis) present in association.

Management

Operative intervention involved a partial talectomy involving the body (corpus tali). The talar neck (collum tali) and head (capitus tali) was left intact. This was performed via a transfibular approach. A plantigrade foot was attained when the body was removed. It allowed complete deformity reduction. The tibia and calcaneus were prepared for arthrodesis and an intramedullary (IM) nail was then used for fixation (Fig. 24.2a). The remaining talar body was removed of cartilage in a curettage fashion. It was then inserted into the remaining void of the tibia and calcaneus.

The navicular then underwent an arthrodesis to the remaining talar neck and head (Fig. 24.2b). Both were prepared in a standard fashion of cartilage curettage, subchondral drilling (2.0 mm drill), and fish scaling. The hallux abductovalgus deformity was managed with an arthrodesis utilizing a locking plate (Fig. 24.2c). Joint compression was attained through the proximal locking slot.

Radiographs show the forefoot well aligned as well as the first metatarsophalangeal joint on the dorsoplantar view. The anteroposterior view of the ankle noted the foot was aligned to the ankle. Fibular impingement was eliminated by excision of the fibula through the transfibular approach and, thus, peroneal tendons were decompressed in the fibular groove. The lateral view notes a plantigrade foot. The longitudinal arch was restored and forefoot pronatus established.

The patient was kept non-weight bearing for 8 weeks. She was then placed in a CAM boot for a further 8 weeks. She returned to shoe wear with a protective total ankle AFO at 20 weeks.

Outcome

The patient did remarkably well considering her obese state. She was extremely compliant. She wore the AFO for a full year. When a complete fusion was noted. She was placed in extra-depth shoe wear. She is not highly ambulatory but she now relates the restoration of normal lifestyle. Her opposite foot notes a peritalar subluxation but is controlled with an accommodative orthotic.

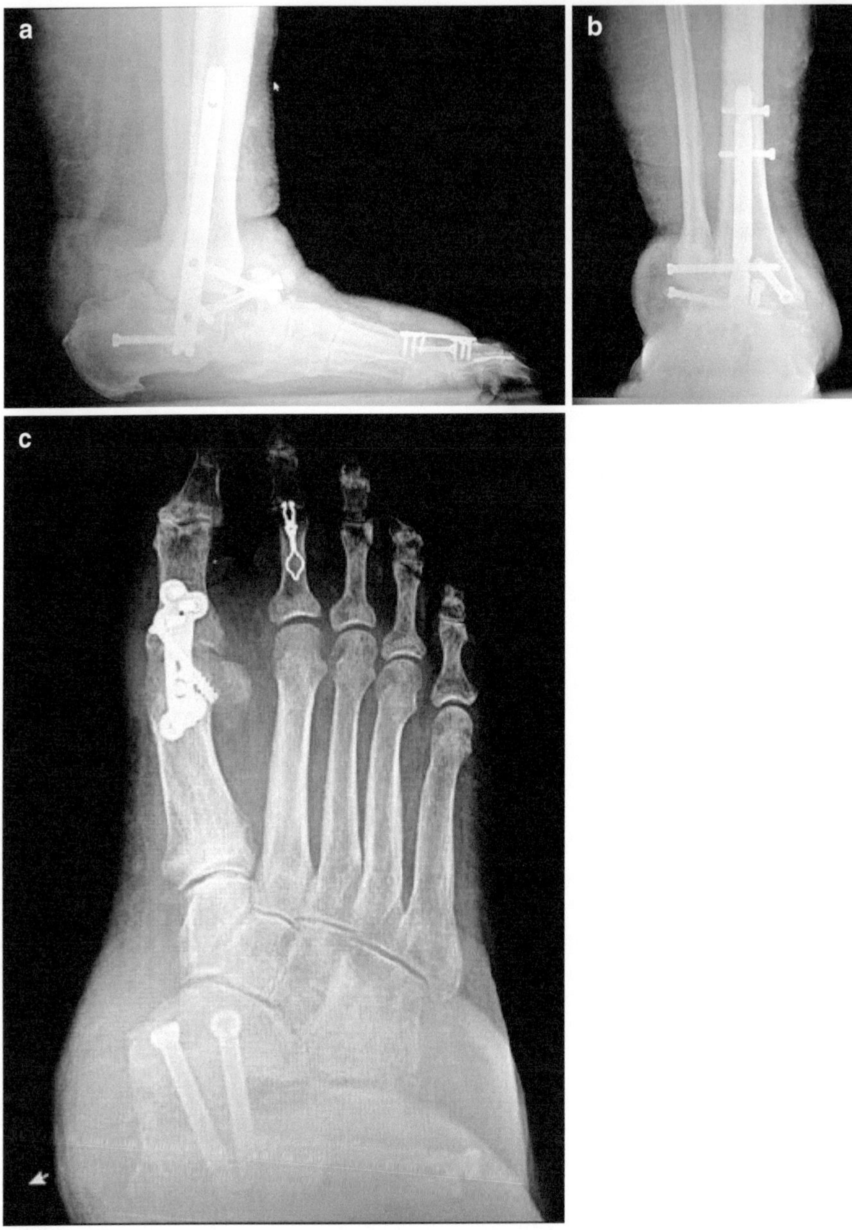

Fig. 24.2 (**a**–**c**) A plantigrade foot was attained with intramedullary fixation via a transfibular approach. Radiographs demonstrate the restoration of the longitudinal arch and the foot well aligned to the ankle joint

Clinical Pearls and Pitfalls

This represents a unique case of a spontaneous peritalar dislocation that was described by Melvin Jahss, MD [1]. This is a biomechanical, non-traumatic, and non-neurologic dislocation [2]. He described this condition that involved patients with a history of long-standing flatfoot deformity and associated obesity. With aging and persistent biomechanical forces, stress on the supporting soft tissue structures that support the talus then become disoptic. Thus the cervical, interosseous, talocalcaneal, and spring ligaments give way and rupture. The talus is then allowed to adduct, plantarflex and fall forward, dislocating from the TN joint. The talus then rests on the sustentaculum tali with complete loss of congruency of the posterior STJ facet. This has also been described by Burns et al. as a sidecar deformity which represents a chronic, lateral STJ dislocation [3].

The long-standing, slow and developmental nature of this condition is noted by an increase in the cuboid abduction angle. This indicates long-standing pronation of the oblique midtarsal joint axis (calcaneocuboid joint). This correlates with the associated significant subtalar pronatory condition. The two joints work in synchrony creating deformity.

With a non-reducible and dislocated TN joint a partial talectomy of the body allows restoration of ankle, subtalar, and midfoot alignment. Leaving the talar neck and head and performing arthrodesis with the navicular aligns the forefoot to the rearfoot. The remaining body is prepared and reinserted as a "cancellous" autograft.

An IM nail is used for added rigidity to withstand significant weight-bearing forces due to the patient's size. This then aligns the rearfoot and ankle.

Case #24A: Management of a Spontaneous Peritalar Dislocation with a Talonavicular Arthrodesis

Addendum

This case of a 75-year-old Caucasian male shows a similar situation of a spontaneous peritalar dislocation that occurred in a much more rapid sequence. The patient stated he had a flatfoot condition from childhood. He states he wore orthotics and never had much trouble with pain. He was also obese but stated that symptoms occurred in his early 50s. He did not have a history of diabetes mellitus and there were no signs of neuropathy, clinically. Vascular supply was normal. Mild pitting edema at the ankle was present. He stated upon presentation and for no reason he began to experience severe right foot pain. He couldn't walk for nearly 2 weeks. He went to urgent care and X-rays were taken. They said he had a "flatfoot" and there were no signs of fracture. Diagnosis was listed as a "sprain." He was placed in a CAM boot and his pain subsided. He then returned to shoe wear. He kept having "discomfort" and noticed his shoe didn't fit quite right. He couldn't wear his orthotics anymore. He presented at 6 months for evaluation after the initial event.

Diagnosis and Assessment

On evaluation, his right foot demonstrated no significant signs of edema. On his arch over the medial foot, there was an isolated tyloma in the vicinity of the talar head (Fig. 24A.1a, b). It appeared to have a normal arch. Looking clinically on a dorsoplantar view of his foot, it appeared to be rectus (Fig. 24A.2a). The second digit aligned with the ankle.

Radiographs noted that on the lateral view the talus migrated anteriorly and was plantarflexed. There was anterior subluxation of the posterior facet (Fig. 24A.2b). The dorsoplantar view noted a complete TN joint dislocation. There were no real significant degenerative changes. His cuboid abduction angle was completely normal.

Here again without neuropathy and no history of trauma, a spontaneous peritalar dislocation was diagnosed. In this case, the process was relatively acute.

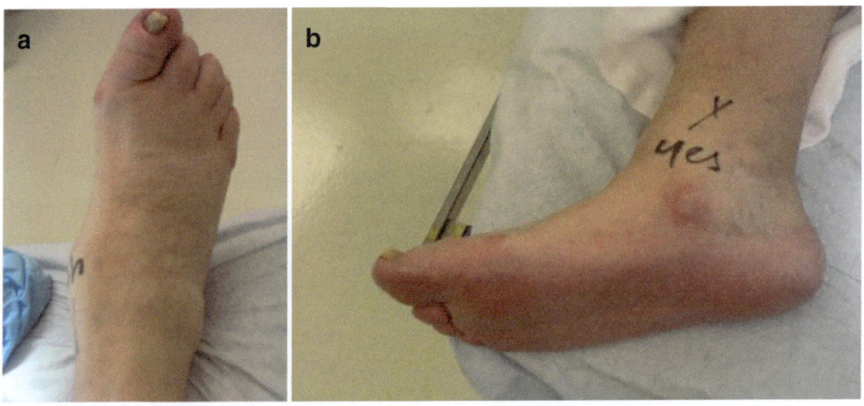

Fig. 24A.1 (**a**) Clinically foot looks relatively rectus, forefoot abduction not present. (**b**) Talar head prominent medially

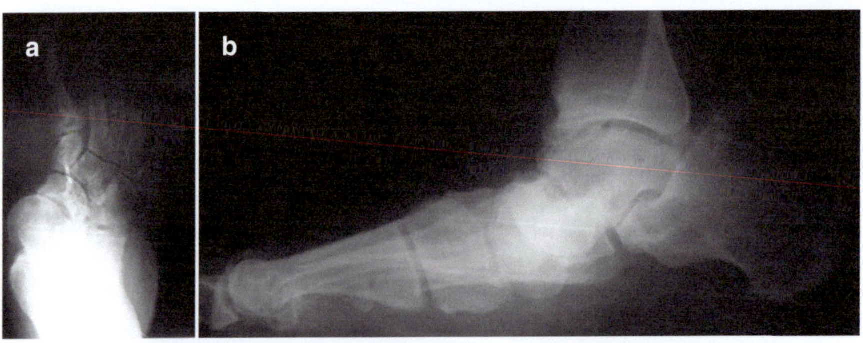

Fig. 24A.2 (**a**) Peritalar dislocation secondary to loss of a ligamentous supporting structures. (**b**) Anterior subluxation of the talus on the posterior facet

Management

The midtarsal joint and subtalar joint could be reduced with clinical stress. Thus, the approach was to address the TN joint dislocation directly. A TN arthrodesis was performed. Intraoperatively when the lamina spreader was placed across the joint, the talus was easily reduced within the STJ mortise. In essence, the talus acted as a "loose tooth" exhibiting no soft tissue ligamentous support (Fig. 24A.3). A TN arthrodesis was performed with three 4.5 mm cannulated screws (Fig. 24A.4a, b, c). He was kept non-weight bearing for 6 weeks. He then ambulated in a controlled ankle motion (CAM) boot for a further 6 weeks. He was then placed in a rigid

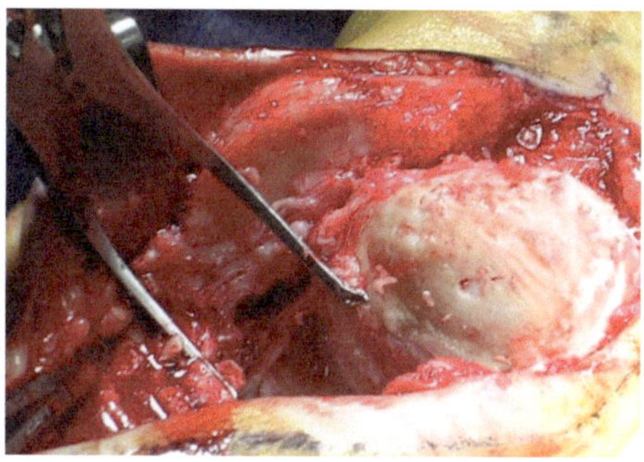

Fig. 24A.3 Utilization of a lamina spreader reduces anterior subluxation of the posterior facet. Talus is like a "loose tooth"

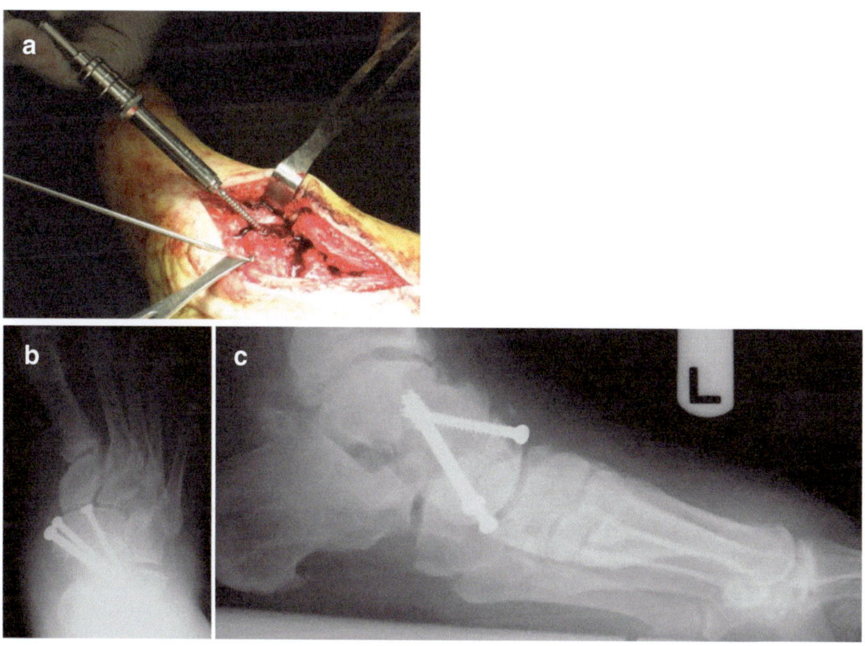

Fig. 24A.4 (**a**) Fixation of talonavicular joint (**b**) Isolated talonavicular arthrodesis. (**c**) Indirect reduction of the posterior facet of the subtalar joint

orthotic with a deep heel seat and high medial flange (a modified University of California biomechanics lab (UCBL) device).

Outcome

The patient did extremely well. At his age and physical condition, he was not highly active. The arthrodesis ultimately consolidated well.

Clinical Pearls and Pitfalls

This is another example of a "spontaneous peritalar dislocation" [2]. The difference in this case was "acuteness" compared to the prior case. The history, plus the radiographs, determine the difference. In this case, the foot appears normal. You can see a longitudinal arch clinically and there was no sign of forefoot abduction. The radiographs show the dislocation. The talus "fell out" of the mortise moving forward, medial and plantar as described by Sangeorzan, "like a screw" [4]. Rotation in the transverse plane about the navicular did not occur. Hence, no increase in the cuboid abduction angle.

The decision to approach the TN joint rather than the ankle was based on the reducibility present clinically. As can be seen intraoperatively the talus had no intrinsic ligamentous support [5]. It could be easily reduced back into its mortise. The lateral view notes excellent restoration of talar position with rearticulation of the posterior facet. Certainly, an addition of subtalar joint fusion and correction of the midfoot at the NC joint could have been added [6–9]. But with his activity level and overall postoperative clinical appearance, the isolated TN joint arthrodesis served him well.

References

1. Jahss MH. Disorders of the Foot & Ankle: Medical and Surgical Management. Saunders. 1991.
2. Specchiulli F, Gabrieli R, Di Carlo V, Maiorana B. Peritalar dislocations. Foot. 2007;17(1):10–4.
3. Elbert DR, Langan TM, Burns PR. Surgical treatment and management for chronic dislocated subtalar joint. J Foot Ankle Surg. 2020;59(2):379–84.
4. Sangeorzan BJ, Hintermann B, de Cesar Netto C, Day J, Deland JT, Ellis SJ, et al. Progressive collapsing foot deformity: consensus on goals for operative correction. Foot Ankle Int. 2020;41(10):1299–302.
5. Michels F, Matricali G, Vereecke E, Dewilde M, Vanrietvelde F, Stockmans F. The intrinsic subtalar ligaments have a consistent presence, location and morphology. Foot Ankle Surg. 2021;27(1):101–9.
6. Merianos P, Papagiannakos K, Hatzis A, Tsafantakis E. Peritalar dislocation: a follow-up report of 21 cases. Injury. 1988;19(6):439–42.
7. Dunn AW. Peritalar dislocation. Orthop Clin N Am. 1974;5(1):7–18.
8. Hörer DI, Fishman J. The early treatment of peritalar dislocation. Int Orthop. 1984;7(4):263–6.
9. Resnick RB, Jahss MH, Choueka J, Kummer F, Hersch JC, Okereke E. Deltoid ligament forces after tibialis posterior tendon rupture: effects of triple arthrodesis and calcaneal displacement osteotomies. Foot Ankle Int. 1995;16(1):14–20.

Case #25: Management of Oblique Talus Deformity with Talar Neck Wedge Osteotomy

25

Case Presentation

This is a 13-year-old African American male who presents with a 2-year history of bilateral painful flatfoot deformities. He has had past conservative treatment that included orthotic care and physical therapy. His mother states that he is unable to participate in sports. He also has difficulty with standing and walking for extended periods when at school.

Diagnosis and Assessment

On clinical examination, he demonstrates bilateral semi-rigid pedal deformity. The subtalar joint (STJ) and talonavicular joint (TNJ) could be reduced but only with manual stress. This was accomplished with the ankle in full plantarflexion. Both feet appear flat with loss of the longitudinal arch height in a non-weight-bearing seated position (Fig. 25.1a). With utilization of the Silfverskiold test he was only able to get to −10 degrees of ankle dorsiflexion [1].

On relaxed calcaneal stance position (RCSP), he notes talar ptosis with significant hallux abductovalgus deformity when viewing the dorsal foot (Fig. 25.1b).

When viewing his calcaneal position posteriorly, a positive Helbing's sign was present with calcaneal valgus being near 30°. Increased girth medially about the STJ was present. The heels themselves did not contact the ground. The talar head was extremely prominent (Fig. 25.1c).

Radiographs note on the lateral view the presence of a significant TNJ fault. Forefoot supinatus was present. The talar neck appeared shortened. There are no signs of talar beaking or a halo sign (Fig. 25.2a).

H. J. Visser, *Challenges in Foot and Ankle Reconstructive Surgery*,
https://doi.org/10.1007/978-3-031-07893-4_25

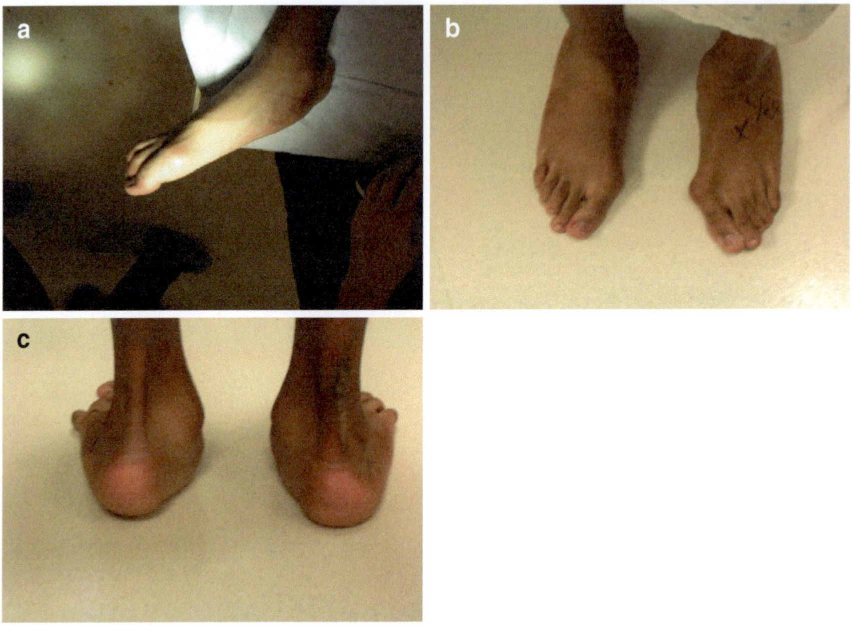

Fig. 25.1 (**a–c**) Flatfoot deformity with forefoot supinatus and hallux abductovalgus

On the dorsoplantar view, there is a significant increase in talar adduction (Harris-Beath angle). Talar uncoverage was near 60%. The cuboid abduction angle was also increased, measuring 12°. There is a severe hallux abductovalgus deformity present. The medial cuneiform is splayed in adduction in reference to the intermediate cuneiform. The joint itself at the first metatarsal base does not display significant atavism (Fig. 25.2b).

The patient exhibits a clinical condition of oblique talus deformity (cribra orbitalia). A CT scan and MRI failed to demonstrate the presence of a medial subtalar joint coalition.

Management

The surgical approach was first to perform an open z-plasty of the Achilles tendon in the frontal plane (Stewart type) (Fig. 25.3a). Second, a biplane calcaneal osteotomy was performed in both the transverse and sagittal planes. Fixation was accomplished with two-stepped nitinol staples. This accommodated the medial shift and inferior translation to reduce heel valgus and restore calcaneal inclination (Fig. 25.3b).

Once the rearfoot deformity had been addressed, correction of the medial arch centered at the talonavicular (TN) fault. A subcapital talar wedge (Grumbine type) osteotomy was performed directly posterior to the talar articular surface

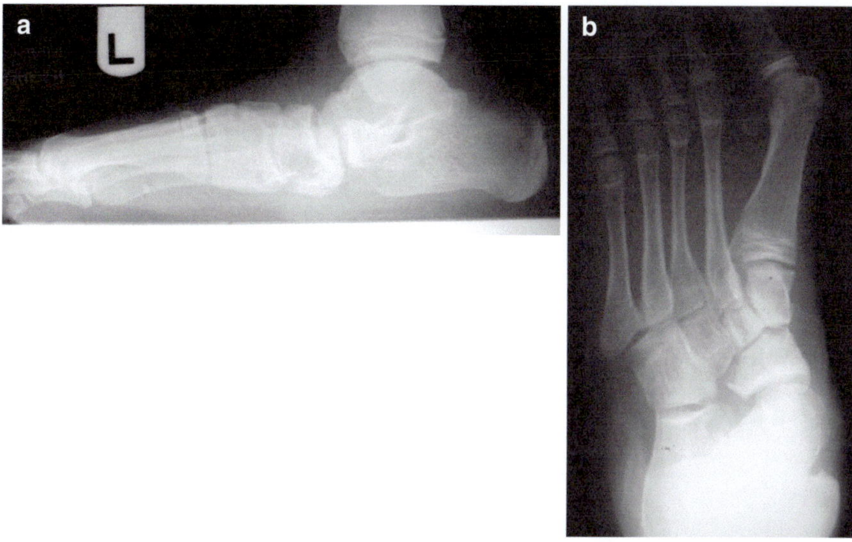

Fig. 25.2 (**a**) TN break with significant forefoot supinatus. There is markedly increased talar inclination angle. (**b**) Dislocation of TN joint, increased cuboid abduction angle

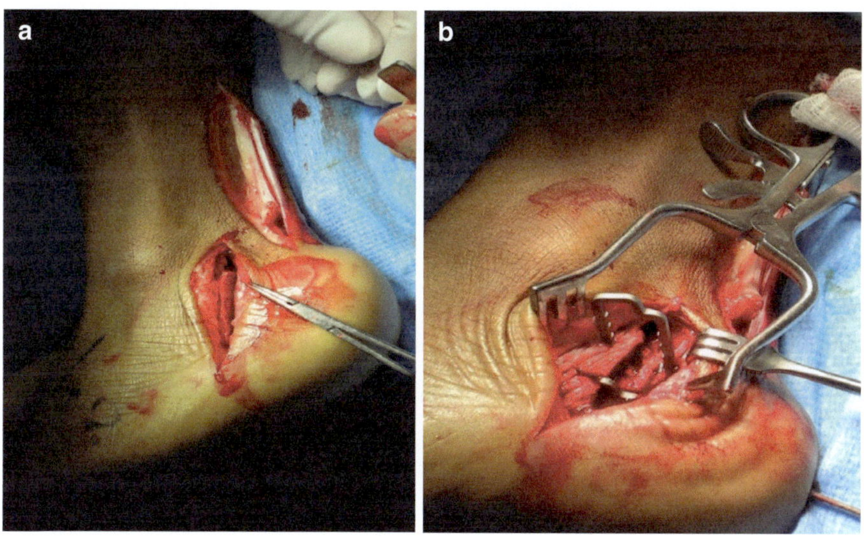

Fig. 25.3 (**a**) Z-plasty lengthening. (**b**) Biplane calcaneal osteotomy

(Fig. 25.4a–g) [2, 3]. Fixation was obtained with a nitinol staple (Fig. 25.4c). A 5/64" Steinmann pin was then used to reduce the residual forefoot supinatus (Fig. 25.5a, b).

The patient was kept non-weight bearing for 6 weeks followed by a weight-bearing boot for a further 6 weeks. The Steinmann pin was removed at 6 weeks.

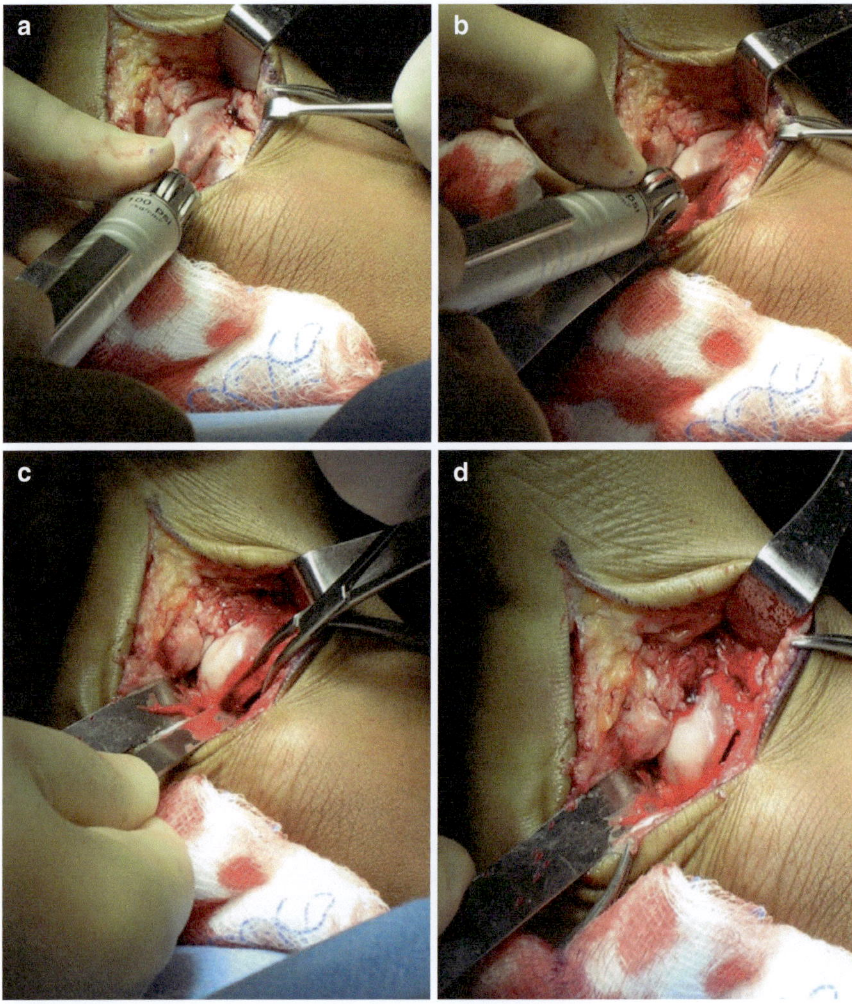

Fig. 25.4 (**a**–**g**) A subcapital talar wedge (Grumbine type) osteotomy was performed directly posterior to the talar articular surface

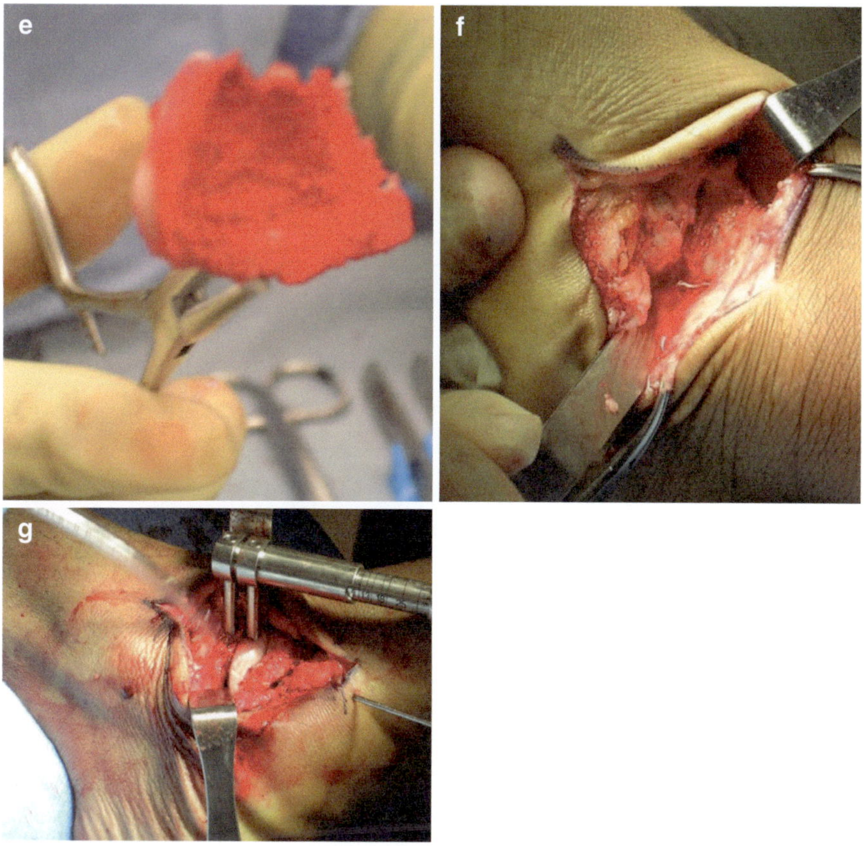

Fig. 25.4 (continued)

Outcome

The post-op radiographs note complete restoration of the TN joint congruity as well as restoration of a normal cuboid abduction angle (Fig. 25.6a). The lateral view notes restoration of the calcaneal inclination angle and correction of talar declination. The TN fault had been corrected as well as the residual forefoot supinatus (Fig. 25.6b). Despite the correction, his overall motion was stiff.

The patient did very well and had the right foot done 6 months later. He did not return for the hallux valgus correction. I had been planning a Lapidus arthrodesis for correction.

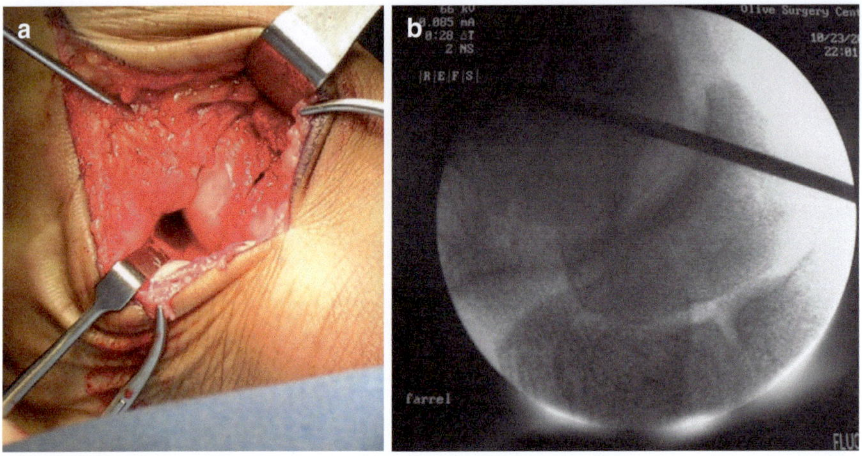

Fig. 25.5 (**a**, **b**) Talus osteotomy fixated with staples. The Steinman pin was to maintain correction of the supinatus deformity at the TN joint.

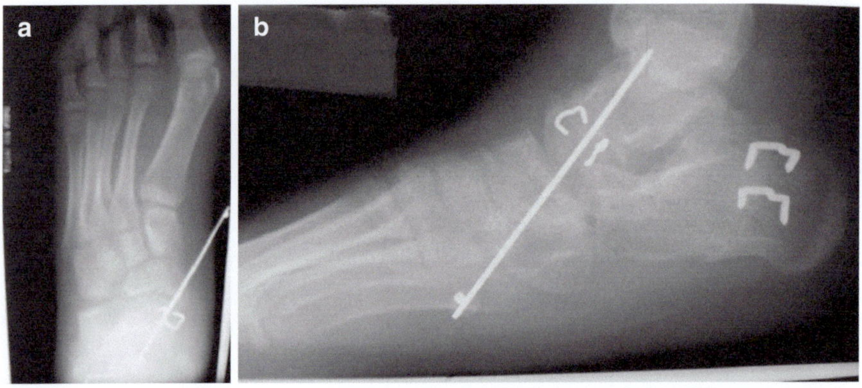

Fig. 25.6 (**a**, **b**) Restoration of cuboid abduction angle as well as correction of calcaneal inclination and talar declination angles

Clinical Pearls and Pitfalls

This is a case of a severe flatfoot (oblique talus) deformity in a child of 13. This is a rare condition and a difficult condition to address surgically. Certainly waiting until the growth plates were closed was a consideration. However, full development of the tarsal bones was present. The hallux abductovalgus deformity was planned to be addressed upon growth plate closure. Thus, a two-staged approach was considered.

As the deformity was reducible but involved stress to reduce it, the following approach was utilized. A z-plasty of the Achilles tendon in the frontal plane was chosen which allows greater contact and less bulk. The equinus was severe, $-10°$, and also restoration of the calcaneal inclination was desired. A biplane calcaneal osteotomy allowed correction of the heel valgus with medial translation and calcaneal inclination with inferior translation.

Addressing the TN fault which is rare in most cases of adolescent flatfoot required an initial work up for a subtalar joint coalition. The pedal appearance, lack of flexible deformity, and increased girth proved suspicious. Other signs of a coalition, however, were absent (talar beaking, halo sign). The MRI and CT scan did not demonstrate a coalition of the medial STJ facet or at the calcaneonavicular interface.

A child in this age group with this degree of deformity could certainly be addressed with a triple arthrodesis. Long term, however, being bilateral one is aware of the consequences. The development of MTJ and ankle joint osteoarthritis [4]. Thus, the approach was to preserve joint motion by talar osteotomy. A subcapital talar neck osteotomy is a powerful procedure. As can be seen the osteotomy is purely triangular. It is performed in the transverse plane. The proximal cut is perpendicular to the neck and the distal to the articular surface. Dissection avoids the talar neck blood supply provided by the dorsalis pedis (anterior tibial) artery. By removal of the wedge, shortening of the medial column, described by Batchelor, occurs. It is extremely powerful in concern to deformity correction. This is demonstrated by the postoperative dorsoplantar and lateral views.

The utilization of a Steinmann pin was performed to reduce the residual forefoot supinatus. This occurs from compensation secondary to ankle equinus and heel valgus created by STJ pronation [5]. The radiographs show this condition by "piling up" of the metatarsals on the lateral view.

In most cases, residual soft tissue contracture about the TNJ will normally reduce when equinus and heel valgus correction is performed. To assure derotation about the TN joint, as demonstrated in this case, a Steinmann pin was utilized to invert (derotate) the navicular about the talus. In some cases, consideration must be given to lengthening of the tibialis anterior tendon. It may become contracted in long-standing and severe cases [6].

References

1. Bouchard M, Mosca VS. Flatfoot deformity in children and adolescents: surgical indications and management. J Am Acad Orthop Surg. 2014;22(10):623–32.
2. Grumbine NA. Talar neck osteotomy for the treatment of severe structural flatfoot deformities. Clin Podiatr Med Surg. 1987;4(1):119–36.
3. Grumbine NA. Talar neck osteotomy for flatfoot reconstruction: a 27-year follow-up study. Clin Podiatr Med Surg. 2006;23(1):41–viii.
4. Vlachou M, Dimitriadis D. Results of triple arthrodesis in children and adolescents. Acta Orthop Belg. 2009;75(3):380–8.
5. Grumbine NA. The varus components of the forefoot in flatfoot deformities. J Am Podiatr Med Assoc. 1987;77(1):14–20.
6. Samaila E, Bonetti I, Bruno C, Argentini E, Magnan B. Navicular tenosuspension with anterior tibialis tendon (young procedure) associated to calcaneo-stop for the treatment of paediatric flexible flatfoot: clinical and ultrasound study. Acta Bio-med. 2016;87(Suppl. 1):69–74.

Case #26: Management of Severe Peritalar Dislocation Secondary to Rheumatoid Arthritis by Double Arthrodesis Utilizing a Medial Incision

26

Case Presentation

This is a 64-year-old male with a history of rheumatoid arthritis. He has had long-term disease and has never, according to his statement, been controlled.

On the initial exam, the anteroposterior ankle X-ray view noted massive soft tissue swelling with the inability to evaluate the osseous structures (Fig. 26.1). He was referred to Rheumatology who with prednisone and the use of the biologic response modifier, Enbrel, was able to control the active synovitis. The residual can be noted on the subsequent lateral and dorsoplantar view of the left foot. The lateral (Fig. 26.2a) noted a subtalar dislocation with residual ankle joint synovitis signified by increased soft tissue density. The dorsoplantar view noted the talonavicular joint (TNJ) dislocation with severe osteopenia (Fig. 26.2b).

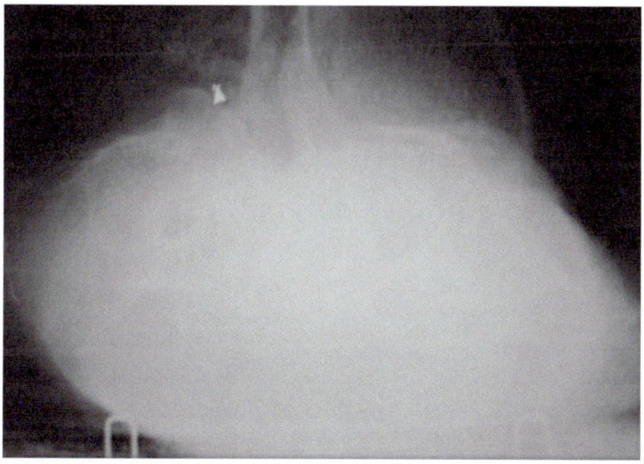

Fig. 26.1 Massive soft tissue swelling with inability to evaluate the osseous structures

H. J. Visser, *Challenges in Foot and Ankle Reconstructive Surgery*,
https://doi.org/10.1007/978-3-031-07893-4_26

Diagnosis

In this case, we see another condition that involves a TNJ dislocation and subtalar joint (STJ) subluxation. In this case, it is secondary to severe rheumatoid synovitis. Destruction of the peritalar soft tissue structures (cervical, interosseous talocalcaneal, and spring ligaments) will not support the talus with weight bearing [1, 2]. The result is a "rocker bottom" flatfoot.

Management

In this case, a double arthrodesis of the TN joint and subtalar joint was performed through a medial incision (Fig. 26.3a). The tibialis posterior tendon sheath was followed to the flexor digitorum longus (FDL) over the STJ (Fig. 26.3b). The TNJ was

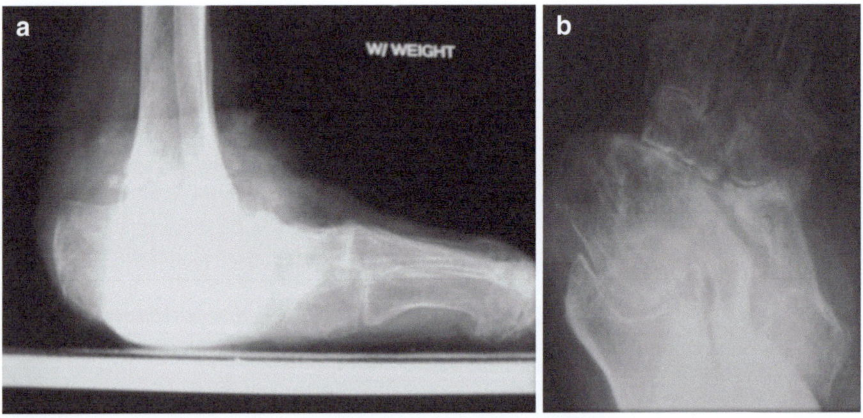

Fig. 26.2 (**a**, **b**) Following medical management of RA, swelling subsided and x-rays demonstrated severe osteopenia, talonavicular and subtalar dislocation with residual ankle joint synovitis signified by increased soft tissue density

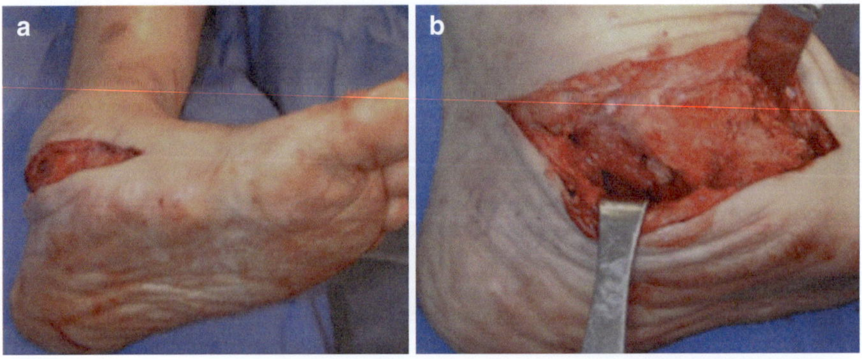

Fig. 26.3 (**a**, **b**) A double arthrodesis of the TN joint and subtalar joint was performed through a medial incision

prepared first with a Hintermann retractor utilizing 0.062" K-wires placed into the navicular tuberosity and anterior talar neck. The anterior, middle, and posterior facets were then prepared again with a Hintermann retractor utilizing 0.062" K-wires placed in the sustentaculum tali and the anterior talar neck [3, 4]. Rigid internal fixation was utilized (Fig. 26.4a–c). The patient was allowed to bear partial weight and immediately had home physical therapy to maintain strength and mobility of the major weight-bearing joints. Arthrodesis occurred at 12 weeks.

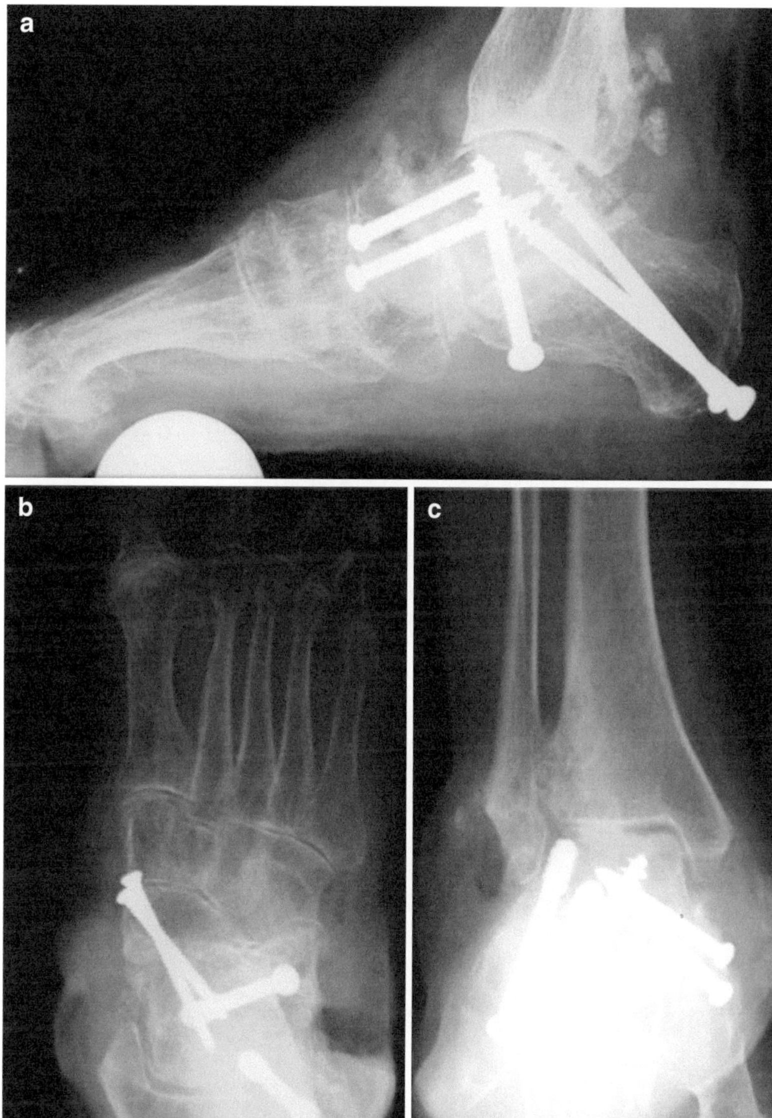

Fig. 26.4 (**a–c**) X-rays note corrected deformities and rigid internal fixation across the subtalar and talonavicular joints

Clinical Pearls and Pitfalls

Control of the rheumatoid disease state has become the norm with biologic response modifiers. On occasion, a patient will be seen that has not had adequate treatment. In this case, control of the synovitis was paramount. These patients are at high risk of infection and wound-healing issues. Failure of arthrodesis can be complicated by extreme osteopenia [5]. A medial approach was utilized for arthrodesis in reduction of the talonavicular and subtalar joint dislocations because of the severe flat foot deformity [6]. A lateral incisional approach for preparation of the subtalar joint is discouraged in these cases. This is due to a high occurrence of wound dehiscence issues. Joint mobilization proved not to be difficult due to loss of soft tissue integrity created by the extreme rheumatoid synovitis. Thus, they are a "loose" bag of bones. Non-cannulated screws are preferred in such cases of severe osteopenia.

References

1. O'Brien TS, Hart TS, Gould JS. Extraosseous manifestations of rheumatoid arthritis in the foot and ankle. Clin Orthop Relat Res. 1997;(340):26–33.
2. D'Amico JC. The pathomechanics of adult rheumatoid arthritis affecting the foot. J Am Podiatry Assoc. 1976;66(4):227–36.
3. Munoz MA, Augoyard R, Canovas F, French Association of Foot Surgery (AFCP). Surgical treatment of hindfoot inflammatory diseases: 107 arthrodesis. Orthop Traumatol Surg Res. 2012;98(6 Suppl):S85–90.
4. Tanaka Y, Takakura Y, Taniguchi A, Sugimoto K, Kumai T, Fukui A. Partial tarsal arthrodesis for rheumatoid feet. Mod Rheumatol. 2004;14(2):130–4.
5. Saleh KJ, Kurdi AJ, El-Othmani MM, Voss BA, Tzeng TH, Saleh J, Lane JM, Mihalko WM. Perioperative treatment of patients with rheumatoid arthritis. J Am Acad Orthop Surg. 2015;23(9):e38–48.
6. Jeng CL, Vora AM, Myerson MS. The medial approach to triple arthrodesis. Indications and technique for management of rigid valgus deformities in high-risk patients. Foot Ankle Clin. 2005;10(3):515–21.

Case #27: Management of a Calcaneal and Subtalar Joint Malunion with Osteotomy and Bone Block Arthrodesis

27

Case Presentation

This is a 60-year-old male who states he suffered a severe fracture of his right heel some 10 years prior. He states that he fell off his roof and landed on the right foot. He suffered no other injuries other than the comminuted intra-articular calcaneal fracture. He states that he was kept in the hospital for 14 days and that he had large hemorrhagic fracture blisters. He stated that after that time the doctors performed surgery. They told him that the fracture was so severe that his foot had to be fused. He then stated the wounds did not completely heal from surgery. He was then placed on intravenous antibiotics for 6 weeks. He was told he did not have osteomyelitis, but there was concern and he was treated as such. The incisional wounds took nearly 3 months to heal. He states he did have one skin graft. Initially, he did have a plantigrade foot, however, over the ensuing 2–3 years, his foot became non-plantigrade and his heel became non-weight bearing.

He further stated that he could never get his heel to the ground. He was placed in a total ankle AFO with a heel wedge. He sought care because he had an increasing amount of anterior ankle pain.

Diagnosis and Assessment

The patient demonstrated a subtalar joint malunion with a severe equinus and loss of calcaneal declination. The midtarsal joint (MTJ) underwent arthrodesis. The calcaneocuboid joint (CCJ) did go on to complete fusion but not the talonavicular joint

H. J. Visser, *Challenges in Foot and Ankle Reconstructive Surgery*,
https://doi.org/10.1007/978-3-031-07893-4_27

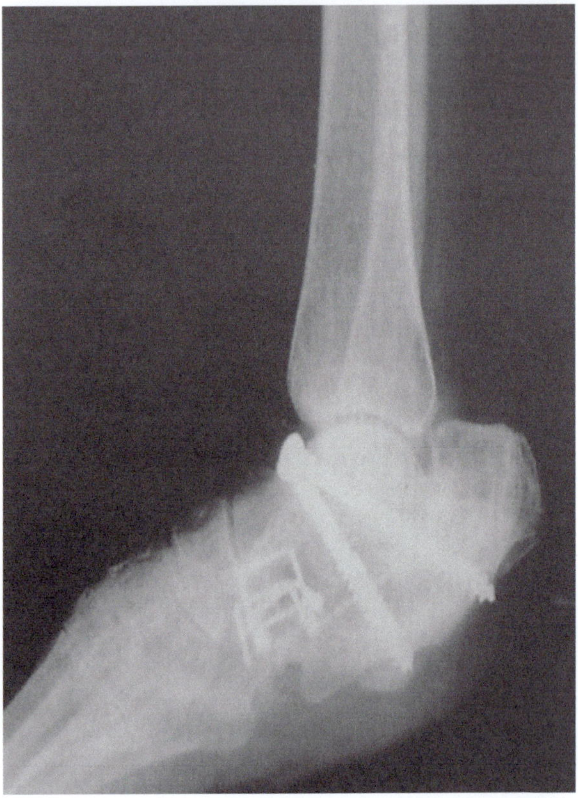

Fig. 27.1 Post ORIF intra-articular calcaneal fracture with severe residual equinus of right foot

(TNJ) (Fig. 27.1). The etiology of his anterior ankle pain was secondary to impingement secondary to the large 6.5 mm screw heads.

He was not able to get his heel to the ground and walked on his toes. His vascular exam was normal. Neurologically, he had sensation loss along the course of the sural nerve. Dermatologically, he had a healed scar running from the distal fibula to the fourth metatarsal base. He had a well-healed scar over the medial TNJ. The lateral incision noted induration and scarring with hyperpigmentation.

Management

A posterior approach (Gallie) in the prone position was utilized (Fig. 27.2a, b) [1, 2]. Due to the lateral scarring a fresh corridor was chosen. Also access to all points of correction could be made. However, prior to prone positioning the two screws in the talar neck were removed in the supine position through a small anterior arthrotomy.

The first procedure involved the Achilles tendon which underwent a z-plasty lengthening in the sagittal place. The posterior ankle was severely scarred. An aggressive release of the posterior scar tissue was performed involving both the

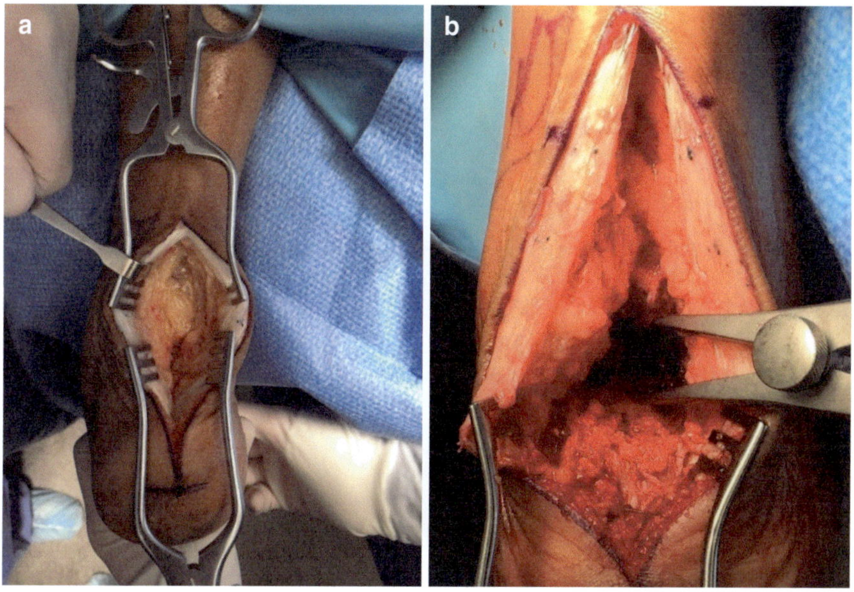

Fig. 27.2 (**a, b**) The subtalar joint was accessed through a Gallie approach with patient in prone position

ankle and the subtalar joint (STJ). The flexor hallucis longus (FHL) muscle was visible proximally and retracted medially to expose the posterior ankle and subtalar joint.

An indirect procedure, a sagittal and medially translating calcaneal osteotomy was performed just posterior to the posterior facet. It was then slid inferior and medial, and with the Achilles tendon lengthening, allowed a plantigrade position. It may also be noted that the heel was in valgus and corrected by the medial slide.

The posterior STJ was then entered under fluoroscopic guidance and a direct procedure to address the malunion was performed with bone block allograft. The allograft was prepared with bone marrow aspirate from the tibia. Two screws were utilized. The first fully threaded 6.5 mm across the bone block allograft acting as a position screw not rendering compression. The second partially threaded 6.5 mm screw was used to provide compression to the anterior subtalar joint (Fig. 27.3).

Outcome

The patient was kept non-weight bearing for 8 weeks. He was then allowed full weight bearing for 6 more weeks in a weight-bearing boot. No wound complications occurred. The patient now has a plantigrade foot. He still has pain with increased activity primarily involving the ankle and midfoot. He is in an Arizona brace. He is happy with the outcome that a plantigrade foot was achieved. However, his activity level remains restricted [3, 4].

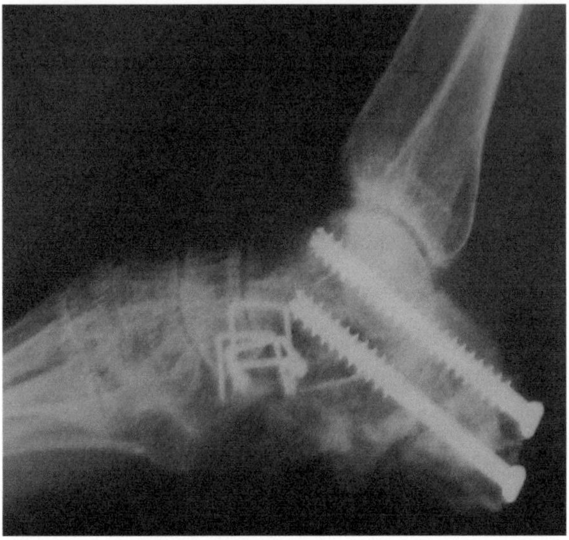

Fig. 27.3 Postoperative x-ray depicts restoration of heel height by way of fixation of bone block allograft with 6.5 mm screws

Clinical Pearls and Pitfalls

This represents a case that was performed years prior when understanding of intra-articular calcaneal fractures was still limited. Computed tomography (CT) scan was not available and was not performed. The attempt here was to perform a triple arthrodesis due to the extreme comminution involving the STJ. Apparently, it represented a Sanders type IV intra-articular calcaneal fracture.

As can be seen, the STJ was fused but the tuberosity portion of the primary fracture line was not addressed. This allowed splinting of the Achilles tendon which pulled the unsupported tuberosity superiorly into severe equinus. This also created a valgus shift. Anterior ankle impingement was secondary to screw prominence. The loss of declination of the talus was created by comminution and posterior facet joint depression. This produced gradual anterior talar neck impingement [5].

This case involved three surgical approaches. (1) soft tissue (Achilles tendon contracture) [6, 7], (2) severe negative calcaneal pitch and valgus (indirect biplane calcaneal osteotomy), and (3) restoring talar inclination (direct bone block arthrodesis). The posterior longitudinal incision allowed accommodation of the restored length of the calcaneus and thus placed no tension on the old incisional scars.

The MTJ was not addressed. The patient's continued discomfort may be secondary to the TNJ nonunion. Post-traumatic ankle joint arthritis was also present.

References

1. Kalamchi A, Evans JG. Posterior subtalar fusion. A preliminary report on a modified Gallie's procedure. J Bone Joint Surg. 1977;59(3):287–9.
2. Laporta G, Bock F, Ghate N. Posterior approach for subtalar joint distraction arthrodesis by compact external fixation: a technique guide. J Foot Ankle Surg. 2013;52(4):547–52.
3. Huang PJ, Fu YC, Cheng YM, Lin SY. Subtalar arthrodesis for late sequelae of calcaneal fractures: fusion in situ versus fusion with sliding corrective osteotomy. Foot Ankle Int. 1999;20(3):166–70.
4. Farouk A, Ibrahim A, Abd-Ella MM, El Ghazali S. Effect of subtalar fusion and calcaneal osteotomy on function, pain, and gait mechanics for calcaneal Malunion. Foot Ankle Int. 2019;40(9):1094–103.
5. Yu GR, Zhang MZ, Yang YF. Corrective osteotomies for Malunited tongue-type calcaneal fractures. Foot Ankle Clin. 2016;21(1):123–34.
6. Rammelt S, Marx C. Managing severely Malunited calcaneal fractures and fracture-dislocations. Foot Ankle Clin. 2020;25(2):239–56.
7. Rammelt S, Zwipp H. Corrective arthrodeses and osteotomies for post-traumatic hindfoot malalignment: indications, techniques, results. Int Orthop. 2013;37(9):1707–17.

Case #28: Revision of Triple Arthrodesis Malunion with Severe Osteopenia

28

Case Presentation

This is a 62-year-old African-American female who presents with a prior history of having undergone a prior triple arthrodesis for post-traumatic osteoarthritis. The patient states that her foot looked well initially but after about 6 months noted that the foot began to collapse. She demonstrated an antalgic gait and complained of plantar midfoot pain. She was in an accommodative orthotic with extra depth shoes.

Diagnosis and Assessment

On examination, the patient demonstrated a rocker bottom foot deformity that was rigid and not reducible. There was no edema and vascular and neurologic exams were completely normal. The patient was not diabetic. She did have a history of stable cardiovascular disease and osteoporosis.

Radiographs note on the lateral view the performance of a triple arthrodesis. There were multiple screws across the talonavicular (TN) and calcaneocuboid (CC) joints. A rocker bottom deformity existed at the midtarsal joint (MTJ) level [1, 2]. The subtalar joint (STJ) demonstrated one screw. All joints had undergone an arthrodesis process. An obvious malunion was present. Also, severe osteopenia was present that involved all osseous structures of the foot and ankle (Fig. 28.1a).

H. J. Visser, *Challenges in Foot and Ankle Reconstructive Surgery*,
https://doi.org/10.1007/978-3-031-07893-4_28

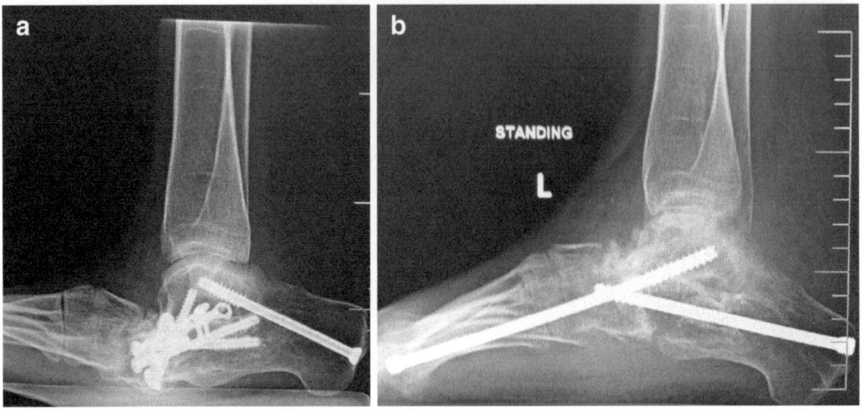

Fig. 28.1 (**a**) Hardware failure secondary to severe osteopenia. (**b**) A large beaming screw was placed through the first metatarsal and spanned the TN joint. The calcaneocuboid joint was secured with a large screw

Management/Outcome

Initial management involved removal of internal fixation. Secondly, an Achilles tendon lengthening was performed. Third, a two-incisional approach utilizing guide pins was performed to create an osteotomy across the TNJ and CCJ. A two-incisional approach was utilized. A plantar triangular midfoot wedge was removed to restore midfoot declination [3]. A beaming screw was then placed medially through the first metatarsal. It also spanned the TNJ. A posterior calcaneal screw was inserted lateral to the Achilles tendon to secure the CCJ (Fig. 28.1b).

The patient was kept non-weight bearing for 4 weeks. She then did 4 weeks in a weight-bearing controlled ankle motion (CAM) boot. The patient was placed in a new accommodative orthotic. She has done quite well now some 3 years postoperatively.

Pearls and Pitfalls

As there were no prior radiographs before the initial procedure was performed, it is difficult to assess the conditions of the foot. By history she was told her foot was extremely arthritic. Utilization of multiple compression screws involving osteopenic bone can lead to accretion and bone mass loss. The Achilles tendon was not addressed and this also may have produced a significant deforming force. Once shortening occurs, the lever arm becomes more proximal and, thus, gives the Achilles tendon a very distinct mechanical advantage.

Correction of the rocker bottom deformity clearly centered at the MTJ which served as the CORA (center of rotation axis). The intact arthrodesis (malunion) can be approached in two ways. An opening wedge osteotomy utilizing bone graft or a corrective closing wedge osteotomy [4, 5]. The closing wedge osteotomy was chosen in this case so as to allow relaxation of the incisions. The same incisions in the original procedure were again utilized.

The fixation involved a single long calcaneal and metatarsal cannulated screws. The long beaming screws serve to create a rebar effect and dissipate force through osteopenic bone.

References

1. Haddad SL, Myerson MS, Pell RF 4th, Schon LC. Clinical and radiographic outcome of revision surgery for failed triple arthrodesis. Foot Ankle Int. 1997;18(8):489–99.
2. Seybold JD. Management of the malunited triple arthrodesis. Foot Ankle Clin. 2017;22(3):625–36.
3. Bibbo C, Anderson RB, Davis WH. Complications of midfoot and hindfoot arthrodesis. Clin Orthop Relat Res. 2001;391:45–58.
4. Toolan BC. Revision of failed triple arthrodesis with an opening-closing wedge osteotomy of the midfoot. Foot Ankle Int. 2004;25(7):456–61.
5. Perez RR, Strash WW. Revision of malaligned triple arthrodesis: a case report. Clin Podiatr Med Surg. 2004;21(3):407–vii.

Part IV

The Charcot Foot and Ankle

Case #29: Revision of Neuropathic Lis Franc Joint Dislocation with Trans-Pedal Wedge Arthrodesis

29

Case Presentation

This is a 46-year-old Caucasian female who has a long history of type I diabetes. She also was on renal dialysis. She has had a past history of coronary stents. She is on Eliquis for a past history of DVT. She initially presented with a hot, swollen midfoot. She denied any history of trauma. She had only mild pain but has a history of neuropathy. She was originally seen by her primary care physician and diagnosed with cellulitis (Fig. 29.1). She was treated with antibiotics, but there was no improvement in her condition. X-rays were taken which showed a subtle neuropathic Lisfranc joint dislocation (Fig. 29.2a, b). She was sent to an orthopedist for treatment.

They placed her non-weight bearing in a contact cast and at 4 weeks performed an open reduction, internal fixation (ORIF) once the soft tissue edema had subsided (Fig. 29.3a, b).

She admitted to not being strictly compliant and she had loss of correction and increasing deformity. She was then placed in a Charcot-restraint orthotic walker (CROW) boot and was told there was nothing more that could be done.

Diagnosis and Assessment

The patient when evaluated and demonstrated a significant varus and abduction rotation of her forefoot. As she was on a waiting list for a kidney transplant, she was required to perform walking on a treadmill to qualify. She stated that she was completely unable to wear a closed shoe and ambulated in a CROW boot (Fig. 29.4a, b).

On review of her initial X-rays, the subtle Lisfranc joint injury included a proximal variant [1, 2]. This was demonstrated by rotation of the medial cuneiform (Fig. 29.2a).

H. J. Visser, *Challenges in Foot and Ankle Reconstructive Surgery*,
https://doi.org/10.1007/978-3-031-07893-4_29

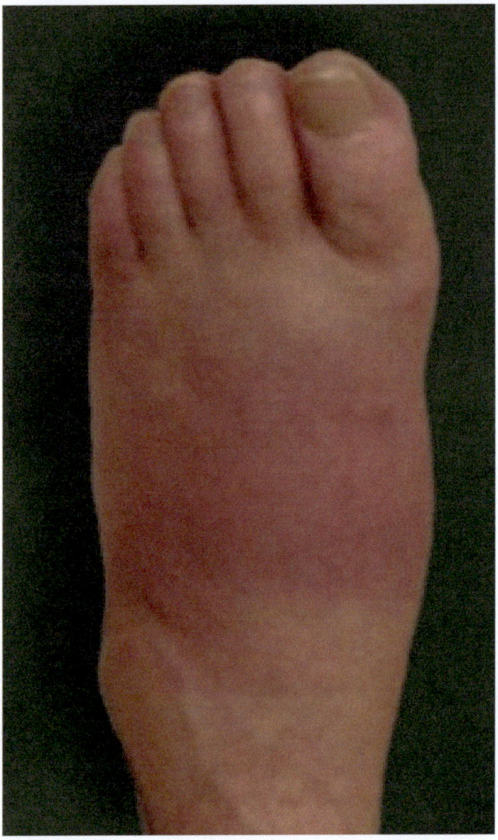

Fig. 29.1 Left foot, diagnosed as cellulitis initially. Eichenholtz Stage 1 Charcot Lisfranc involvement

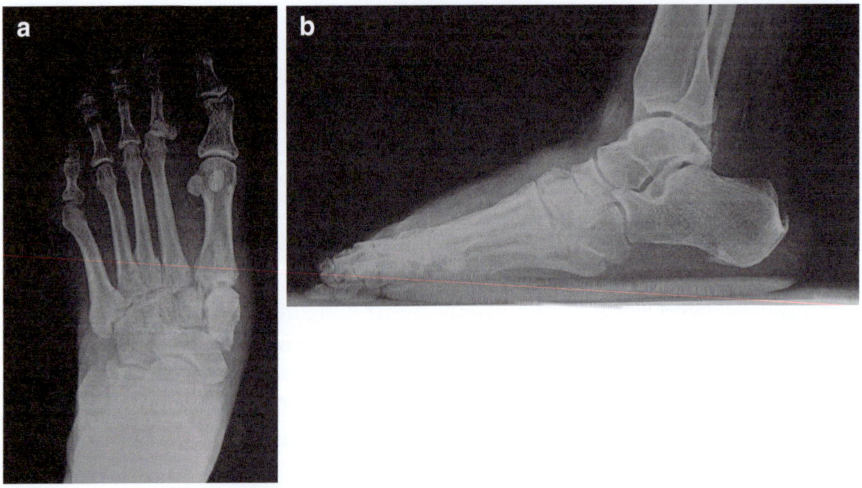

Fig. 29.2 (**a**) Lisfranc "subtle" spontaneous dislocation of left foot. (**b**) First metatarsal medial cuneiform articulation notes mild plantar gapping

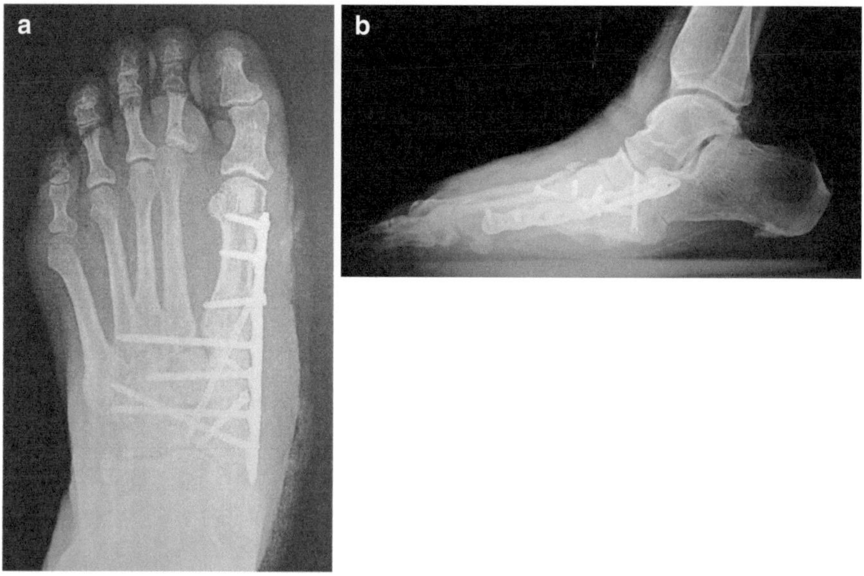

Fig. 29.3 (**a**) ORIF with medial locking plate, 3.5 mm spanning screws. (**b**) Note marked instability of the medial column, Meary's angle not restored

It exhibited a positive notch sign. Postoperative alignment appeared excellent in the dorsoplantar view. On the lateral view, however, a significant naviculocuneiform (NC) joint fault was present (Fig. 29.2b). A posterior group lengthening had not been performed [3].

Radiographs viewed some 6 months later show complete loss of fixation. Significant abduction of the forefoot at the tarsometatarsal joint (TMTJ) 1, 2, 3 exists (Fig. 29.5a). There was avascular necrosis of the medial cuneiform. The intermediate cuneiform was dislocated. The lateral view showed a persistent NC joint fault and forefoot supinatus (Fig. 29.5b).

Management

The hardware was then removed. Initially, a long medial incision from the tip of the medial malleolus to the first metatarsal was made along the medial aspect of the foot. The tibialis anterior tendon was then detached. It was later reattached with a suture anchor with closure. A gastrocnemius recession was performed. A posterior (Koutsogiannis type) calcaneal osteotomy was performed to address the heel valgus. A transpedal wedge osteotomy was then performed through the cuneonavicular and cuboid structures (Fig. 29.6a, b). Arthrodesis of the first metatarsal cuneiform and TN joint were done next. They were fixated with an intramedullary 6.5 mm bolt. A long, one-third tubular rigid locking plate and spanning screws were placed across these joint structures (Fig. 29.7a–c) [4].

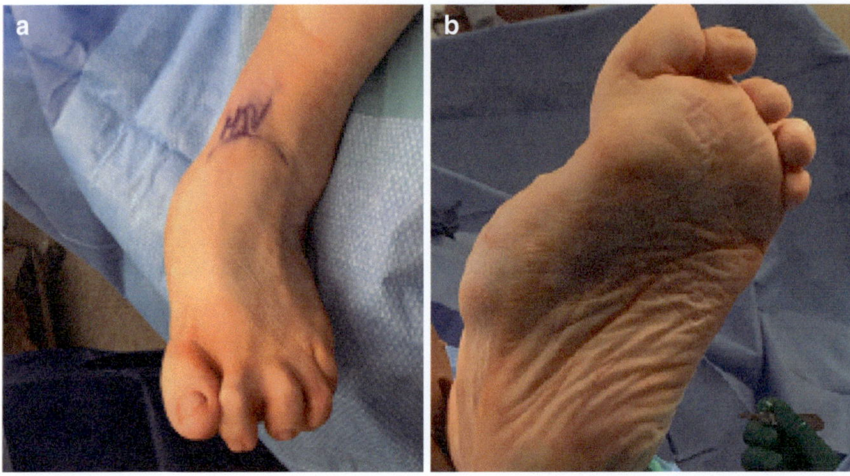

Fig. 29.4 (**a**, **b**) Clinical appearance, severe rigid midfoot abduction

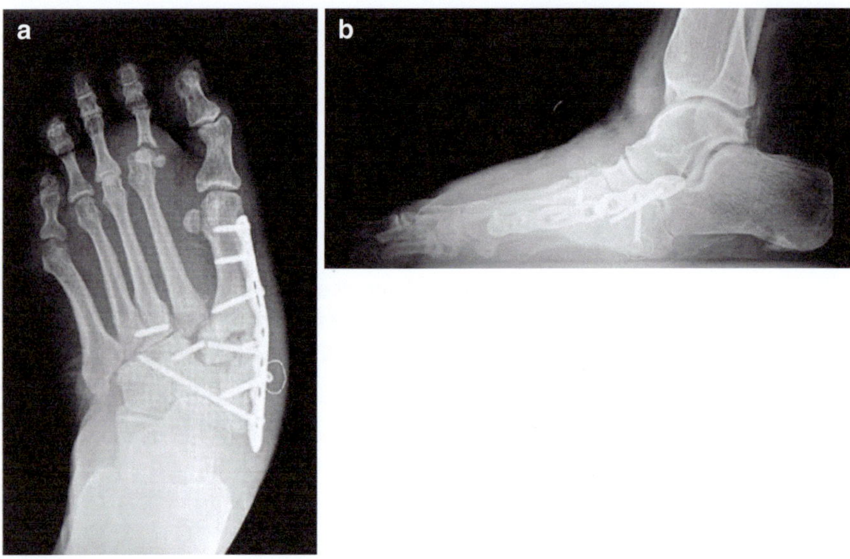

Fig. 29.5 (**a**) Radiographs demonstrate significant abduction of the forefoot, with avascular necrosis of the medial cuneiform, and dislocation of the intermediate cuneiform. (**b**) Persistent NC fault with forefoot supinatus

Excellent deformity correction was accomplished. A static circular frame external fixator was applied (Fig. 29.8) [5].

Post-op course was 12 weeks of non-weight bearing. The external fixator was then removed. The patient was then placed for 12 weeks in a controlled ankle motion (CAM) boot weight bearing with walker assistance. She was then converted to an Arizona brace.

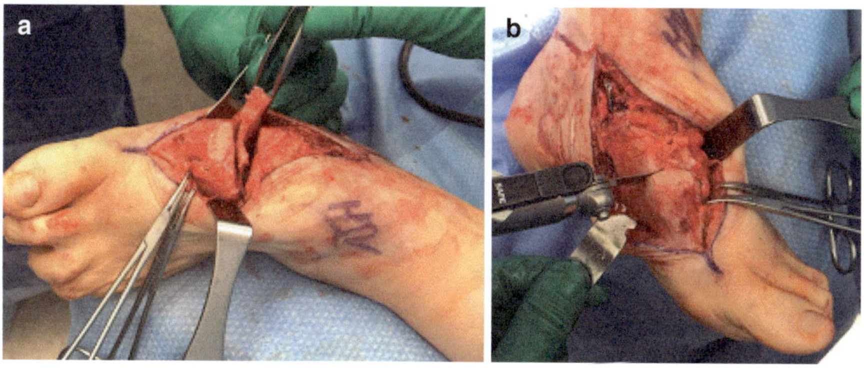

Fig. 29.6 (**a**, **b**) Transpedal wedge osteotomy performed through the cuneonavicular and cuboid structure

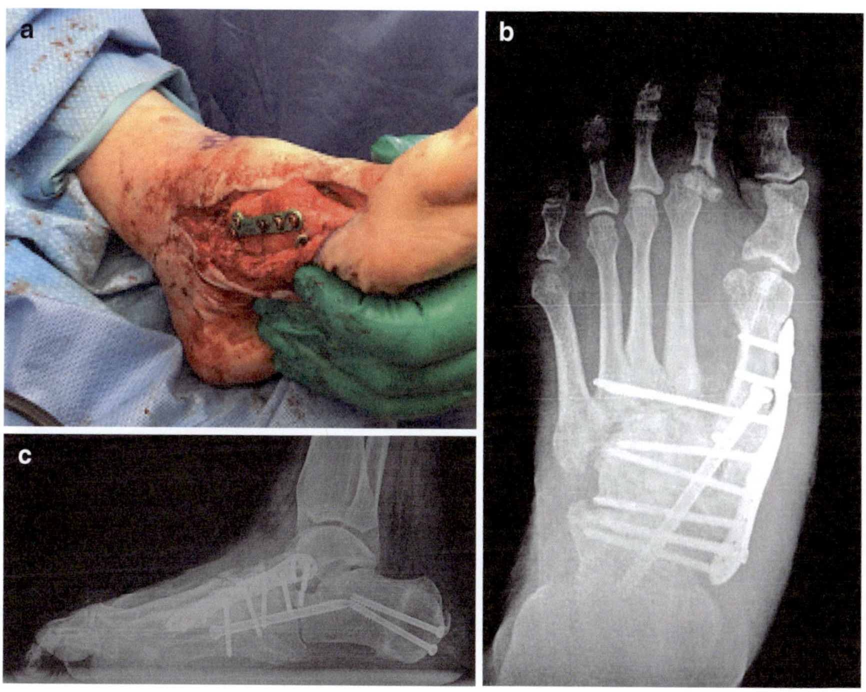

Fig. 29.7 (**a**, **b**) Fixation of osteotomy was performed with 1/3 tubular rigid locking plate and spanning screws with included TN arthrodesis. (**c**) Meary's angle restored

Outcome

The patient demonstrated an uneventful course. There were no wound problems or pin tract infections. She was able to pass her treadmill test at 8 months postoperatively and received a kidney.

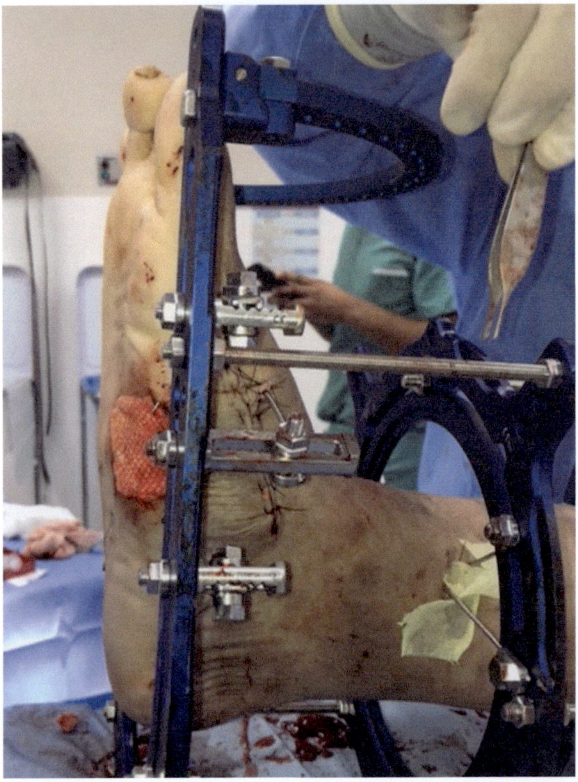

Fig. 29.8 Static circular frame applied

Clinical Pearls and Pitfalls

As can be seen involving this case, a controversy exists as to what is the best course of management of Eichenholtz stage I Charcot foot. Current thought often remains to initiate immediate non-weight bearing. Weight bearing is normally not allowed until stage III occurs. Calcitonin, bisphosphonates, and bone stimulation have been considered as adjuncts. They, however, have not shown any true alteration of stage progression. The Lisfranc type "subtle" neuropathic joint injury represents an early finding of a spontaneous dislocation. In stage III, this condition often remains unstable. And weight bearing often leads to a midfoot rocker bottom foot deformity. More current thought is to manage this condition similar to a non-neuropathic state. This involves "ramped up" ORIF and represents super construct. In this case, this was done. Certain issues must be addressed. (1) Equinus with stiffness due to glycosylation offers increased stress generated on a shorter lever arm centered at the Lisfranc midfoot joints [3, 6].

(2) An attempted anatomic ORIF was performed. As was in this case, a ligamentous lesion, expectation of stability healing is uncertain in the neuropathic foot. Extended fixation beyond the zone of involvement and arthrodesis must be

considered. In this case, it includes the entire medial column [5]. (3) With the presence of the proximal variant, stability of the medial and central column can only be achieved by arthrodesis.

Protection of the internal fixation construct must be supplemented with a circular fixator. This protects the foot and allows protected weight bearing.

References

1. Myerson M. The diagnosis and treatment of injuries to the Lisfranc joint complex. Orthop Clin North Am. 1989;20(4):655–64.
2. Faciszewski T, Burks RT, Manaster BJ. Subtle injuries of the Lisfranc joint. J Bone Joint Surg Am. 1990;72(10):1519–22.
3. Alrashidi Y, Hügle T, Wiewiorski M, Herrera-Perez M, Valderrabano V. Surgical treatment options for the diabetic Charcot midfoot deformity. Clin Podiatr Med Surg. 2017;34(1):43–51.
4. Grant WP, Garcia-Lavin S, Sabo R. Beaming the columns for Charcot diabetic foot reconstruction: a retrospective analysis. J Foot Ankle Surg. 2011;50(2):182–9.
5. Brandão RA, Weber JS, Larson D, Prissel MA, Bull PE, Berlet GC, Hyer CF. New fixation methods for the treatment of the diabetic foot: beaming, external fixation, and beyond. Clin Podiatr Med Surg. 2018;35(1):63–76.
6. Ahmed N. Advanced glycation endproducts—role in pathology of diabetic complications. Diabetes Res Clin Pract. 2005;67(1):3–21.

Case #30: Management of Charcot Midfoot Deformity with Trans-cuneonaviculocuboid Wedge

30

Case Presentation

This is a 46-year-old Caucasian male who presents with a history of long-term swelling and left foot pain. He noted foot swelling some 9 months prior to evaluation. He notes that he slipped and twisted his foot. He was seen in a local ER and told that there were no abnormalities on X-ray. He was diagnosed with a sprain. After continued swelling and low-grade pain, he sought podiatric care. He was diagnosed with a Charcot foot deformity. He was managed by a non-weight bearing and placed on a knee scooter. This was some 8 weeks after the initial injury. He states that he often walked on it during that time frame.

His medical history was significant for insulin-dependent diabetes mellitus (IDDM). He had received a kidney via renal transplant some 2 years prior. He was on warfarin secondary to a history of past left leg deep vein thrombosis and pulmonary embolism after his renal transplant. He had no further events but an inferior vena cava filter had been placed.

Neurologic exam noted profound sensory, autonomic, and motor neuropathy at the ankle/pedal level. He was unable to feel a 5.09 Semmes-Weinstein monofilament to the lower leg bilaterally. His Lewis flare test was abnormal. Vascular exam noted a good dorsalis pedis and posterior tibial artery pulse at 2/4 with normal perfusion. Doppler exam noted triphasic waveforms and normal arterial digital pressures.

H. J. Visser, *Challenges in Foot and Ankle Reconstructive Surgery*,
https://doi.org/10.1007/978-3-031-07893-4_30

Diagnosis and Assessment

On evaluation, the patient was diagnosed with Eichenholtz stage III Charcot foot deformity. He was referred for treatment as he had developed an ulceration over the plantar aspect of his medial cuneiform [1]. The ulceration was 4 × 3.2 cm and extended to the capsule. On his radiographs, he demonstrated a Schoen I Charcot deformity. The first metatarsal-medial cuneiform dislocation exhibited an angle of 24 degrees of abduction. A complete neuropathic homolateral dislocation with avascular necrotic resorption of the metatarsal bases 1–4 and cuneiform and cuboid was present (Fig. 30.1a, b) [2, 3]. His rearfoot was in rectus alignment but clinically

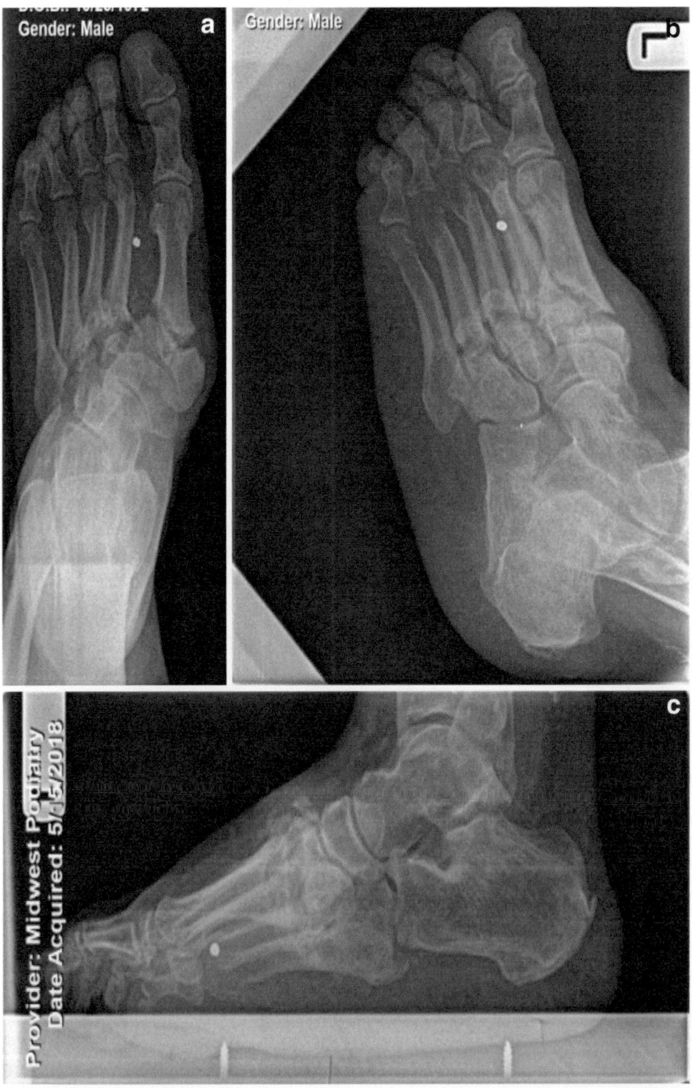

Fig. 30.1 (**a–c**) Abducted foot deformity caused by neuropathic homolateral dislocation with avascular necrotic resorption of the metatarsal bases 1–4

the midfoot was not plantigrade. Also the degree of abduction would not accommodate shoe wear (Fig. 30.1b, c).

Management

Warfarin therapy was stopped 5 days preoperatively. Lovenox was used as a bridge for anticoagulation. The tourniquet was used at the ankle level. The ulceration was managed with wound care and a contact cast. After 6 weeks, it had healed. Surgery was then planned to realign the midfoot and stabilize the proximal midtarsal and subtalar joints.

Initially, a gastrocnemius recession was performed. Secondly, a trans-cuneionaviculo cuboid wedge was performed. The proximal cut was made parallel to the midtarsal joint (MTJ). The distal cut was made through the cuneometatarsal bases. Beaming screws were then placed in the first (7.0 beam) and fourth (5.5 beam) metatarsals (Fig. 30.2a, b) [4, 5]. A locking plate was placed dorsomedial spanning from the first metatarsal to the talus. The medial column osteotomy corrected the rocker bottom deformity. The talonavicular (TN) and calcaneocuboid (CC) joints subsequently underwent arthrodesis (Fig. 30.3a–c).

The patient was placed in a static circular frame (Fig. 30.4) and allowed protected weight bearing for 12 weeks [4]. The frame was then removed. He was then placed in a controlled ankle motion (CAM) boot and allowed full weight bearing for 12 weeks. He was subsequently placed in a total ankle foot orthosis (AFO).

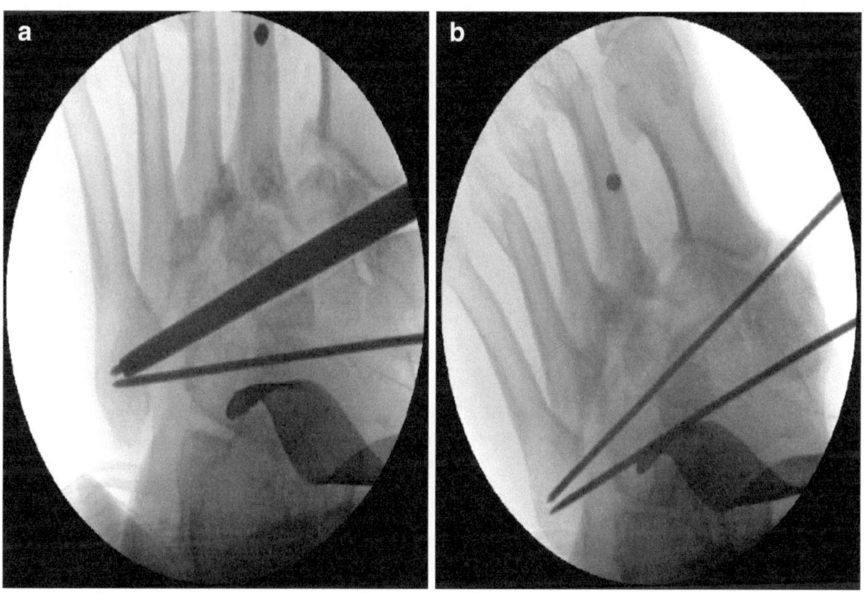

Fig. 30.2 (**a**, **b**) A trans-cuneionaviculocuboid wedge was performed

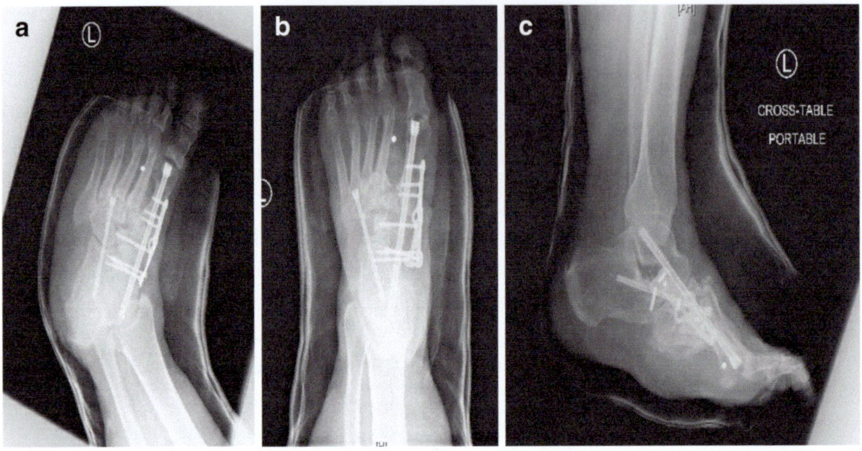

Fig. 30.3 (**a**–**c**) Correction of the deformity achieved by arthrodesis of the calcaneocuboid and talonavicular joints. Beaming screws were placed in the first and fourth metatarsals along with a dorsal medial spanning plate

Fig. 30.4 A static frame was applied

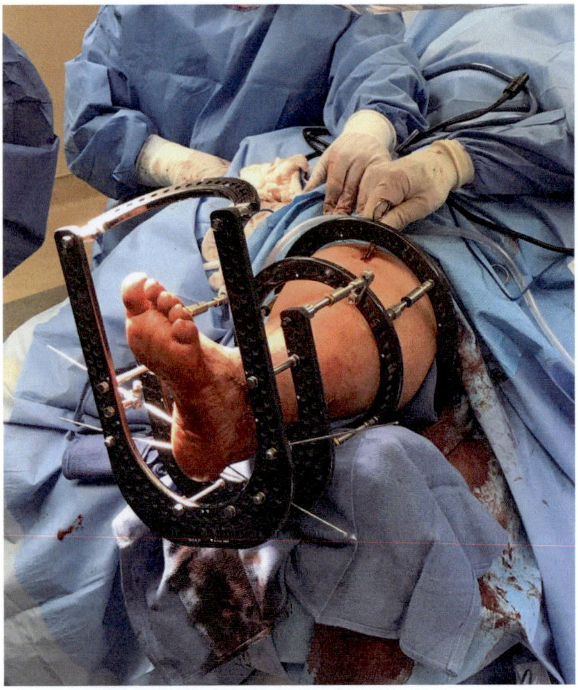

Outcome

The patient had an excellent recovery. A plantigrade foot was attained. The CC joint did not undergo arthrodesis but was asymptomatic.

Clinical Pearls and Pitfalls

The deformity presented here represents a paradox. On lateral X-ray view, it appeared to be plantigrade, with excellent longitudinal arch structure. Clinically, the midfoot was weight bearing at the medial cuneiform due to loss of stability of the first metatarsal-medial cuneiform joint.

When abduction deformity at the first metatarsal-medial cuneiform exceeds 15 degrees a midfoot wedge osteotomy is preferred over anatomic joint alignment. Attempted anatomic alignment in these large abduction deformities require bone grafting. This leads often to nonunion and destabilization in a neuropathic foot.

Extending fixation and fusion beyond the zone of injury in a neuropathic foot is a principle described by Sammarco and must be strictly adhered to [5]. “Locking” the beams is often a valuable adjunct to provide medial column stability by resisting torsion and bending forces. This includes the beaming screw supported by the locking plate.

References

1. Kavarthapu V, Vris A. Charcot midfoot reconstruction—surgical technique based on deformity patterns. Ann Joint. 2020;5:28.
2. Schon LC, Easley ME, Weinfeld SB. Charcot neuroarthropathy of the foot and ankle. Clin Orthop Relat Res. 1998;349:116–31.
3. Schon LC, Weinfeld SB, Horton GA, Resch S. Radiographic and clinical classification of acquired midtarsus deformities. Foot Ankle Int. 1998;19(6):394–404.
4. Siddiqui NA, LaPorta GA. Midfoot charcot reconstruction. Clin Podiatr Med Surg. 2018;35(4):509–20.
5. Sammarco VJ. Superconstructs in the treatment of charcot foot deformity: plantar plating, locked plating, and axial screw fixation. Foot Ankle Clin. 2009;14(3):393–407.

Case #31: Management of Severe Charcot Foot and Ankle Deformity with Posterior Tendon Group Lengthening and Capsulotomies with Arthrodesis and Tarsometatarsal Joint 4 and 5

31

Case Presentation

This is a 68-year-old Caucasian female who presents with a long-term history of Charcot osteoarthropathy. She has had a long history of plantar ulcerations plantar to the cuboid. The patient had long-term conservative care involving a Charcot restraint orthotic walker (CROW) boot with heel elevation. She was an insulin-dependent diabetes mellitus (IDDM) with a HgA1c of 7.6%. On neurological examination, there was loss of protective sensation. She was unable to perceive a 5.07 Semmes-Weinstein (SW) monofilament to her lower leg. Her vascular perfusion was adequate with palpable 2/4 dorsalis pedis (DP) and posterior tibial (PT) pulses. Triphasic waveforms were present on Doppler assessment.

Diagnosis and Assessment

Her foot was non-plantar grade in fixed equinus (Fig. 31.1a). Her heel was not in contact with the ground. A rocker bottom deformity was present with WB occurring at the cuboid (Fig. 31.1b). She had an ulceration present that measured 2 × 2 cm and was shallow in depth. She states that it had been draining recently. It had not healed for over 2 years. Workup for presence osteomyelitis was found negative. Her serology was within normal range.

H. J. Visser, *Challenges in Foot and Ankle Reconstructive Surgery*,
https://doi.org/10.1007/978-3-031-07893-4_31

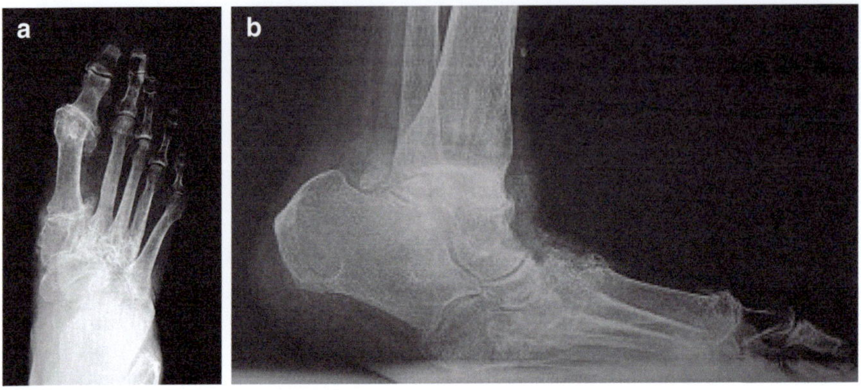

Fig. 31.1 (**a**, **b**) Non-plantargrade foot with rocker bottom deformity in fixed equinus

Management

The patient had a non-plantigrade foot with severe gastrocnemius soleus equinus. Prior to the first initial incision, the plantar ulcer was barriered off with tegaderm. The first procedure addressed the equinus with an open z-plasty in the frontal plane [1, 2]. The second procedure involved aggressive release of the posterior capsule of the ankle and STJ [3]. The third procedure in the sagittal plane calcaneal osteotomy (Mitchell) was also performed (Fig. 31.2a, b) [4]. The issue now once the heel was made plantar grade was to address the tarsometatarsal (TMT) 4, 5 metatarsal-cuboid dislocation. The cuboid was at the center of the rotational axis (CORA) thus the cuboid was the area of plantar WB pressure. This was addressed with TMT 4, 5 cuboid arthrodesis (Fig. 31.2c) [5, 6]. All wounds were closed with 1 g of vancomycin powder.

The patient was kept on non-weight bearing (NWB) for 12 weeks, she was then placed in a controlled ankle motion (CAM) boot for a further 12 weeks. She was then sent to physical therapy (PT) and had to be trained to ambulate again.

Outcome

This was an extreme success. The patient states that she had gotten her "life back." She was placed in an Arizona brace initially. However with PT, she was eventually allowed to ambulate in an accommodative foot orthotic

Clinical Pearls and Pitfalls

This represents a rather unusual case of Charcot foot deformity. A severe rocker bottom deformity was created secondary to glycosylation of the Achilles tendon via the Maillard reaction [7]. This led to resultant stiffness and contracture. The apex

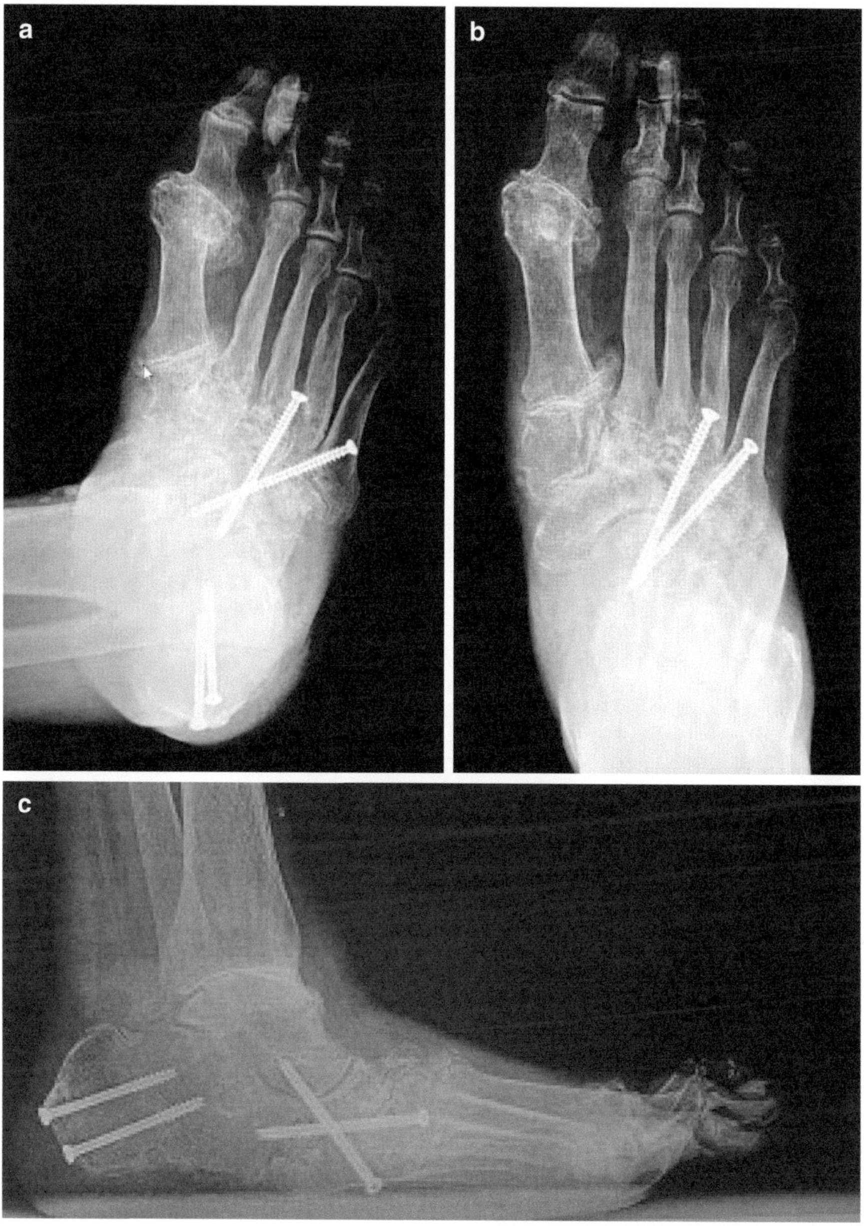

Fig. 31.2 (**a**–**c**) Radiographs following release of Achilles tendon, ankle and STJ capsules. A sagittal plane calcaneal osteotomy and arthrodesis of the TMTs 4 and 5

(CORA) of the rocker bottom foot deformity was the cuboid. In this case to allow weight bearing (WB) of the heel addressing the equinus required an aggressive soft tissue release of the posterior ankle and subtalar joint (STJ) capsule. This allowed the foot to become plantar grade. Radiographically, a navicular cuneiform (NC) fault of the medial column persists. The foot however was plantar grade; there were no further plantar prominences. This was accomplished by the joint resection arthrodesis at metatarsals 4 and 5 with the cuboid. The metatarsals 4 and 5 are always dorsally subluxed to the cuboid. Thus, resection is required for proper alignment of the joint. The elevated medial column became parallel to the lateral WB portion of the foot.

References

1. Downey MS. Ankle equinus. In: McGlamry ED, editor. Comprehensive textbook of foot surgery, vol. 1. Baltimore: Williams & Wilkins; 1987. p. 368–402.
2. Sakurai M, Kokubun S. Coronal plane lengthening of Achilles tendon. Orthop Traumatol. 1993;2:188–92.
3. Jauregui JJ, Zamani S, Abawi HH, Herzenberg JE. Ankle range of motion after posterior subtalar and ankle capsulotomy for relapsed Equinus in idiopathic clubfoot. J Pediatr Orthop. 2017;37(3):199–203.
4. Mitchell GP. Posterior displacement osteotomy of the calcaneus. J Bone Joint Surg. 1977;59(2):233–5.
5. Yu X, Pang QJ, Yu GR. The injuries to the fourth and fifth tarsometatarsal joints: a review of the surgical management by internal fixation, arthrodesis and arthroplasty. Pak J Med Sci. 2013;29(2):687–92.
6. Raikin S, Schon L. Arthrodesis of the fourth and fifth tarsometatarsal joints of the midfoot. Foot Ankle Int. 2003;24(8):584–90.
7. Couppé C, Svensson RB, Kongsgaard M, Kovanen V, Grosset JF, Snorgaard O, Bencke J, Larsen JO, Bandholm T, Christensen TM, Boesen A, Helmark IC, Aagaard P, Kjaer M, Magnusson SP. Human Achilles tendon glycation and function in diabetes. J Appl Physiol (Bethesda, MD 1985). 2016;120(2):130–7.

Case #32: ORIF of Neuropathic Ankle Fracture Utilizing Multiple Tetracortical Syndesmotic Screw Fixation

32

Case Presentation

This is a 61-year-old insulin-dependent diabetes mellitus (IDDM) female who had presented to the emergency room (ER) after sustaining a fall in her garden as she misstepped on the sidewalk. She sustained an initial pronation abduction injury or bimalleolar (Pott's) fracture to her right ankle (Fig. 32.1a–c). She was an IDDM and her HgA1c was 9.6%. A closed reduction was performed in the ER. The patient was then placed in a posterior splint (Fig. 32.2a, b). She was admitted to the hospital and the surgeon on call decided not to operate. He felt there was an adequate reduction and had her transferred to a skilled nursing facility (SNF). His concern was to perform surgery with the elevated HgA1c. He made the decision to place her in a contact cast.

The patient was then seen at 3 weeks, the contact cast removed and the new X-rays were taken. They showed a complete loss of reduction. An ulceration had developed over the medial malleolus (Fig. 32.3a, b).

Neurologically, she had loss of protective sensation, unable to perceive a Semmes-Weinstein monofilament (SWMF) 5.09 to her lower leg. Her vascular perfusion was deemed normal. A doppler evaluation noted normal triphasic waveforms. She gave a history of a myocardial infarction (MI) 4 years prior. Drug eluting stents were placed. Cardiology had deemed her stable.

Diagnosis and Assessment

This patient demonstrates a case of a neuropathic bimalleolar fracture that was unstable. It was difficult to understand the decision of not performing open reduction internal fixation (ORIF). The elevated HgA1c of 9.6% would only be a factor in an elective case.

H. J. Visser, *Challenges in Foot and Ankle Reconstructive Surgery*,
https://doi.org/10.1007/978-3-031-07893-4_32

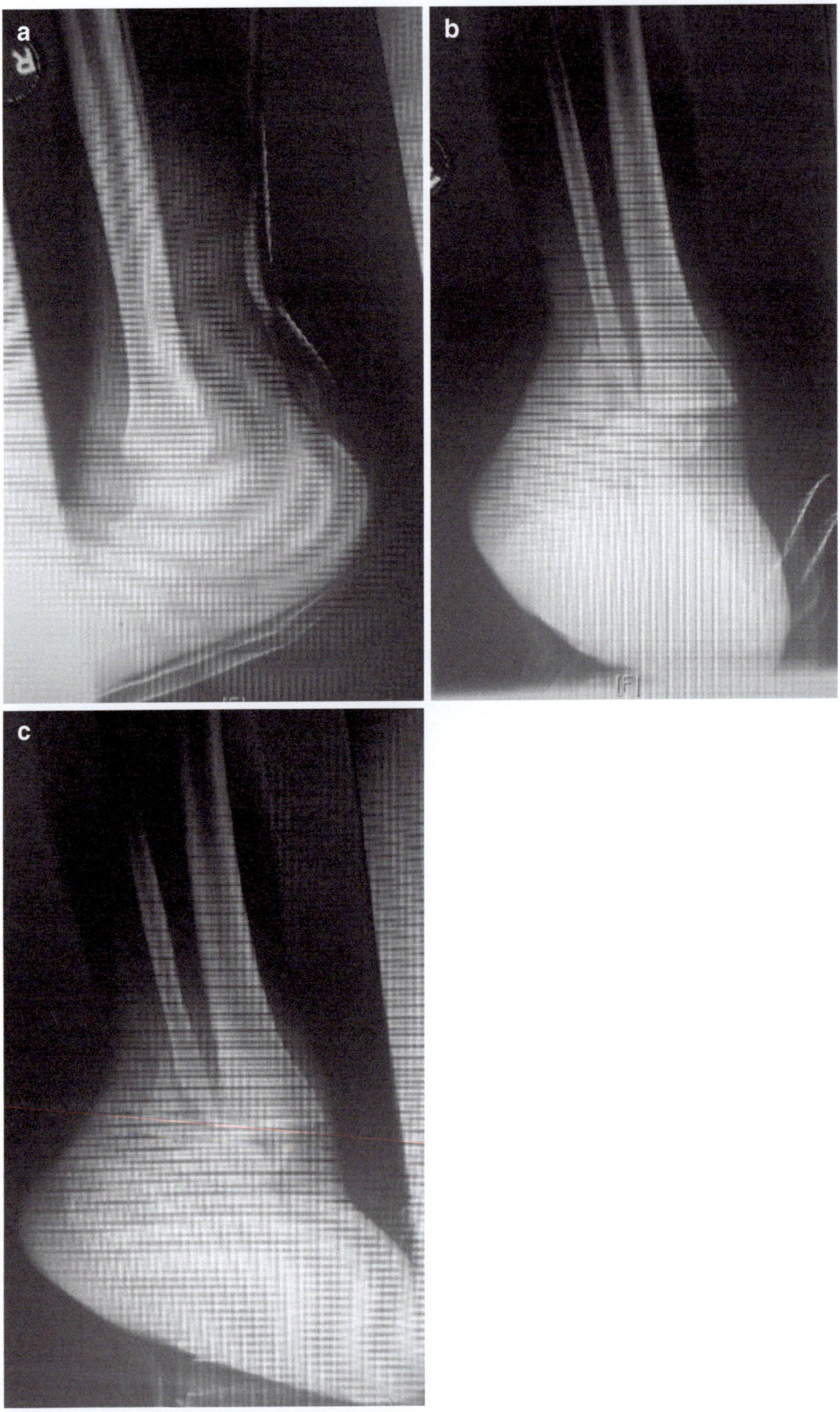

Fig. 32.1 (**a**–**c**) Neuropathic bimalleolar ankle fracture dislocation

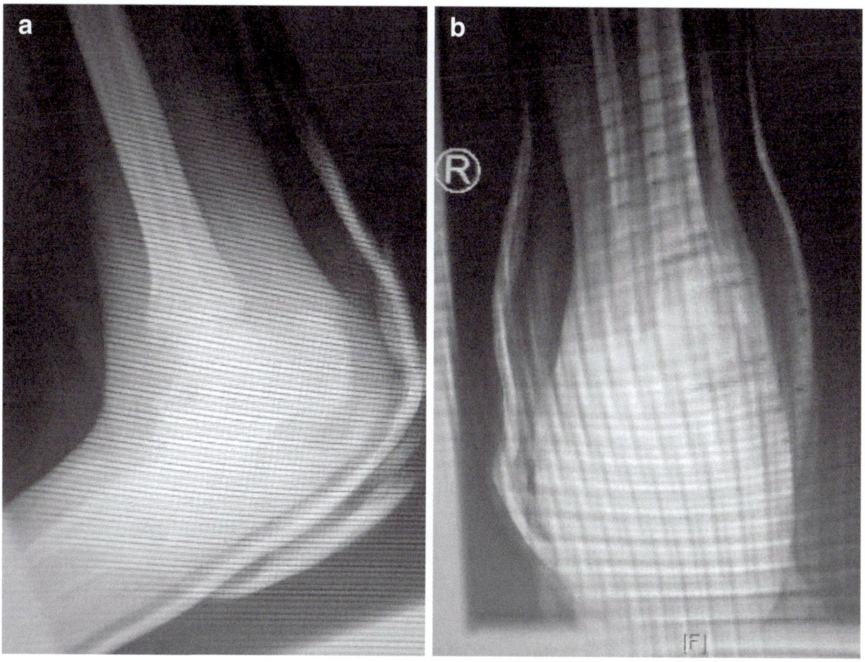

Fig. 32.2 (**a**, **b**) Immediate post closed reduction with splint application

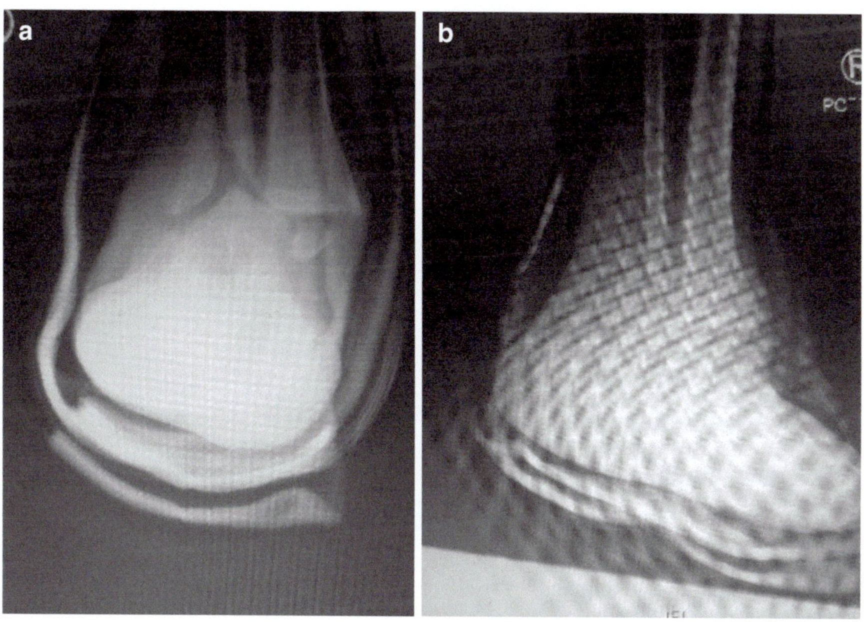

Fig. 32.3 (**a**, **b**) Complete loss of reduction 3 weeks post injury

Her elevated HgA1c and profound neuropathic state required aggressive ORIF. This involved extension of ORIF well beyond the zone of injury. Critical stabilization of the ankle joint mortise was required.

Management

The approach was to reduce the fibula with an extended 8-hole anatomical locking plate. Reduction was difficult due to the fracture being 5 weeks old. Complete dissection of fibula was required. A 5/64″ Steinman pin was utilized to secure the talus in the ankle mortise [1]. Multiple points of tetra cortical screw fixation through the plate with 3.5 mm screws were utilized to secure the syndesmosis [2]. A large reduction clamp was utilized with the ankle placed at 90°. The medial malleolus was secured with extended long 4.0 mm screws of 60 mm in length. This was performed percutaneously to avoid the ulceration over the medial malleolus (Fig. 32.4a–c). The ulceration measured 4.5 × 3.5 cm to the level of periosteum. It had dry/eschar with no drainage noted. A barrier technique with tegaderm was utilized. The lateral fibular incision was closed with 2 g of vancomycin powder. The patient was kept at non-weight bearing (NWB) for 16 weeks. The Steinman pin was removed at 8 weeks. NWB isometric strengthening exercises began at 8 weeks. She was then placed in a weight-bearing (WB) cast for 6 more weeks and converted to an Arizona brace.

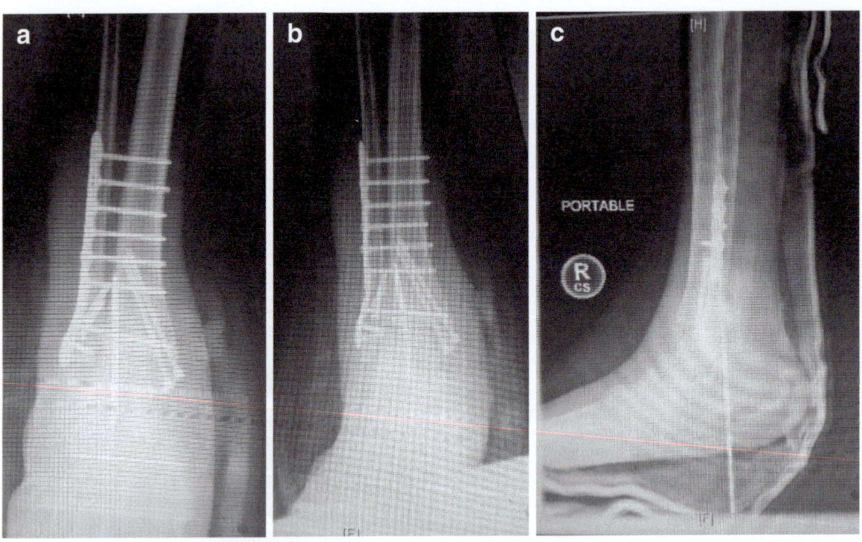

Fig. 32.4 (**a**, **b**) Syndesmosis secured with large one-third tubular locking plate and tetracortical screw fixation. The medial malleolus was fixated with two parallel screws in percutaneous fashion. (**c**) Utilization of 5/64″ Steinmann pin to secure the talus to the ankle and STJ

Outcome

Despite her elevated HgA1c, she developed no signs of infection or a wound dehiscence. This patient did extremely well. It signifies the complexity of this limb-threatening fracture. She ambulates near normally but is unprotected from bracing in her home. She wears the Arizona brace when outside her home.

Clinical Pearls and Pitfalls

Neuropathic ankle fractures represent a complex situation. They require a more aggressive approach to fixation than would be normally required in the sensate limb [3–6]. Traditional syndesmotic fixation in this type of injury would require one point of fixation in a tricortical manner.

It is of utmost importance that in the presence of neuropathic loss of protective sensation (LOPS) that injury to the syndesmosis and stability of the talus be protected by extended forms of fixation [1]. When operative intervention is 5 weeks out, full mobilization of the fibula is required. This brings it to length. It serves to re-establish anatomic alignment of the incisura. Although it is best to "open" the medial malleolus to remove debris at the fracture site anatomic reduction was attained in this case. Insertion of medial malleolar screws should extend if possible to the lateral tibial cortex. The first screw should be in the anterior colliculus, and then only placed halfway. The second screw is then placed near the intra-articular groove [7]. Then a back-and-forth insertion is done to avoid rotation of the fracture fragment. Long fibular locking plates, multiple tetra, and tricortical syndesmotic screws, splinting the talus to the tibia with large 5/64 in. Steinmann pins and long bicortical malleolar screw fixation is necessary.

NWB, with isometric exercises, proves critical in the rehabilitation process.

References

1. Jani MM, Ricci WM, Borrelli J Jr, Barrett SE, Johnson JE. A protocol for treatment of unstable ankle fractures using transarticular fixation in patients with diabetes mellitus and loss of protective sensibility. Foot Ankle Int. 2003;24(11):838–44.
2. Perry MD, Taranow WS, Manoli A 2nd, Carr JB. Salvage of failed neuropathic ankle fractures: use of large-fragment fibular plating and multiple syndesmotic screws. J Surg Orthop Adv. 2005;14(2):85–91.
3. Tucker A, Craig Stone N. Neuropathic ankle fractures. CJEM. 2012;14(2):128–32.
4. Wukich DK, Kline AJ. The management of ankle fractures in patients with diabetes. J Bone Joint Surg. 2008;90(7):1570–8.
5. Schon LC, Marks RM. The management of neuroarthropathic fracture-dislocations in the diabetic patient. Orthop Clin N Am. 1995;26(2):375–92.
6. Costigan W, Thordarson DB, Debnath UK. Operative management of ankle fractures in patients with diabetes mellitus. Foot Ankle Int. 2007;28(1):32–7.
7. Femino JE, Gruber BF, Karunakar MA. Safe zone for the placement of medial malleolar screws. J Bone Joint Surg. 2007;89(1):133–8.

Case #33: Management of a Neuropathic Ankle Fracture with Ankle Arthrodesis Utilizing an Intramedullary Nail

33

Case Presentation

This is an 84-year-old Caucasian white female who presented to the emergency (ER) with a left ankle injury occurring at home in her garden. She states that she misstepped awkwardly off an edge of a flower bed and felt a "pop" but experienced no significant pain. She noted that her foot was dangling and began to swell. She then contacted one of her daughters who brought her to the ER.

Her past medical history was significant for type II diabetes mellitus (DM). She also had a history of coronary artery disease and cardiac stents placed some 12 years prior. She had quit smoking only 6 years prior. Her HgA1c was 9.2%.

On the lower extremity (LE) exam, she had ecchymosis and 3+ edema. Her pulses were intact and cap refill was less than 3 s. Her neurological exam noted loss of protective sensation (LOPS) to the lower leg via Semmes-Weinstein monofilament (SWMF) 5.07 g [1]. The ankle appeared dislocated and the foot was flail.

Diagnosis and Assessment

Radiographs noted a dislocated trimalleolar fracture (Cotton type) involving the left ankle. The present mechanism appeared as a Lauge-Hansen supination external rotation (SER IV) (Fig. 33.1a, b) [2]. There was considerable osteopenia. A computed tomography (CT) scan noted a Volkmann type posterior malleolar fracture [3]. It involved greater than 40% of the tibial articular surface with superior displacement (Fig. 33.2).

H. J. Visser, *Challenges in Foot and Ankle Reconstructive Surgery*,
https://doi.org/10.1007/978-3-031-07893-4_33

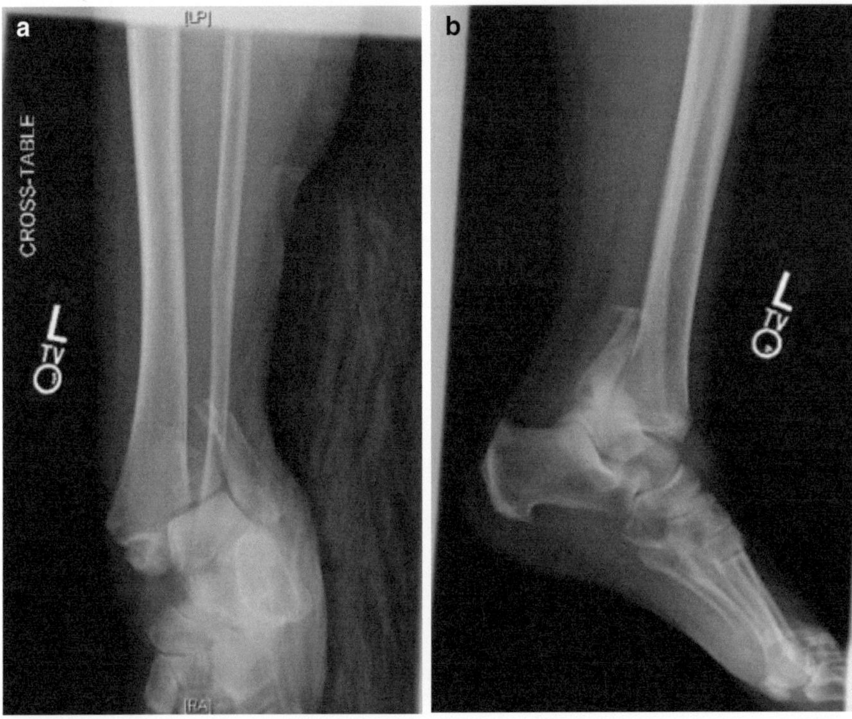

Fig. 33.1 (**a**, **b**) Tri-malleolar neuropathic ankle fractur

A closed reduction was attempted leading to a partial reduction (Fig. 33.3a, b) [4]. Due to her age, profound neuropathy, elevated HgA1c and significant osteopenia a primary ankle arthrodesis was performed.

Management

The procedure was performed within 24 h of injury. Initially, a limited medial anterior arthrotomy was performed. The tibial and talar articular surfaces were prepared by curettage of cartilage, subchondral drilling, and fish scaling of the surfaces. This along with laminal spreader distraction allowed reasonable reduction of the malleoli and anatomic alignment of the ankle joint.

A percutaneous intramedullary nail was performed to attain an ankle arthrodesis. It was a 300 mm straight nail. The subtalar joint (STJ) was not prepared (Fig. 33.4a–h).

The patient was kept on non-weight bearing (NWB) for 12 weeks, followed by a weight-bearing (WB) controlled ankle motion (CAM) boot for a further 12 weeks. A total ankle foot orthosis (AFO) was then prescribed.

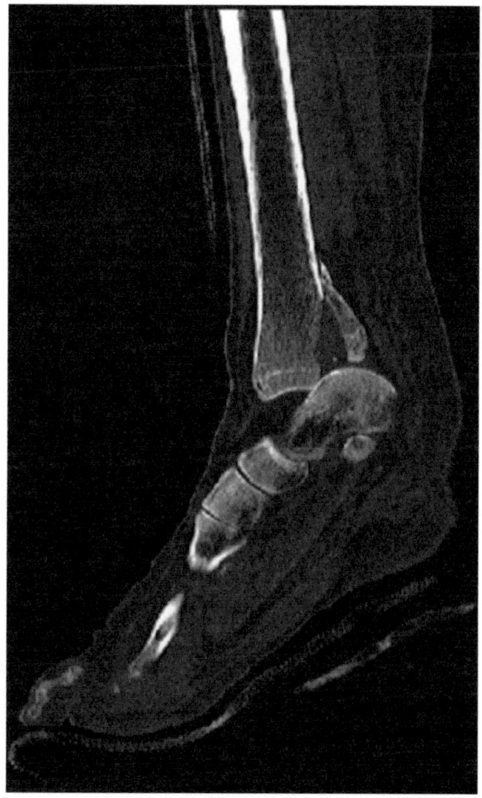

Fig. 33.2 CT image depicts posterior talar displacement of greater than 40% of the tibial articular surface

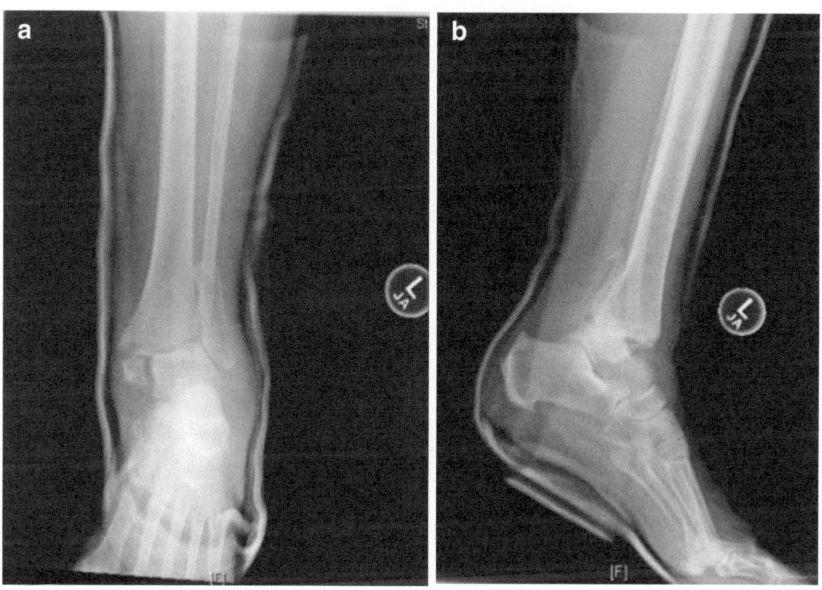

Fig. 33.3 (**a**, **b**) Failed attempted closed reduction

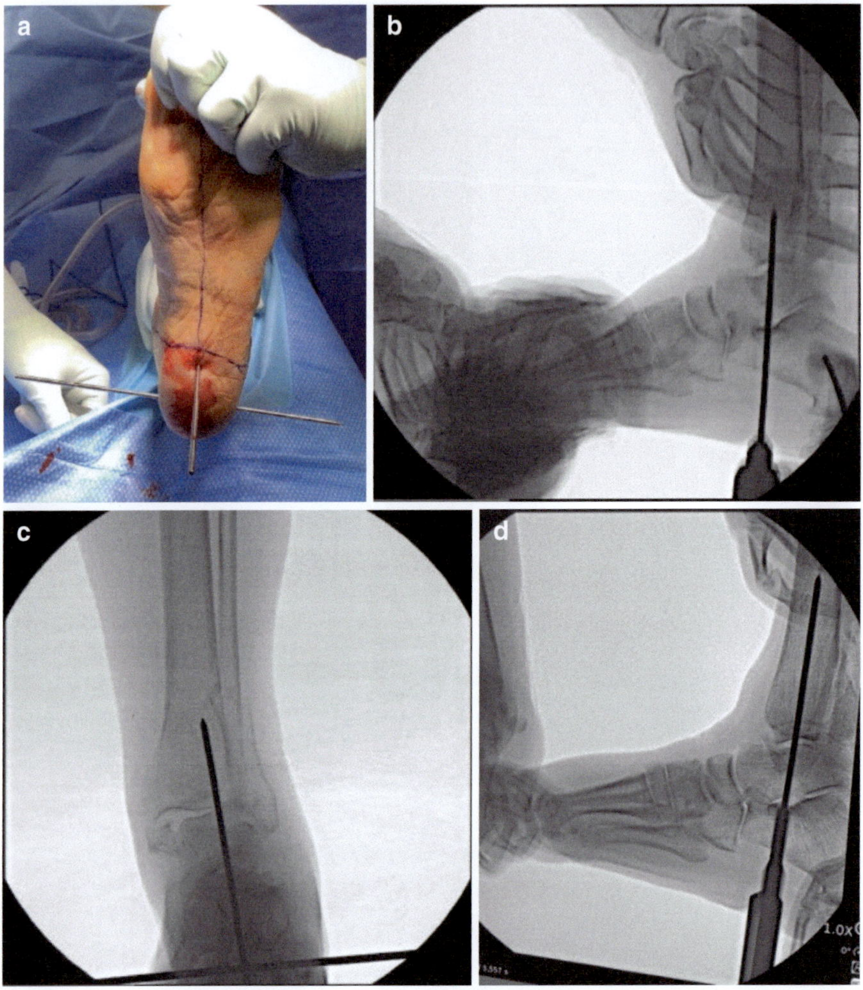

Fig. 33.4 (**a–h**) Percutaneous placement of guide pin followed by reaming and placement of intramedullary nail. The subtalar joint was not prepared

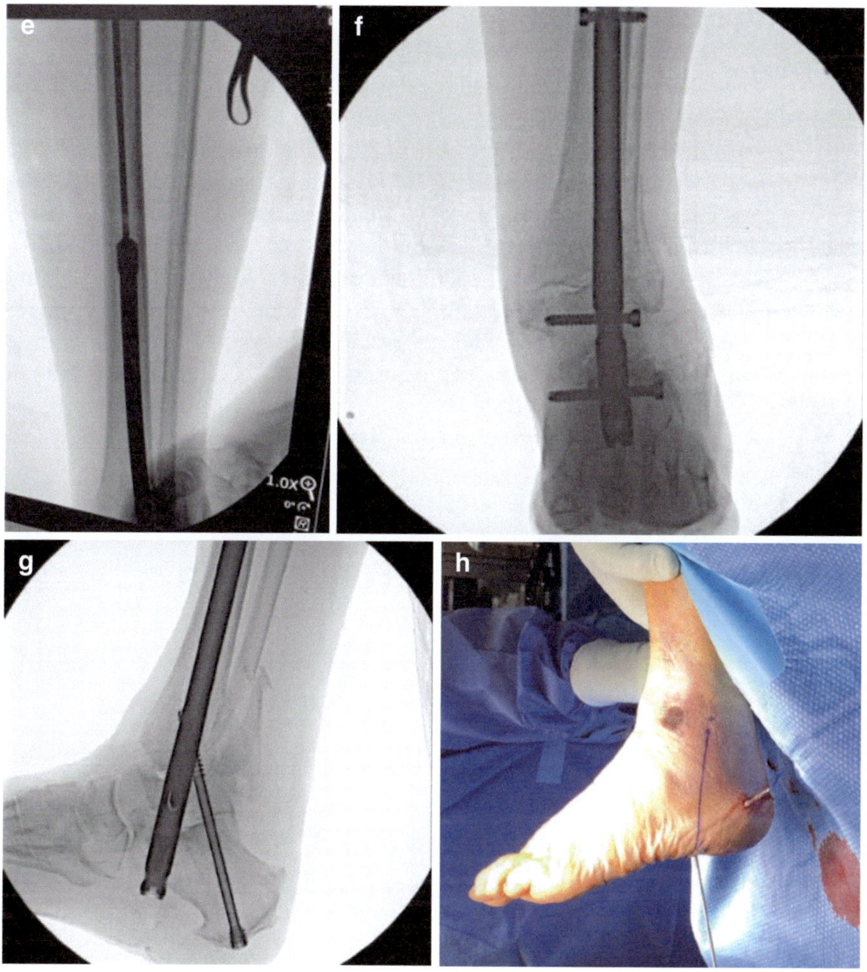

Fig. 33.4 (continued)

Outcome

The patient has done quite well. Her primary concern was to return to gardening which she is able to do. There were no post-op wound complications and an arthrodesis was accomplished at the ankle joint level.

Clinical Pearls and Pitfalls

A severe potential limb-threatening neuropathic ankle injury must be assessed in a different light as opposed to standard surgical management. With the patient's age (84), degree of neuropathy, elevated HgA1c of 9.2% and associated osteopenia, the standard open reduction internal fixation (ORIF) is a complicated option [5–8]. This requires three large incisions. In this case, the goal was to establish a stable, plantar grade foot. Thus, a primary arthrodesis with minimal exposure and dissection provides a viable option. The main issue with neuropathic ankle fractures is stability and healing and protection of the talus [9]. If fracture fixation fails, then re-dislocation and further emergence of an acute neuropathic process can compromise the talus. This can often lead to a rapidly reabsorbing avascular necrotic condition of the talus. This further endangers the overall foot and ankle stability [9, 10]. In these cases, extensive dissection leads to an increased risk of infection and wound healing also complicated by an elevated HgA1c [11–13]. Performing surgical correction (within 24 h) can subvert more extensive soft tissue edema (fracture blisters) caused by non-reduced intra-articular fractures with large cancellous interface. The incision serves to decompress the interstitial spaces and thus reduce strain on capillary flow to the skin.

References

1. Weinstein S. Fifty years of somatosensory research. J Hand Ther. 1993;6(1):11–22. https://doi.org/10.1016/s0894-1130(12)80176-1.
2. Hansen H. Lague. In: Ankelbrud I, editor. Genetisk diagnose og reposition. Diss Munksgaard, Kbhn; 1942.
3. Donohoe S, Alluri RK, Hill JR, Fleming M, Tan E, Marecek G. Impact of computed tomography on operative planning for ankle fractures involving the posterior malleolus. Foot Ankle Int. 2017;38(12):1337–42. https://doi.org/10.1177/1071100717731568.
4. Sarkisian JS, Cody GW. Closed treatment of ankle fractures. J Trauma: Injury Infect Crit Care, 1976;16(4):323–26. https://doi.org/10.1097/00005373-197604000-00014.
5. Hoogervorst P, Bergen CV, Van den Bekerom M. Management of osteoporotic and neuropathic ankle fractures in the elderly. Curr Geriatr Rep. 2017;6(1):9–14. https://doi.org/10.1007/s13670-017-0196-y.
6. Rbia N, van der Vlies CH, Cleffken BI, Selles RW, Hovius S, Nijhuis T. High prevalence of chronic pain with neuropathic characteristics after open reduction and internal fixation of ankle fractures. Foot Ankle Int. 2017;38(9):987–96. https://doi.org/10.1177/1071100717712432.
7. Manchanda K, Nakonezny P, Sathy AK, Sanders DT, Starr AJ, Wukich DK. A systematic review of ankle fracture treatment modalities in diabetic patients. J Clin Orthop Trauma. 2020;16:7–15. https://doi.org/10.1016/j.jcot.2020.12.013.
8. Hanas R, John G. 2010 consensus statement on the worldwide standardization of the hemoglobin a1c measurement. Diabetes Care. 2010;33(8):1903–4. https://doi.org/10.2337/dc10-0953.
9. Tucker A, Craig Stone N. Neuropathic ankle fractures. CJEM. 2012;14(2):128–32. https://doi.org/10.2310/8000.2011.110338.
10. Bonnel F, Toullec E, Mabit C, Tourné Y, Sofcot. Chronic ankle instability: biomechanics and pathomechanics of ligaments injury and associated lesions. Orthop Traumatol Surg Res. 2010;96(4):424–32. https://doi.org/10.1016/j.otsr.2010.04.003.

11. Lambert LA, Falconer L, Mason L. Ankle stability in ankle fracture. J Clin Orthop Trauma. 2020;11(3):375–9. https://doi.org/10.1016/j.jcot.2020.03.010.
12. Tarabichi M, Shohat N, Kheir MM, Adelani M, Brigati D, Kearns SM, Patel P, Clohisy JC, Higuera CA, Levine BR, Schwarzkopf R, Parvizi J, Jiranek WA. Determining the threshold for HbA1c as a predictor for adverse outcomes after total joint arthroplasty: a multicenter, retrospective study. J Arthroplast. 2017;32(9S):S263–S267. e1. https://doi.org/10.1016/j.arth.2017.04.065.
13. Shohat N, Muhsen K, Gilat R, Rondon AJ, Chen AF, Parvizi J. Inadequate glycemic control is associated with increased surgical site infection in total joint arthroplasty: a systematic review and meta-analysis. J Arthroplast. 2018;33(7):2312–2321.e3. https://doi.org/10.1016/j.arth.2018.02.020.

Case #34: Management of End-Stage Rigid Equinoadductovarus Foot and Ankle Deformity Secondary to Charcot-Marie-Tooth Disease with Talectomy and Tibiocalcaneal Arthrodesis

34

Case Presentation

This is a 73-year-old Caucasian male who presents with a severe equinoadductovarus foot and ankle deformity. The patient was not a diabetic and overall had little medical issues other than hypertension and hyperlipidemia. He states that his foot began to become "high arched" in his late 20s and began to progress over the ensuing years [1]. His first issue was the development of a plantar ulceration. First, over the fifth metatarsal head. This required the fifth metatarsal head resection. The second was for an ulceration over his styloid process at the fifth metatarsal for osteomyelitis. He states that he was on IV antibiotics for 6 weeks. He states that his foot had "rolled over" before the surgeries. There was no real change in his position after the bone excision. He ambulated with a controlled ankle motion (CAM) boot and had been in it since his first operation 4 years ago. He was referred for possible reconstruction.

Diagnosis and Assessment

Evaluation of vascular supply noted 2/4 dorsalis pedis (DP) and posterior tibialis (PT) pulses. Arterial studies with Doppler evaluation noted triphasic waveforms. Neurologically, he had loss of protection sensation (LOPS) to the lower leg as identified with a Semmes-Weinstein monofilament (SWMF) 5.09 [2]. He was not initially diagnosed but neurologic referral revealed degenerative Charcot Marie Tooth (CMT) [3, 4].

Radiographs involving the DP and oblique views reveal adductovarus deformity and a remaining portion of the midshaft of the fifth metatarsal (Fig. 34.1a, b). His lateral view showed a midfoot cavus with a posterior component (Fig. 34.1c). His Meary's angle intersected at the talonavicular (TN) joint (Fig. 34.1a, b). His AP

H. J. Visser, *Challenges in Foot and Ankle Reconstructive Surgery*,
https://doi.org/10.1007/978-3-031-07893-4_34

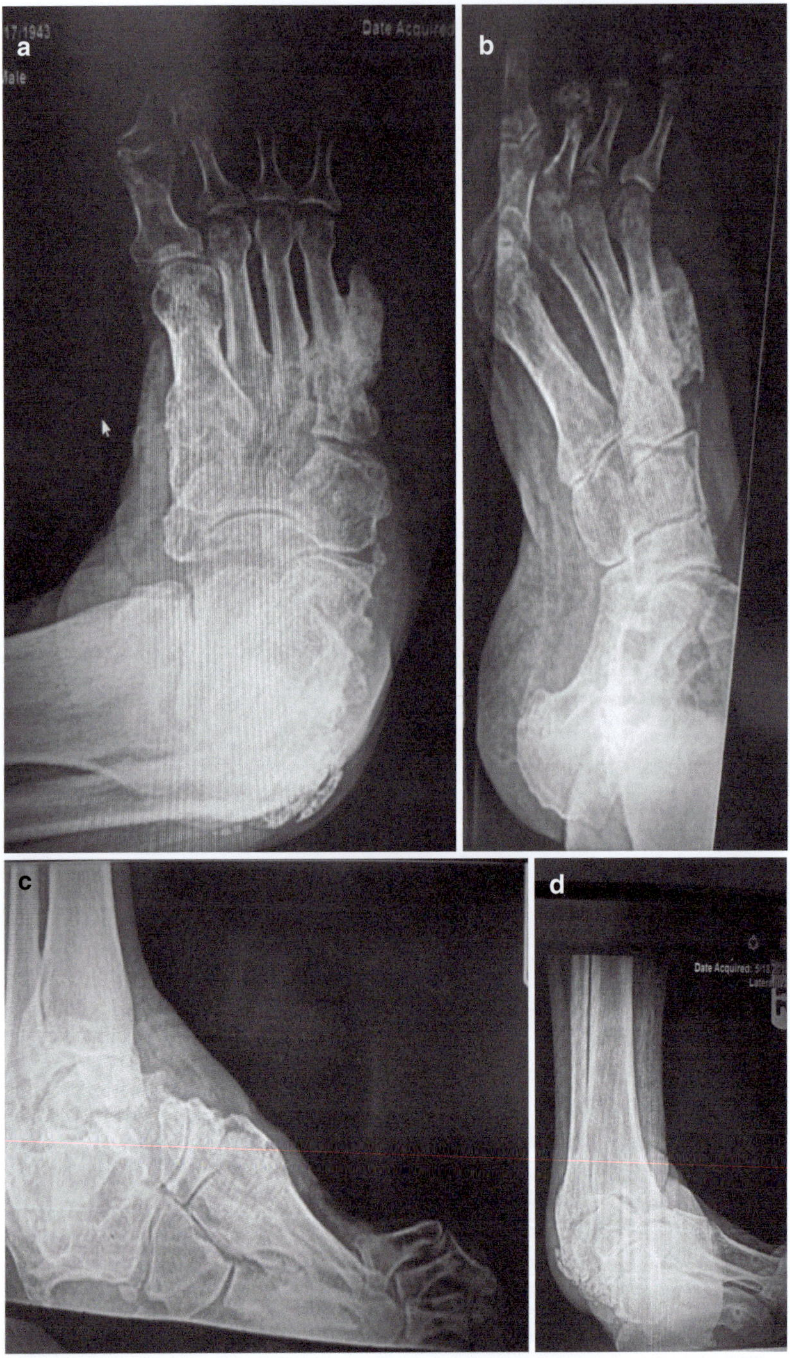

Fig. 34.1 (**a–d**) Rigid adductovarus deformity of the foot and ankle. Cavus deformity is present at the midfoot. The ankle joint was severely incongruous with advanced degenerative changes present

ankle view (Fig. 34.1d) showed a severe incongruous talar tilt with significant degenerative joint disease (DJD). His clinical pictures reflect the radiographic deformity (Fig. 34.2a–d).

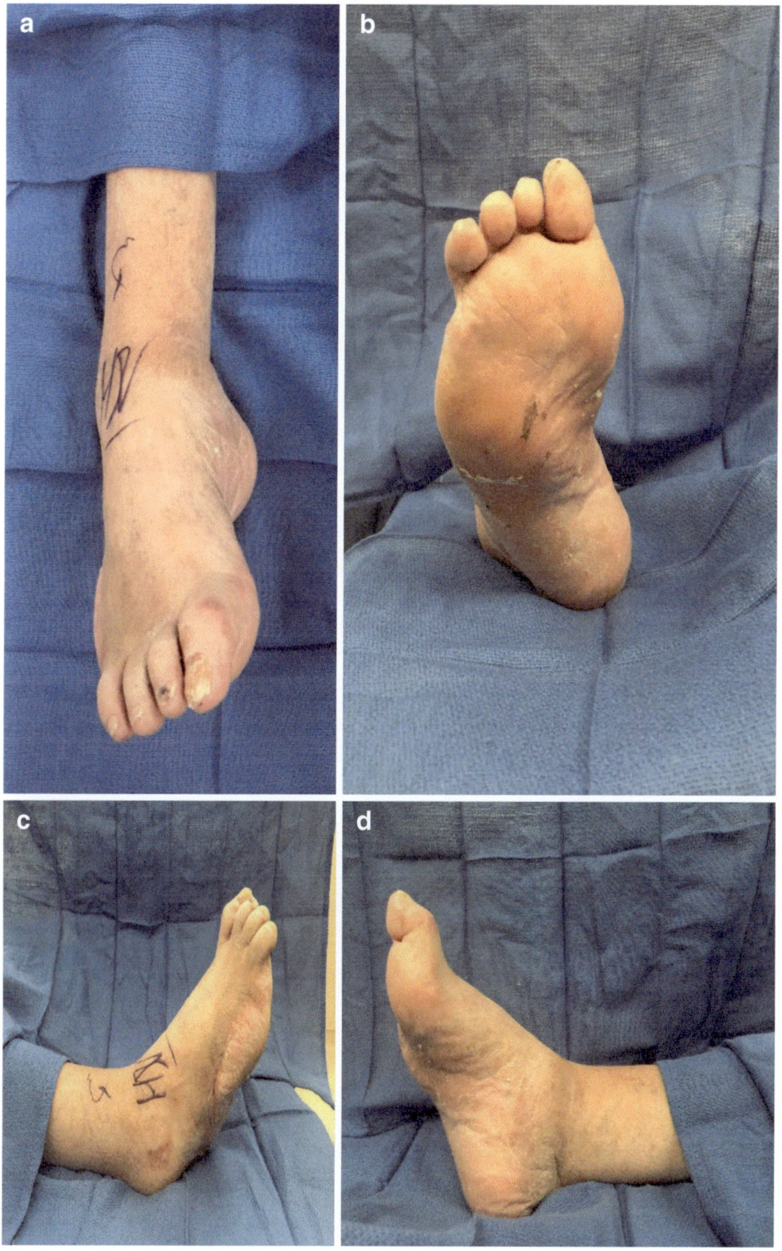

Fig. 34.2 (**a**–**d**) Clinical images of the rigid adductovarus foot and ankle deformity. Prior partial amputation noted secondary to bony prominences which produced subsequent ulcerations and infections

The diagnosis was a severe rigid equinoadductocavovarus foot and ankle deformity. This was secondary to CMT-1 compounded by sensory and motor neuropathy [5, 6].

Management

As the deformity was fixed and rigid, the goal was to perform a talectomy via a transfibular approach [7]. The initial first procedure involved resection of the fibular malleolus to allow exposure of the talar body. The fibula was subsequently then used as an autograft. It was morselized in a bone mill (Fig. 34.3a–c).

The second procedure involved a complete talectomy, which allowed reduction of the deformity at the ankle and subtalar joint (STJ) level (Fig. 34.4a–d) [8–10]. This created a plantar grade foot. A tibiocalcaneal arthrodesis was performed. Autograft and allograft supplemented with bone marrow aspirate was tightly packed at the tibial-calcaneal interface (Fig. 34.5a–c). The defect between the anterior tibia and navicular was also back filled tightly with bone graft (Fig. 34.5d).

A cannulated 6.5 mm position screw was placed in a compression mode from the calcaneus to the tibia (Fig. 34.6a, b). The construct was then further secured with a lateral anatomical locking plate. It contoured to the tibial calcaneal lateral surface with only limited lateral bone resection (Fig. 34.7a–c).

The patient was kept at non-weight bearing (NWB) for 14 weeks and was allowed to weight bear (WB) in a CAM boot for a further 16 weeks (Fig. 34.8). Radiographs show well-aligned and plantigrade foot and ankle. Tibio-navicular calcaneal arthrodesis with lateral locking plate and 6.5 mm cannulated positioning screw

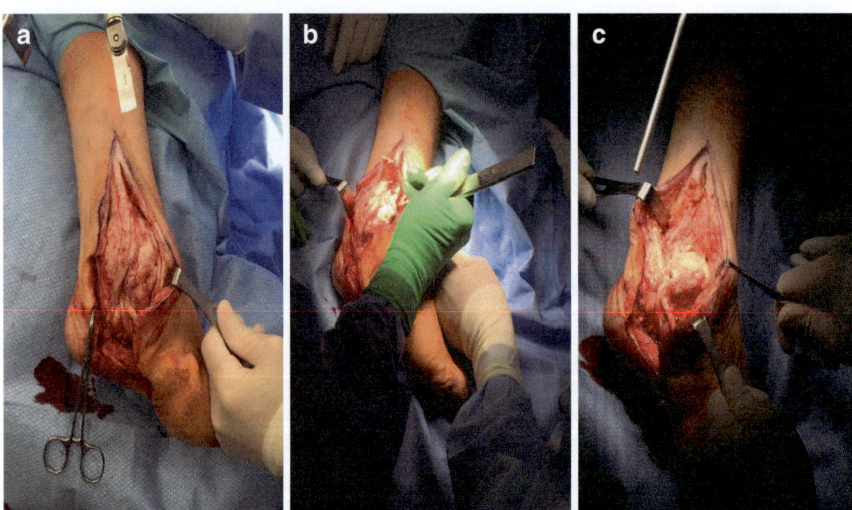

Fig. 34.3 (**a**) Lateral transfibular approach, right ankle. (**b**) Osteotome used to osteotomize the distal fibula. (**c**) Exposure of lateral ankle and talus

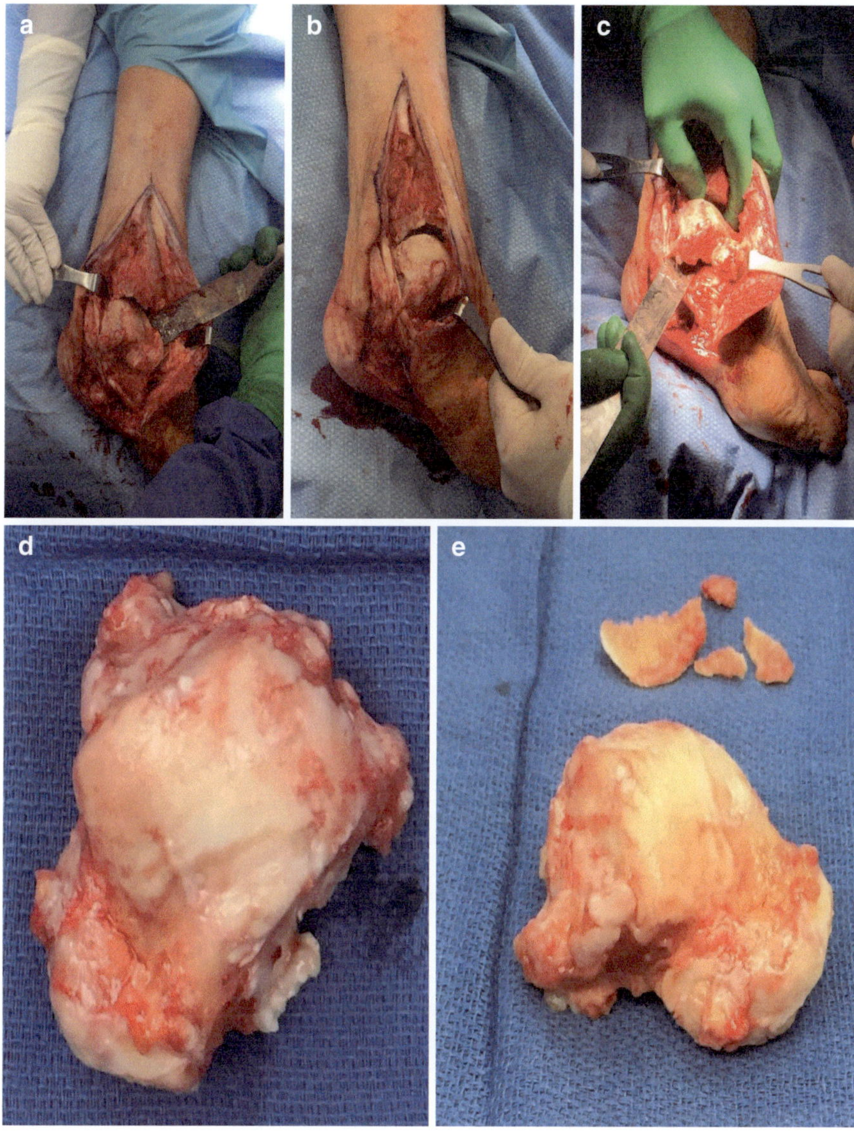

Fig. 34.4 (**a**) Talar body exposed. (**b**) Talar body exposed. (**c**) Extirpation of talar body. (**d**, **e**) Excision of complete talar body

(Fig. 34.9a–c). A total ankle foot orthosis (AFO) was then constructed. A 2 in. wedge was placed in the ipsilateral shoe sole. This served to offset the leg length discrepancy (anisomelia).

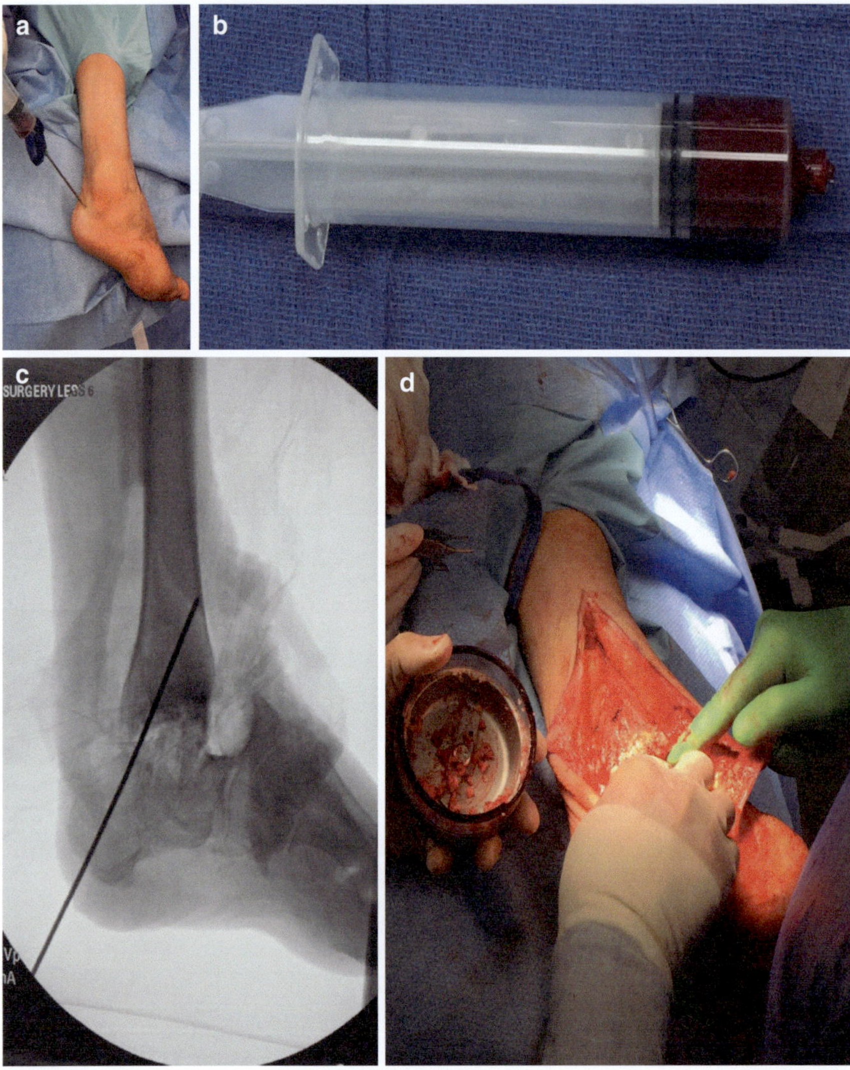

Fig. 34.5 (**a**) Aspiration bone marrow from calcaneus with Jamshidi needle. (**b**) Calcaneal bone marrow aspirate. (**c**) Tight back filling with autograft and bone marrow aspirate. (**d**) Packing autograft with bone marrow aspiration at tibial-navicular interface

Outcome

This patient did extremely well and was very happy with his outcome. He had no further recurrent ulcerations, and he was extremely grateful that he could ambulate with a brace and accommodative shoe wear.

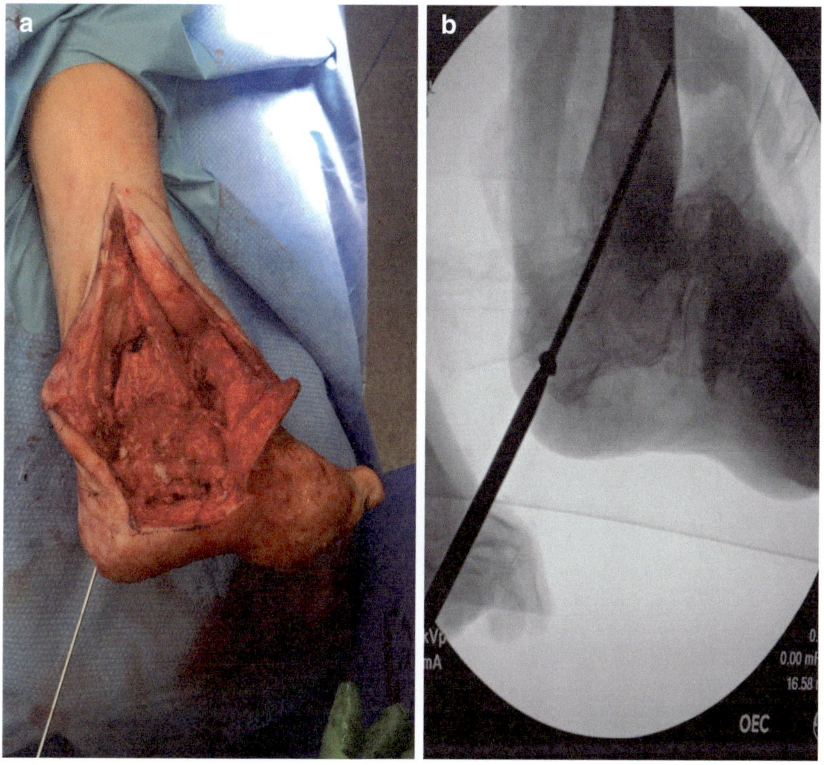

Fig. 34.6 (**a**) 6.5 mm position screw. (**b**) Compression with 6.5 mm position screw

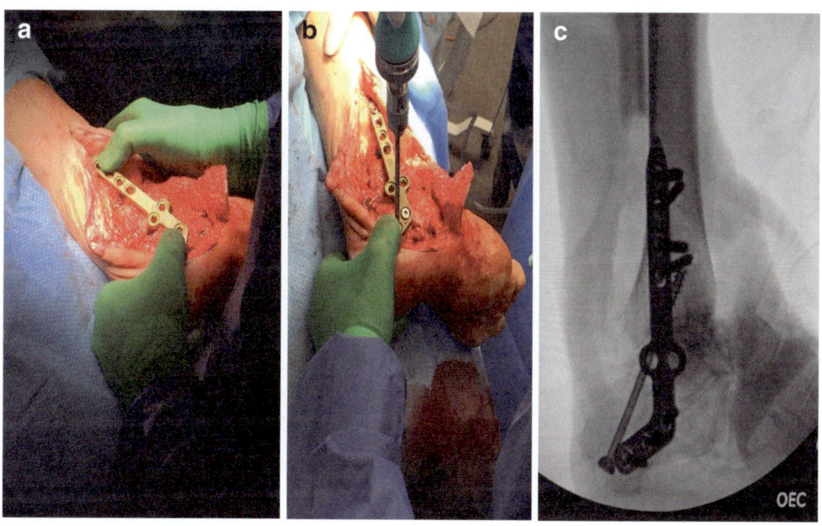

Fig. 34.7 (**a**) Lateral anatomic locking plate. (**b**) Anatomic contoured lateral ankle locking plate. (**c**) Post-operative radiograph with plantigrade foot

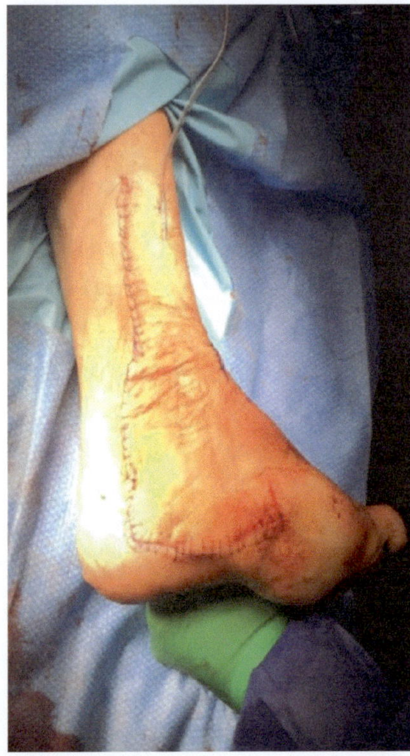

Fig. 34.8 Anatomically aligned and plantigrade right foot and ankle

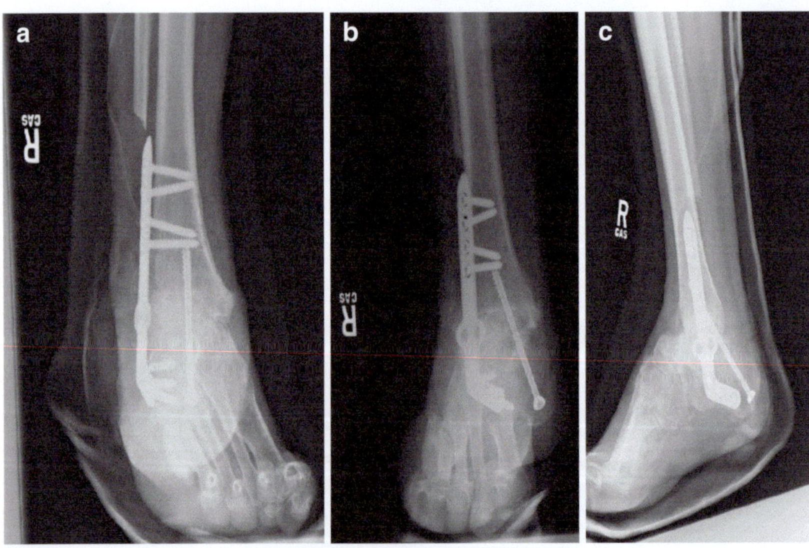

Fig. 34.9 (**a**–**c**) Tibio-navicular calcaneal arthrodesis with lateral locking plate and 6.5 mm cannulated positioning screw

Clinical Pearls and Pitfalls

This patient interestingly when referred was told that he had a Charcot foot deformity. Despite the fact that he was not diabetic, certainly Charcot foot deformity can be seen with idiopathic forms of peripheral neuropathy. In this case, he did demonstrate a neuropathic foot but was secondary to undiagnosed CMT-1. As can be seen when reviewing the radiographs, there were no signs of bony destruction other than the resected portions of the fifth metatarsal.

In cases of long-standing CMT-1 as was seen in this patient, demonstration of symptoms in his late 20s created by muscle and tendon imbalance noted the development of a cavus foot deformity [3]. This was created by a strong tibialis posterior and peroneus longus overpowering the paralyzed peroneus brevis and tibialis anterior which was seen in this case. The brevis had been detached when the fifth metatarsal and styloid process had been excised for osteomyelitis. These two situations lead to the development of a rigid adductocavovarus foot and ankle deformity.

As can be seen, on the radiographs meary's angle intersects at the TN joint. This indicates a midfoot cavus with a posterior component [11]. In CMT, the intersection of meary's angle will never be more proximal than the talonavicular (TN) joint; this is due to the continued restraint of the unaffected gastrocnemius soleus muscle group.

With the always functional Achilles (gastroc-soleus) muscle group, the unopposed tibialis posterior and peroneus longus muscles produce a severe varus deformity at the STJ. Also adductus occurs at the midtarsal joint (MTJ) level. The peroneus longus now is able to fully plantarflex the first metatarsal. The talus abducts and dorsiflexes (closed kinetic chain supination) and the ankle malleoli become more externally rotated. This is noted by the posterior position of the fibula radiographically. This dynamic literally subluxes the talus out of the ankle mortise.

Along with the muscle dynamics involving CMT, it often coincides with that distal symmetrical sensory peripheral neuropathy that leads to loss of protective sensation. In this case, creation of a plantar grade foot by arthrodesis was the best option.

Anatomic lateral locking plates offer neutralization to screw compression. Also there is intrinsic compression available within the plate. This construct serves to resist shearing and long-standing rotational and distracting forces.

References

1. Piazza S, Ricci G, Caldarazzo Ienco E, Carlesi C, Volpi L, Siciliano G, Mancuso M. Pes cavus and hereditary neuropathies: when a relationship should be suspected. J Orthop Traumatol. 2010;11(4):195–201. https://doi.org/10.1007/s10195-010-0114-y.
2. Weinstein S. Fifty years of somatosensory research. J Hand Ther. 1993;6(1):11–22. https://doi.org/10.1016/s0894-1130(12)80176-1.
3. Pareyson D, Marchesi C. Diagnosis, natural history, and management of Charcot–Marie–tooth disease. Lancet Neurol. 2009;8(7):654–67. https://doi.org/10.1016/s1474-4422(09)70110-3.

4. Reilly MM, Rossor AM. Charcot–Marie–tooth disease. In: Oxford textbook of neuromuscular disorders. UK: Oxford University Press; 2014. p. 61–74. https://doi.org/10.1093/med/9780199698073.003.0008.
5. Venance S, Tawil R. Neuromuscular diseases: approach to clinical diagnosis. Neuromuscul Disord. 2011:1–5. https://doi.org/10.1002/9781119973331.ch1.
6. Visser HJ, Wolfe J, Kouri R, Aviles R. Neurologic conditions associated with cavus foot deformity. Clin Podiatr Med Surg. 2021;38(3):323–42.
7. Menelaus MB. Talectomy for equinovarus deformity in arthrogryposis and spina bifida. J Bone Joint Surg. 1971;53-B(3):468–73. https://doi.org/10.1302/0301-620x.53b3.468.
8. Cooper RR, Capello W. Talectomy a long-term follow-up evaluation. Clin Orthop Relat Res. 1985;201 https://doi.org/10.1097/00003086-198512000-00005.
9. Joseph TN, Myerson MS. Use of talectomy in modern foot and ankle surgery. Foot Ankle Clin. 2004;9(4):775–85.
10. Dias LS, Stern LS. Talectomy in the treatment of resistant talipes equinovarus deformity in myelomeningocele and arthrogryposis. J Pediatr Orthop. 1987;7(1):39–41.
11. Neri T, Barthelemy R, Tourné Y. Radiologic analysis of hindfoot alignment: comparison of Méary, long axial, and hindfoot alignment views. Orthop Traumatol Surg Res. 2017;103(8):1211–6.

Case #35: Management of Neuropathic Avascular Necrosis of the Talus and Severe Ankle Varus Dislocation with Femoral Head Allograft and Lateral Anatomic Locking Plate

35

Case Presentation

This is a 54-year-old the past Caucasian male who gives a history of long-term type II diabetes mellitus (DM). He has been insulin dependent for the past 14 years. He was obese but otherwise no hx of cardiac issues. He was hypertensive and demonstrated hypercholesterolemia. He was seen in the past with plantar ulceration (5 years on and off), but all these healed with wound care and offloading techniques. On this particular presentation, he noted about 6 months of chronic ankle edema but says he was only mildly painful. He stated he did not recall an injury; it just was swollen. He sought medical care when he became alarmed that when he stood down and bore weight, his ankle gave out in inversion. The vascular examination was normal. He had 2–3 plus pitting edema involving the right ankle. His ankle was unstable and he was unable to further ambulate.

Diagnosis and Assessment

Radiographs noted advanced vascular necrosis of the talus (Fig. 35.1a, b). There was significant resorption of the talar neck (collum tali) and head (capitus tali). On the AP ankle view, there was lateral talar translation and varus tilt of the ankle and subtalar joint (STJ). This represented a limb-threatening condition of neuropathic avascular necrosis (AVN) of the talus secondary to Charcot osteoarthropathy [1–3].

H. J. Visser, *Challenges in Foot and Ankle Reconstructive Surgery*,
https://doi.org/10.1007/978-3-031-07893-4_35

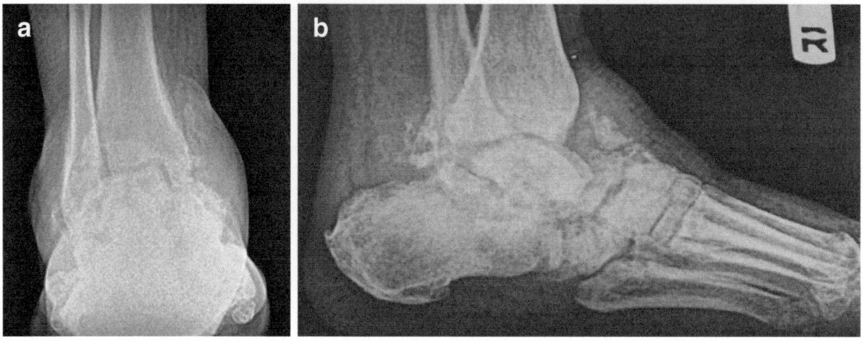

Fig. 35.1 (**a**) AVN of talus secondary to Charcot deformity, lateral destabilization of right ankle. (**b**) Advanced AVN of the right talus

Management

In this case, the approach was to remove the talus through a transfibular approach (Fig. 35.2a). The talus was easily explanted (Fig. 35.2b). Acetabular reamers were utilized to prepare the tibial and calcaneal surfaces (Fig. 35.2c–f). A fresh frozen femoral head allograft was utilized to stabilize the tibia to the calcaneus. The femoral head allograft was then constructed to the void and allowed the established length and ligamentotaxis. This was done with a rotary burr (Fig. 35.3).

The graft was then fenestrated and soaked with bone marrow aspirate. The femoral head was then placed in the void and a 6.5 mm cannulated position screw placed was from the calcaneus to the tibia and through the graft (Fig. 35.4a–c). A blade plate was then placed laterally (Fig. 35.5). The blade was inserted with a mallet into the calcaneus. The proximal portion was then secured to the tibia with 3.5 mm non-locking screws. Anatomic alignment and a plantar grade foot was attained.

An intrinsic bone stimulator was applied with the anode wrapped around the graft, tibial, and calcaneal surfaces (Fig. 35.4b, c). The cathode was placed subcutaneously in the lower leg.

The patient was kept at non-weight bearing (NWB) for 16 weeks and transferred to a controlled ankle motion (CAM) boot until 6 months postoperative. He was then placed in an Arizona brace.

Outcome

The patient obtained partial arthrodesis on the talar side. There was graft resorption and the foot and ankle ultimately positioned into a mild varus.

He returned 1.5 years later saying he had food poisoning. On exam, he had developed fifth metatarsal head ulceration and plantar lateral space abscess. An incision and drainage were performed along with the fifth metatarsal head resection and he

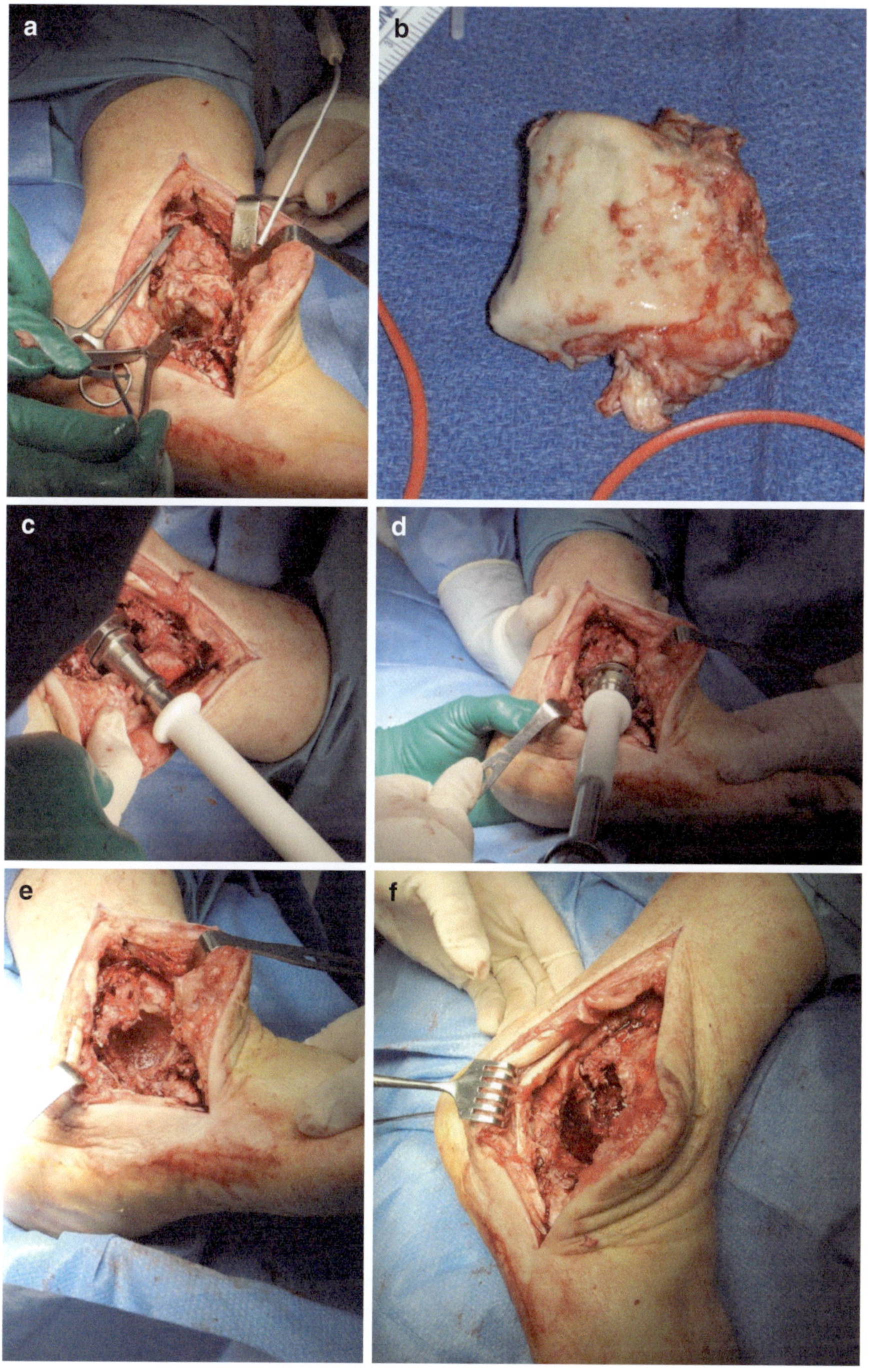

Fig. 35.2 (**a**) Transfibular approach, right ankle. (**b**) Excised remaining talar body. (**c**) Acetabular reamer preparation of calcaneus. (**d**) Acetabular reamer preparation of tibia. (**e**) Prepared canals of calcaneus. (**f**) Prepared canals of tibia with exposed cancellous bone

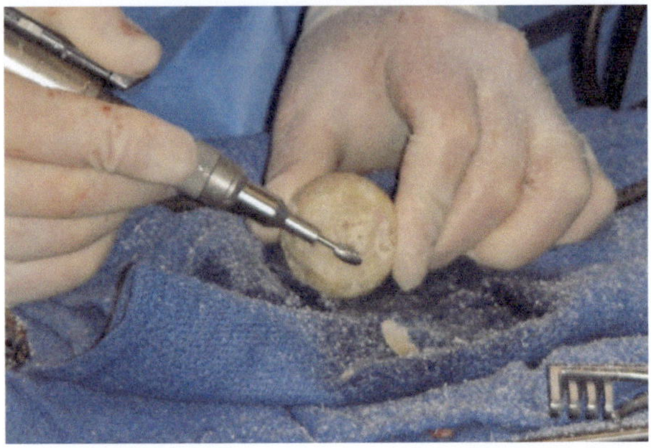

Fig. 35.3 Femoral head remodeling of allograft

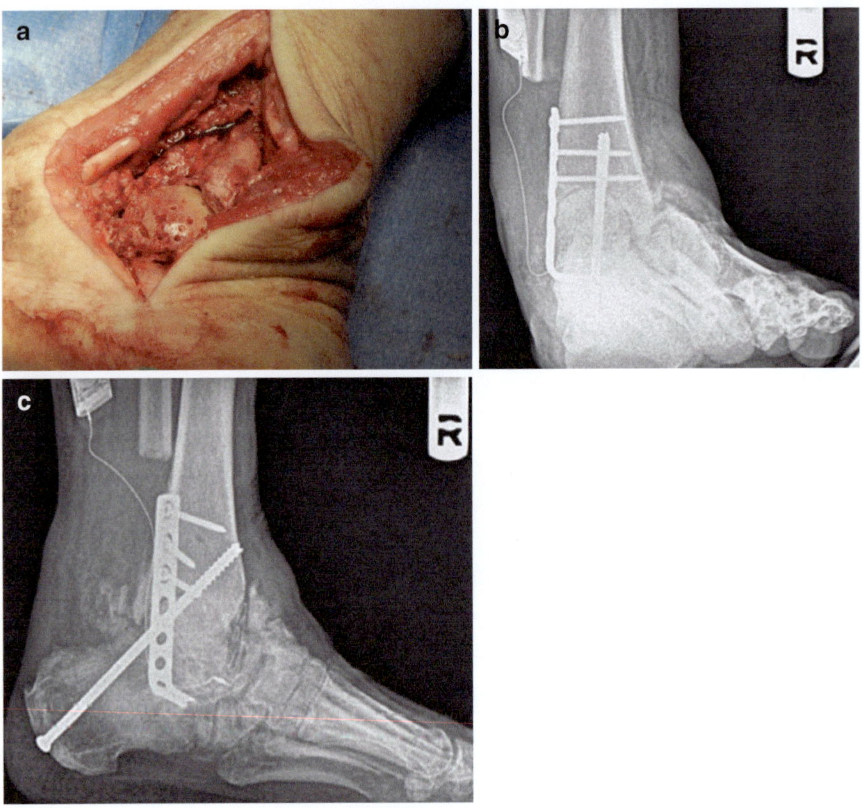

Fig. 35.4 (**a**) Placement of femoral head allograft into contoured prepared tibia and calcaneus. (**b**) Plantigrade foot with 6.5 mm position screw, lateral blade plate and internal bone stimulator. (**c**) 6.5 mm position screw in femoral head allograft with blade plate

subsequently healed. However, he developed a deep vein thrombosis (DVT) at the femoral vein level and a pulmonary embolism, despite DVT prophylaxis. An inferior vena cava (IVC) filter (green field) was placed. The patient was bridged from

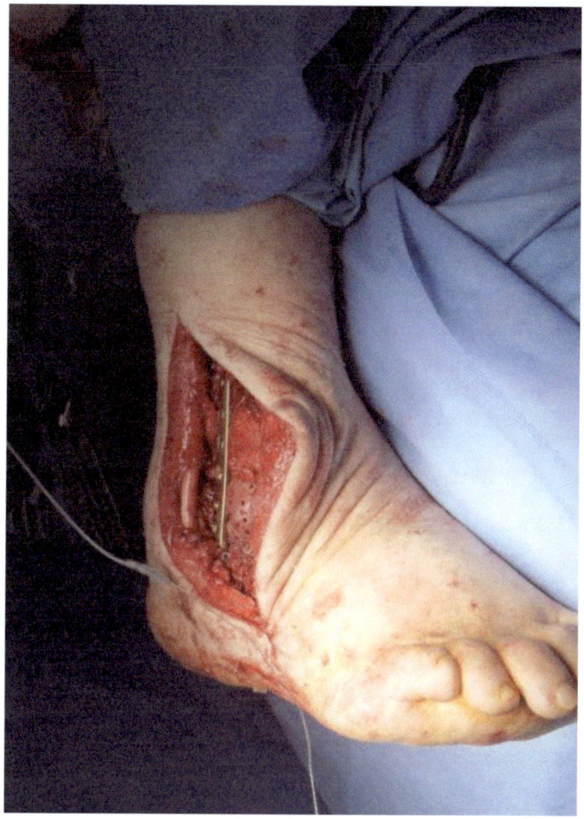

Fig. 35.5 Blade plate application

coumadin with Lovenox. He then, 3 months later presented with loosening of the lateral plate. The graft had resorbed significantly and a nonunion was present. The hardware was removed along with the cathode from the bone stimulator and much of the anode wire was possible. The patient became infected. An attempt at limb salvage with intravenous (IV) antibiotics and further debridement of bone was performed. These measures ultimately failed and a below knee (BK) amputation was performed.

Clinical Pearls and Pitfalls

The Charcot ankle deformity with loss of talar integrity poses a significant surgical challenge for limb salvage [4, 5]. Certainly, amputations have been commonly chosen as a form of management. Morbidity is high with death at 5 years in a significant majority [5–7].

Attempt at limb salvage can be with a talocalcaneal (TC) arthrodesis, but this leads to significant limb shortening. This can place an excessive stress on the contralateral limb [8, 9]. This could serve to generate a Charcot osteoarthropathic process. In this patient, he was reasonably active and young. Allograft of a femoral head is a reasonable option. The downside was seen here with resorption and thus loosening and loss of fixation. The hope is that creeping substitution would reconstitute the graft and provide enough stability. Probably, a longer term of NWB may be needed up to 6 months. This serves to protect the graft. The center of the graft often is not replaced by creeping substitution [10, 11]. The result is the collapse of the graft. In this case, an internal bone stimulator was used. Ultimately, the construct failed.

References

1. Subramaniam B, Pomposelli F, Talmor D, Park KW. Perioperative and long-term morbidity and mortality after above-knee and below-knee amputations in diabetics and nondiabetics. Anesth Analg. 2005;100(5). https://doi.org/10.1213/01.ANE.0000147705.94738.31.
2. Taylor CE, Zhang Y, Qiu Y, Henninger HB, Foreman KB, Bachus KN. Estimated forces and moments experienced by osseointegrated endoprostheses for lower extremity amputees. Gait Posture. 2020;80:49–55. https://doi.org/10.1016/j.gaitpost.2020.05.018.
3. Khamis S, Carmeli E. The effect of simulated leg length discrepancy on lower limb biomechanics during gait. Gait Posture. 2018;61:73–80. https://doi.org/10.1016/j.gaitpost.2017.12.024.
4. Steele JR, Kadakia RJ, Cunningham DJ, Dekker TJ, Kildow BJ, Adams SB. Comparison of 3d printed spherical implants versus femoral head allografts for tibiotalocalcaneal arthrodesis. J Foot Ankle Surg. 2020;59(6):1167–70. https://doi.org/10.1053/j.jfas.2019.10.015.
5. Alshahrani H. Treatment of avascular necrosis of the femoral head with bone graft and interference screw. MOJ Orthop Rheumatol. 2016;4(6). https://doi.org/10.15406/mojor.2016.04.00159.
6. Adelaar RS, Madrian JR. Avascular necrosis of the talus. Orthop Clin North Am. 2004;35(3):383–95.
7. Gross CE, et al. Treatments for avascular necrosis of the talus: a systematic review. Foot Ankle Spec. 2014;7(5):387–97.
8. Horst F, Gilbert BJ, Nunley JA. Avascular necrosis of the talus: current treatment options. Foot Ankle Clin. 2004;9(4):757–73.
9. Lowery NJ, et al. Surgical management of Charcot neuroarthropathy of the foot and ankle: a systematic review. Foot Ankle Int. 2012;33(2):113–21.
10. Blume PA, et al. Charcot neuroarthropathy of the foot and ankle: diagnosis and management strategies. Clin Podiatr Med Surg. 2014;31(1):151–72.
11. Aulivola B, Hile CN, Hamdan AD, Sheahan MG, Veraldi JR, Skillman JJ, Campbell DR, Scovell SD, LoGerfo FW, Pomposelli FB Jr. Major lower extremity amputation: outcome of a modern series. Arch Surg. 2004;139(4):395–9. https://doi.org/10.1001/archsurg.139.4.395.

Case #36: Management of Neuropathic Talar Avascular Necrosis with Talectomy and Arthrodesis Utilizing a Femoral Locking Plate

36

Case Presentation

This is a 46-year-old Caucasian female who presents as a long-term fragile diabetic that is insulin dependent and on renal dialysis. She also had demonstrated cardiac issues requiring drug eluting stents. She had a prior procedure performed that was diagnosed as osteomyelitis involving the navicular bone. She had continuous nocturnal fever. The osteomyelitis was diagnosed on magnetic resonance imaging (MRI) [1]. However, her serology did not really support it. The navicular was resected and a polymethylmethacrylate antibiotic (PMMA) spacer with vancomycin was placed at the resection site (Fig. 36.1a, b). The plan was to then do a second-stage arthrodesis with bone graft. She then sought another opinion.

She was grossly swollen at the foot and ankle level. Pulses couldn't be felt. Vascular studies were performed which showed triphasic pulsatile flow. Her digital pressures were also normal. Neurologically, she had profound motor sensory, and autonomic neuropathy with loss of protective sensation (LOPS) to the level of the knee. The mid foot was positioned, due to resulting instability in an adductovarus position.

Diagnosis and Assessment

Radiographs (Fig. 36.1a, b) show the presence of a large spacer (PMMA) that had replaced the navicular bone. The talar head and neck showed complete reabsorption. This was secondary to resultant instability and autonomic neuropathy. There was partial avascular necrosis (AVN) of the remaining talus. Clinically, the foot was unstable and with weight bearing (WB) tilting into varus. This is confirmed by the WB anterior posterior (AP) ankle view (Fig. 36.1c).

H. J. Visser, *Challenges in Foot and Ankle Reconstructive Surgery*,
https://doi.org/10.1007/978-3-031-07893-4_36

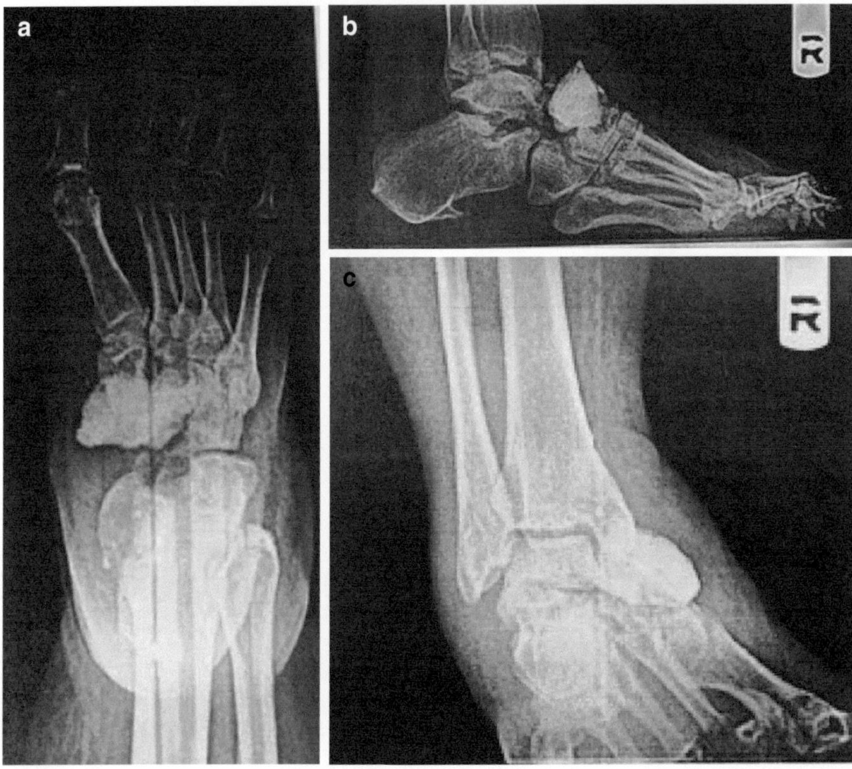

Fig. 36.1 (**a**) PMMA spacer for presumed osteomyelitis of navicular. (**b**) Talar neck AVN with resorption and application of PMMA spacer. (**c**) Varus foot and ankle instability secondary to Charcot osteoarthropathy

The assessment was Charcot osteoarthropathy involving the talus with a retained PMMA spacer at the navicular, cuneiform level [2, 3]. There was resultant foot and ankle varus instability.

Management

In this case, a transfibular approach was again utilized (Fig. 36.2a). As the talar body was unstable as well as primarily avascular, it was excised (Fig. 36.2b). In this case, once the talar body and PMMA spacer were removed, it was manually distracted to full length. This was as much as allowed by the soft tissue envelope. This was secured by two guide pins for two 8.0 mm screws. The two large 8.0 mm fully threaded screws were then placed in a parallel manner from the calcaneus to the anterior tibia (Fig. 36.3a, b). These served to act as struts to preserve the newly acquired length. Bone graft (resected fibula) was then morselized via bone mill. It was then packed as tightly as possible to fill the large void (Fig. 36.4a, b). All

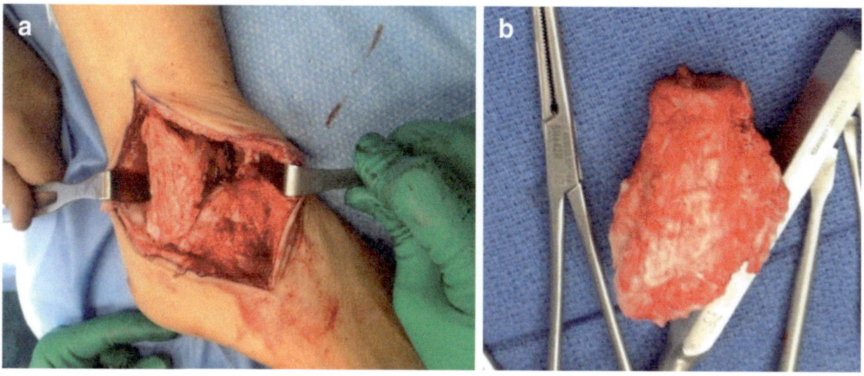

Fig. 36.2 (**a**) Transfibular approach. (**b**) Excised remaining talar body

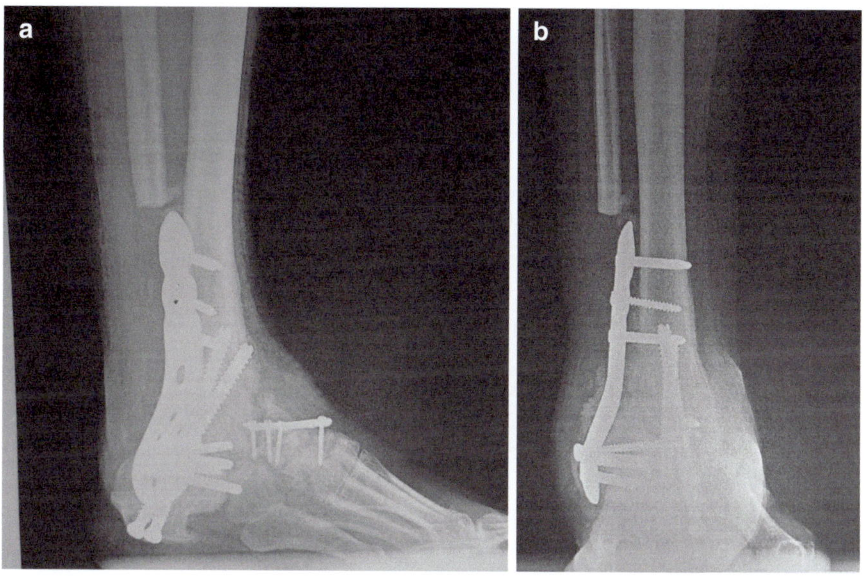

Fig. 36.3 (**a**, **b**) Utilization of 8.0 mm screws as struts with application of femoral locking plate

remaining cartilage was removed from the tibia and calcaneus. A large femoral locking plate was then applied to the lateral tibial/graft/calcaneus interface. This provided further rigidity to the construct. The interface at the PMMA spacer site was also back filled tightly and the cuneiforms prepared distally. It was secured with a one-third tubular plate (Fig. 36.3a, b). The proximal screw engaged to the tibia. The patient was kept non-weight bearing (NWB) on a knee scooter for 16 weeks. Protected WB in a controlled ankle motion (CAM) boot was continued for 6 months. An Arizona brace was prescribed. The patient attained a solid arthrodesis.

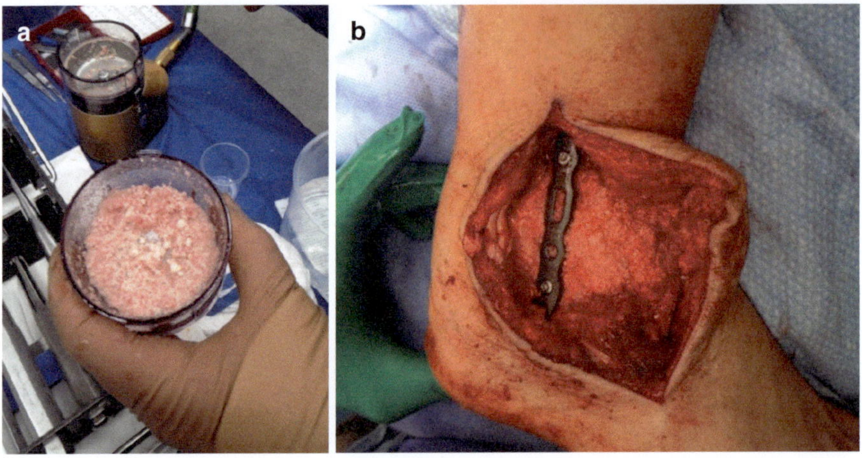

Fig. 36.4 (**a**) Allograft with bone marrow aspirate. (**b**) Tight back fill of allograft with bone marrow aspirate at resection site

Outcome

The patient acquired a stable plantar grade foot. However, during healing of the arthrodesis, a mild residual varus occurred. 2 years later, she lost her opposite leg to osteomyelitis. She was seen just 3 months ago with a chronic styloid ulceration of the fifth metatarsal. She had been seen in a wound clinic for 8 months, and they were able to heal the ulceration with a contact cast [4, 5]. She was then referred again for care. She had re-ulcerated after only 1 week out of the contact cast. With the varus positioning of the fusion (2°) and the overload from loss of her opposite leg ambulating in a prosthesis break down was inevitable. As her ankle and midfoot were secure via prior arthrodesis, a resection of the fifth metatarsal styloid was performed. She is now again ambulatory without recurrent ulceration.

Clinical Pearls and Pitfalls

This case again represents the dilemma of loss of the talus and in this case the navicular secondary to Charcot deformity. As is known, this represents a limb and possible life-threatening condition. The degree of instability cannot be managed by a Charcot restraint orthotic walking (CROW) boot. Most often with loss of the talus a valgus or varus positioning leads to pressure over the remaining medial or lateral malleolus. The result is ulceration and often osteomyelitis in rapid order [6–8]. Thus despite WB in an external bracing support. Often Charcot disease is mistaken for osteomyelitis [9]. Osteomyelitis is extremely rare without the presence of an ulceration. Chronic edema and pain with associated systemic signs of fever can be seen in a Charcot patient [10, 11]. Despite LOPS, systemic fever and a positive MRI led to a diagnosis of osteomyelitis. This despite no bone biopsy or bone cultures being performed. Also her erythrocyte sedimentation rate (ESR) was 15 mm/h and C-reactive protein (CRP) of 1.2 mg/dL. Utilizing the pathology report in reference to the navicular related avascular changes. Bone cultures were negative. Thus, indeed, she demonstrated Charcot disease.

The concept of a rigid construct with a large femoral locking plate and 8.0 mm screws can be a good option in cases of talar loss in a younger patient. Back filling of morselized bone graft is critical [12, 13]. Concerning the PMMA spacer, a Masquelet technique was employed [14]. The membrane formed over the spacer offered a high level of growth factors to enhance incorporation of the tightly packed graft [15–17].

References

1. Nawaz A, et al. Diagnostic performance of FDG-PET, MRI, and plain film radiography (PFR) for the diagnosis of osteomyelitis in the diabetic foot. Mol Imaging Biol. 2010;12(3):335–42.
2. Elmarsafi T, et al. Long-term outcomes of permanent cement spacers in the infected foot. J Foot Ankle Surg. 2017;56(2):287–90.
3. Elmarsafi T, et al. Viability of permanent PMMA spacer with combined free fasciocutaneous tissue transfer for failed Charcot reconstruction: a 38 month prospective case report. Int J Surg Case Rep. 2017;41:174–9.
4. Nabuurs-Franssen MH, et al. Total contact casting of the diabetic foot in daily practice: a prospective follow-up study. Diabetes Care. 2005;28(2):243–7.
5. Frigg A, et al. Recurrence and prevention of diabetic foot ulcers after total contact casting. Foot Ankle Int. 2007;28(1):64–9.
6. Mueller MJ, Minor SD, Diamond JE, Blair VP 3rd. Relationship of foot deformity to ulcer location in patients with diabetes mellitus. Phys Therapy. 1990;70(6):356–62. https://doi.org/10.1093/ptj/70.6.356.
7. Pinzur MS, Schiff AP. Deformity and clinical outcomes following operative correction of Charcot foot: a new classification with implications for treatment. Foot Ankle Int. 2018;39(3):265–70. https://doi.org/10.1177/1071100717742371.
8. Wong TM, Lau TW, Li X, Fang C, Yeung K, Leung F. Masquelet technique for treatment of posttraumatic bone defects. Scientific World J. 2014;2014:710302. https://doi.org/10.1155/2014/710302.
9. Wukich DK, Raspovic KM, Hobizal KB, Sadoskas D. Surgical management of Charcot neuroarthropathy of the ankle and hindfoot in patients with diabetes. Diab/Metab Res Rev. 2016;32(Suppl 1):292–6. https://doi.org/10.1002/dmrr.2748.
10. Ledermann HP, Morrison WB. Differential diagnosis of pedal osteomyelitis and diabetic neuroarthropathy: MR Imaging. Semin Musculoskelet Radiol. 2005;9(3):272–83. https://doi.org/10.1055/s-2005-921945.
11. Jude EB, Boulton AJ. Update on Charcot neuroarthropathy. Curr Diab Rep. 2001;1(3):228–32. https://doi.org/10.1007/s11892-001-0038-2.
12. Rogers LC, Bevilacqua NJ. The diagnosis of Charcot foot. Clin Podiatr Med Surg. 2008;25(1):43–vi. https://doi.org/10.1016/j.cpm.2007.10.006.
13. Brown CH. A technique for distal tibial bone graft for arthrodesis of the foot and ankle. Foot Ankle Int. 2000;21(9):780–1. https://doi.org/10.1177/107110070002100913.
14. Bullens P, de Waal Malefijt M, Louwerens JW. Conversion of failed ankle arthroplasty to an arthrodesis. Technique using an arthrodesis nail and a cage filled with morsellized bone graft. Foot Ankle Surg. 2010;16(2):101–4. https://doi.org/10.1016/j.fas.2009.01.001.

15. Morelli I, Drago L, George DA, Gallazzi E, Scarponi S, Romanò CL. Masquelet technique: myth or reality? A systematic review and meta-analysis. Injury. 2016;47(Suppl. 6):S68–76. https://doi.org/10.1016/S0020-1383(16)30842-7.
16. Olesen UK, Eckardt H, Bosemark P, Paulsen AW, Dahl B, Hede A. The Masquelet technique of induced membrane for healing of bone defects. A review of 8 cases. Injury. 2015;46(Suppl. 8):S44–7. https://doi.org/10.1016/S0020-1383(15)30054-1.
17. Saxer F, Eckardt H. Rekonstruktion ossärer Defekte mit der Masquelet-Technik [Reconstruction of osseous defects using the Masquelet technique]. Der Orthopade. 2017;46(8):665–72. https://doi.org/10.1007/s00132-017-3443-1.

Case #37: Talocalcaneal Arthrodesis with Severe Neuropathic Equinoadductovarus Foot and Ankle Deformity Secondary to L5-S1 Radiculopathy

37

Case Presentation

This is a 57-year-old female with rheumatoid arthritis (RA) presents with severe fixed, rigid talipes equinovarus secondary to apparent Charcot disease [1, 2]. The patient has been in a wheelchair for 9 years. She has had chronic ulceration on the lateral malleolus and cuboid from her ankle foot orthosis (AFO) (Fig. 37.1a–c). She had been admitted multiple times to the hospital with sepsis. She had been in the intensive care unit (ICU) also multiple times for septicemia. Weight bearing (WB) is only for transfer and both legs are affected. Her vascular exam is normal and her neurological status shows loss of protective (LOPS) to the knee. This was secondary to the L3 to S1 fusion. She exhibits severe equinus with pedal adductovarus which is fixed. She has at this current time a large ulceration over the left malleolus 4 × 3 cm and over the cuboid 1 × 2 cm. Both have been ruled out for osteomyelitis.

Diagnosis and Management

As can be seen by the left foot radiographs, there has been resection of the styloid process and thus detachment of the peroneus brevis tendon . She shows degenerative and cystic changes about the talonavicular (TN) joint (Fig. 37.2a–c). This could be secondary to the RA. Patient was in a wheelchair and maintained non-weight bearing (NWB). Transfer occurred on the opposite limb. The surgical goal was to attain a plantar grade foot. This was to be accomplished by talectomy and talocalcaneal (TC) arthrodesis [3, 4]. Elimination of the chronic ulcerations would be accomplished by surgical excision. A talectomy was performed and a 200 mm intramedullary (IM) nail placed across the prepared tibial calcaneal surface (Figs. 37.3a–g, 37.4a–e, 37.5a, b, and 37.6a, b) [5, 6].

H. J. Visser, *Challenges in Foot and Ankle Reconstructive Surgery*,
https://doi.org/10.1007/978-3-031-07893-4_37

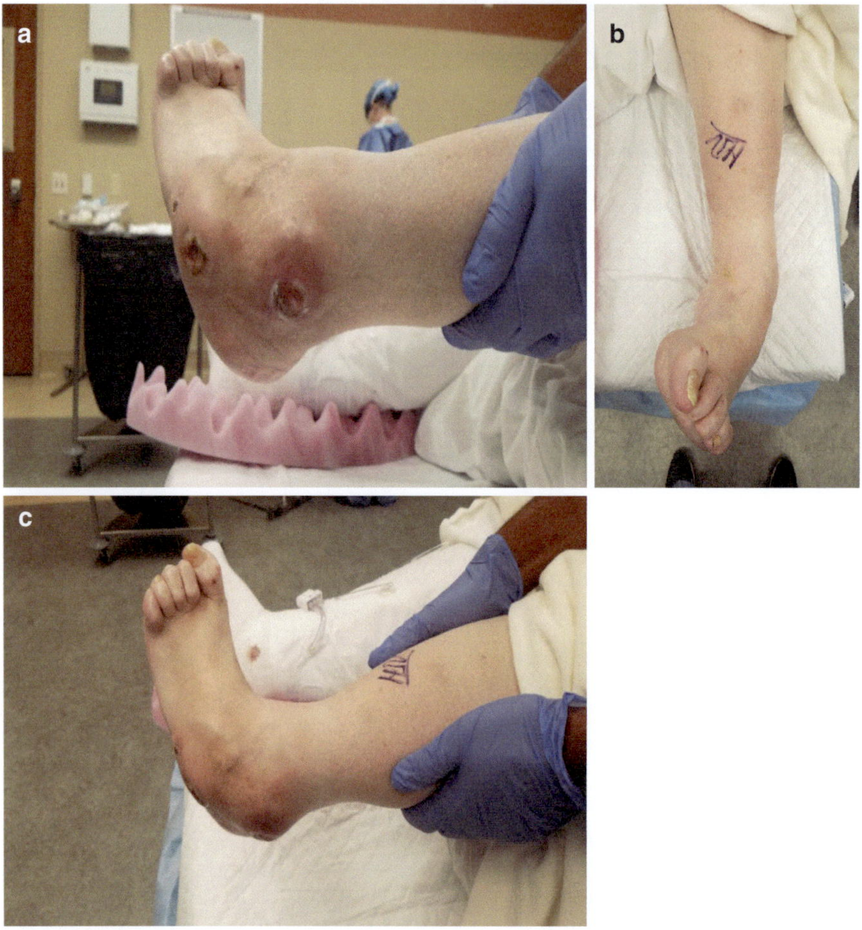

Fig. 37.1 (**a–c**) Severe fixed rigid talipes equinovarus secondary to apparent Charcot disease

Outcome

The patient developed wound drainage and ultimately a deep infection at 3 weeks post operative [7]. The nail had become loose and was removed. A polymethyl methacrylate antibiotic (PMMA) spacer impregnated with vancomycin and gentamicin was placed at the TC interface (Fig. 37.7). This was done in combination with an aggressive debridement. Soft tissue and cultures bone grew methicillin-resistant staph aureus (MRSA), 6 weeks of intravenous (IV) antibiotics was performed. She now remains stable, no further surgery has been planned. Her right foot was then done 6 months later. A large ulceration (6 × 8 cm) was excised and talectomy with

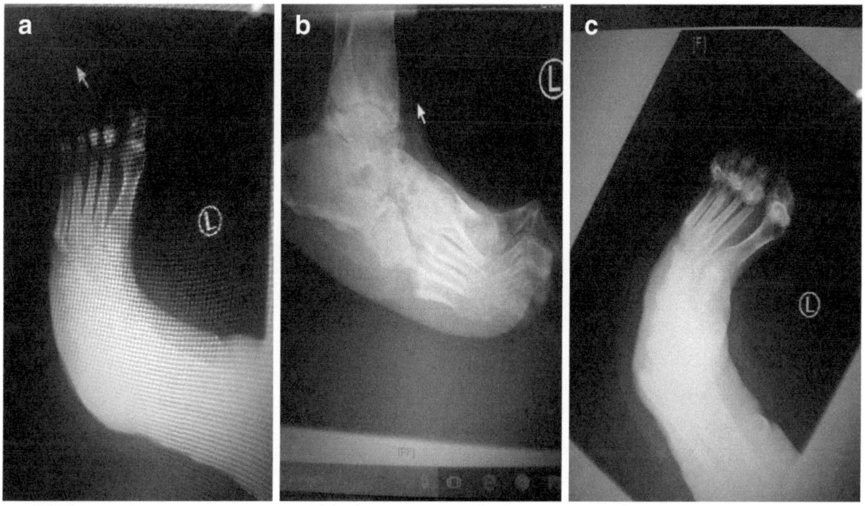

Fig. 37.2 (**a**–**c**) Degenerative and cystic changes about the talonavicular joint

TC arthrodesis performed. On this occasion, an anatomic lateral locking plate was utilized. It also became infected 2 weeks postoperatively and the hardware removed. A PMMA (vancomycin and gentamicin) spacer was placed at the talocalcaneal site. The deep infection healed. 1 year later, the right foot which was her dominant transfer foot showed the spacer to have buckled out of the joint. Another PMMA spacer was replaced and secured with 5/64 in. threaded Steinmann pins. She is now demonstrating a plantar grade foot and ankle. She was placed in a well-fitting Arizona style brace. She has been infection free for 12 months.

Clinical Pearls and Pitfalls

This issue in this case was to address both the severe deformity and chronic ulcerations. They had been present for nearly 2 years. The ulceration provided a constant source of bacteremia. This was complicated by her immunosuppression from her RA. Also she was on Enbrel and Xarelto. Bridging with Lovenox was needed with each case. She had severe anemia from chronic disease. After the first surgery, her Hgb dropped under 7 mg/dL. This required transfusion of two units of packed red blood cells. The goal was to attain healing of the chronic neuropathic ulceration. This was never possible from a wound healing standpoint. In this case, I chose to excise them. Recently, I have chosen to use vancomycin powder for wound closure. I did not in these cases. I have had great success with this technique. Whether infection could have been prevented in these cases is hard to know. The patient was urged to have bilateral below knee amputation (BKA) on multiple occasions. Fortunately

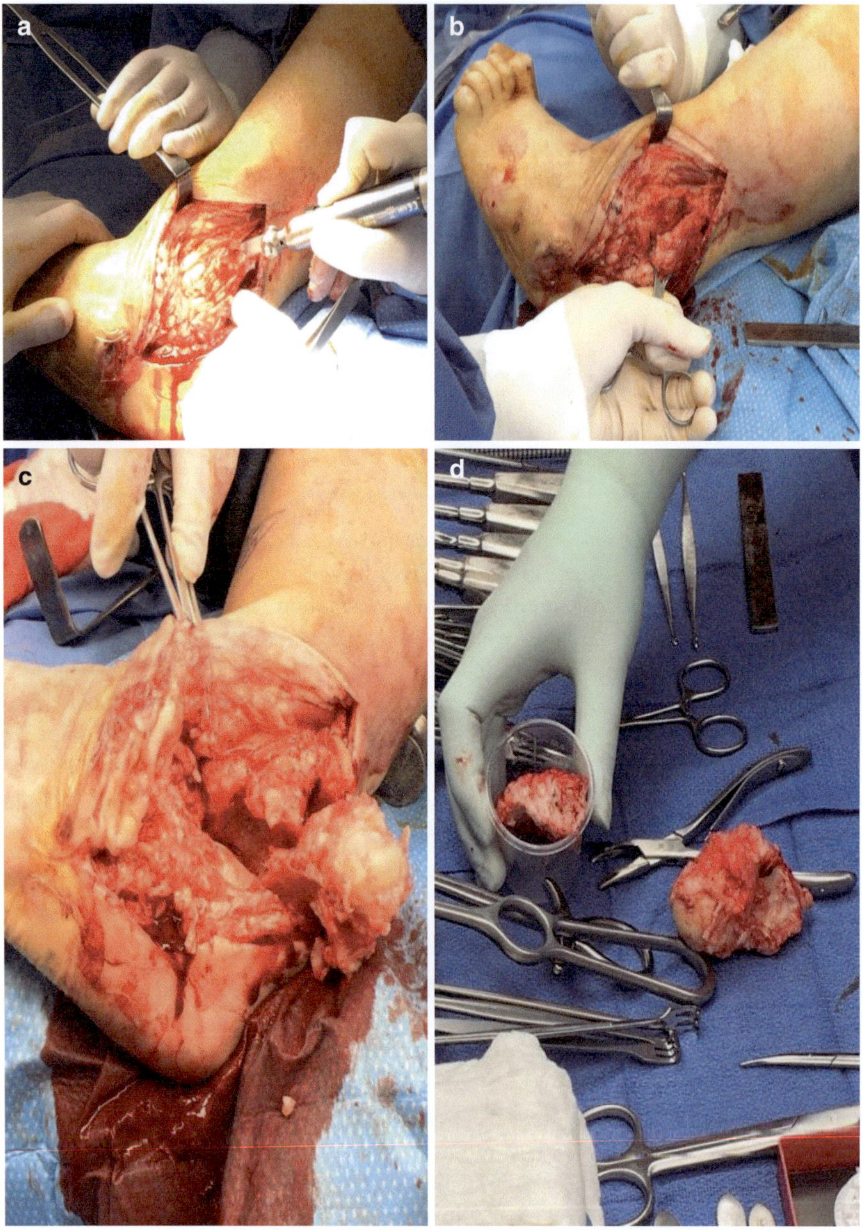

Fig. 37.3 (**a**) A lateral transfibular approach with fibular osteotomy, left foot. (**b**) Removal of fibular malleolus and partial shaft to create a window to the ankle joint. (**c**) Resection of the talus. (**d**) Resected talus, fibula to be used for autograft. (**e**) Preparation of tibial and calcaneal joint surface for arthrodesis. (**f**) Remaining defect of ankle joint with resected talus. (**g**) Realignment of foot to leg with backfilled bone graft

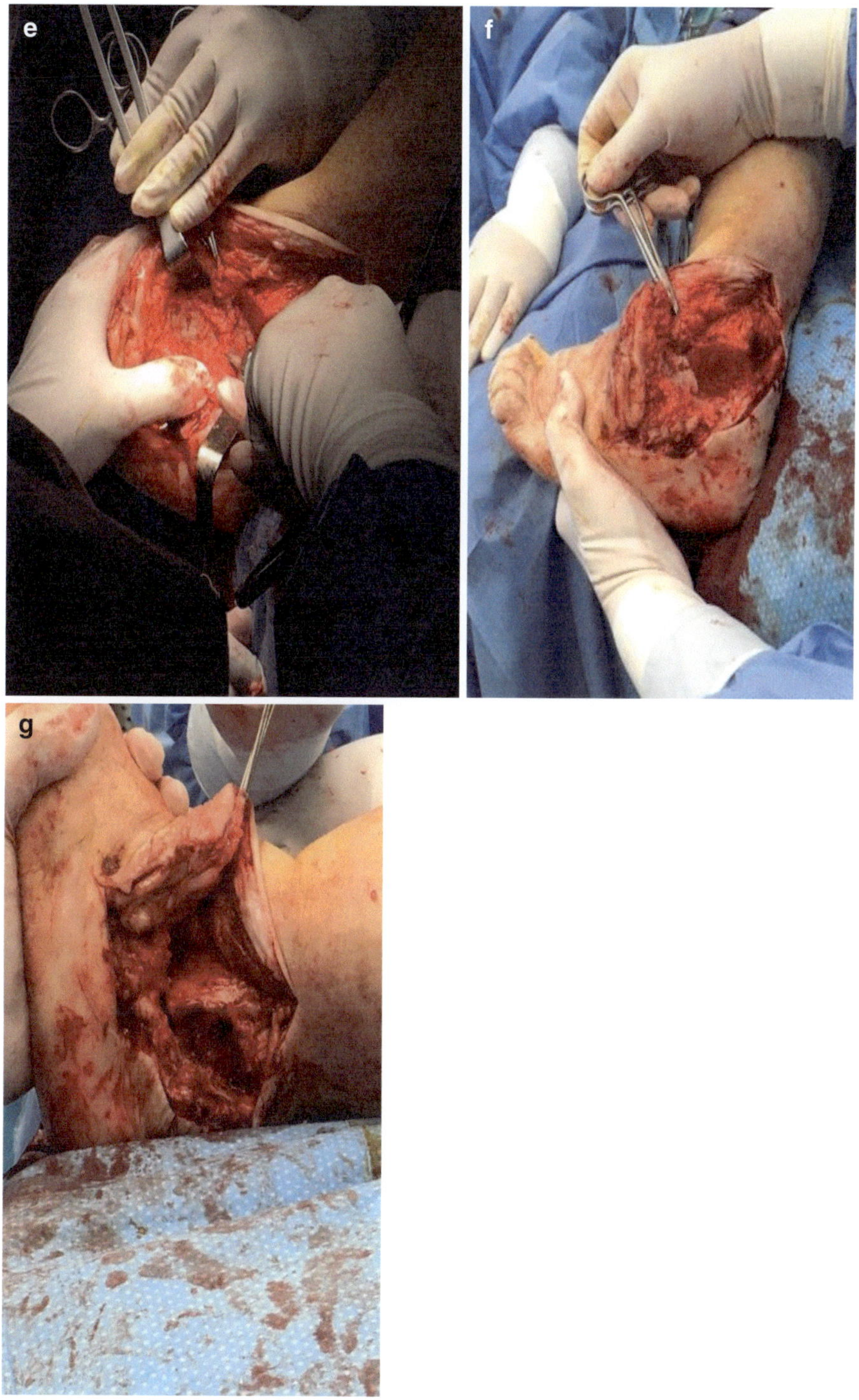

Fig. 37.3 (continued)

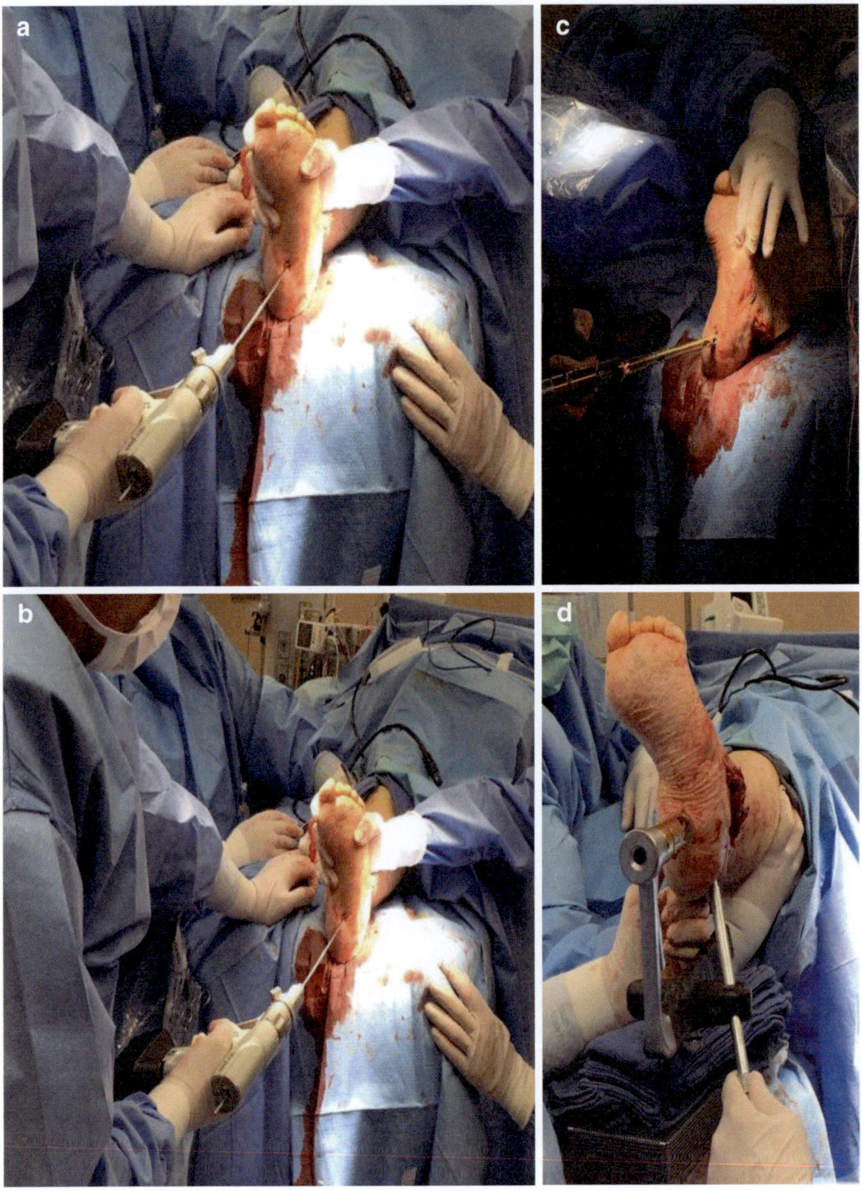

Fig. 37.4 (**a**, **b**) Guide pin for IM nail. (**c**) Reaming osseous canal. (**d**) Preparation for IM nail. (**e**) Insertion of IM nail

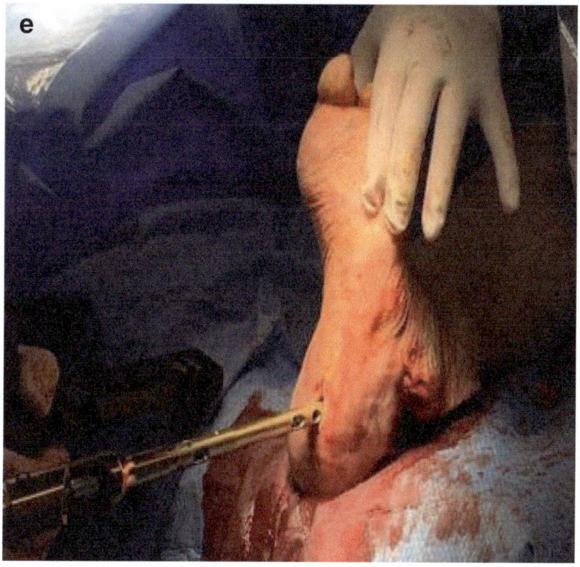

Fig. 37.4 (continued)

in both cases, a plantar grade foot was obtained and made braceable. No further infections have occurred. In cases of deep infection, hardware removal, bone cultures and placement of an antibiotic loaded polymethyl methacrylate (PMM) spacer is required [8–11]. Culture-specific antibiotics for 6 weeks are an adjutant [9]. The spacer reinforced with threaded Steinmann pins should be done to provide stability as was done in this case. If the patient was to be WB, a staged bone grafting would be needed [12, 13]. This would fill the remaining defect at the TC interface by removal of the PMMA spacer. Further cultures utilizing frozen sections would be needed prior to utilization of internal fixation. This is a long process. The etiology of neuropathy was secondary to lumbar surgery. The fusion extended from L3 to S1. This allowed her to sit upright in her wheelchair. Her radiographs were not consistent with Charcot disease. The source of her equinoadductovarus foot deformity was secondary to her L4 to S1 radiculopathy [14, 15]. It also was the source of her sensory disturbances and ulcer manifestations.

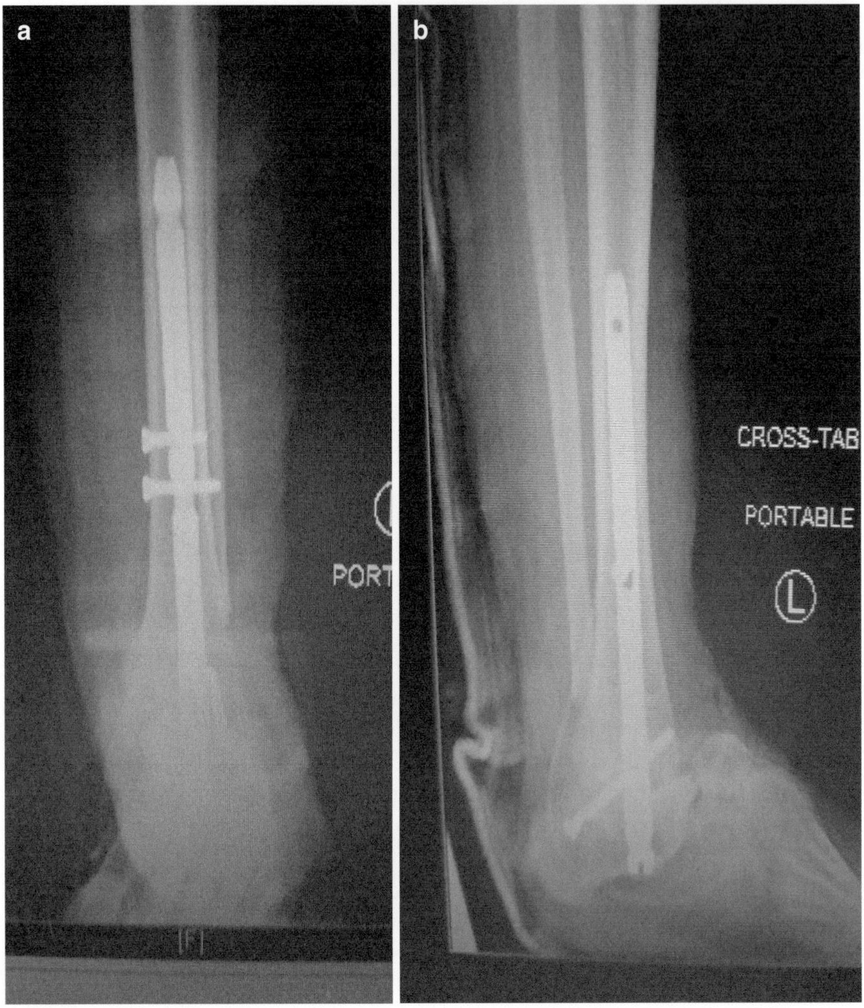

Fig. 37.5 (**a, b**) Tibiocalcaneal arthrodesis with IM nail, creation of plantigrade foot

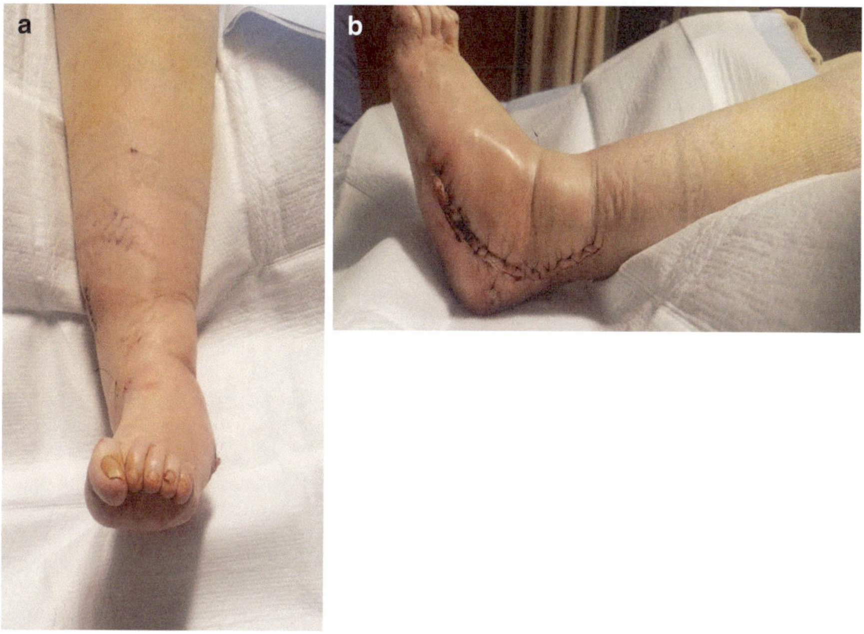

Fig. 37.6 (**a**, **b**) Creation of plantigrade foot

Fig. 37.7 An antibiotic impregnated polymethylmethacrylate antibiotic (PMMA) spacer was placed at the TC interface

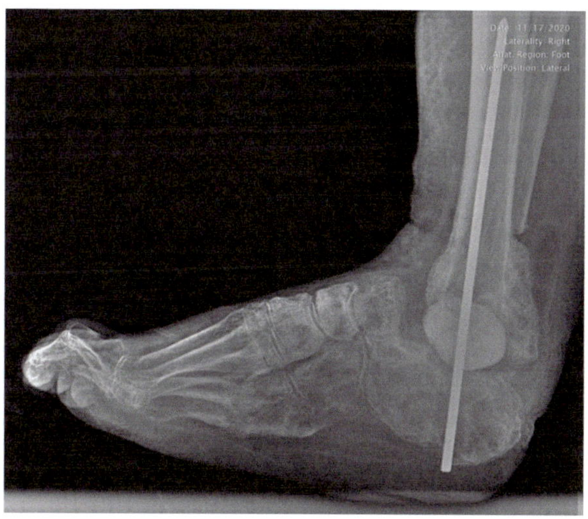

References

1. Bacino CA, Hecht JT. Etiopathogenesis of equinovarus foot malformations. Eur J Med Genet. 2014;57(8):473–9.
2. Lawrence SJ, Botte MJ. Management of the adult, spastic, equinovarus foot deformity. Foot Ankle Int. 1994;15(6):340–6.
3. Joseph TN, Myerson MS. Use of talectomy in modern foot and ankle surgery. Foot Ankle Clin. 2004;9(4):775–85.
4. Tom RK, Pupp GR. Talectomy for diabetic Charcot foot. An alternative to amputation. J Am Podiatr Med Assoc. 1992;82(9):447–53.
5. Klos K, et al. The use of a retrograde fixed-angle intramedullary nail for tibiocalcaneal arthrodesis after severe loss of the talus. Strategies Trauma Limb Reconstr. 2009;4(2):95–102.
6. Jehan S, et al. The success of tibiotalocalcaneal arthrodesis with intramedullary nailing: a systematic review of the literature. Acta Orthop Belg. 2011;77(5):644.
7. Bibbo C, Goldberg JW. Infectious and healing complications after elective orthopaedic foot and ankle surgery during tumor necrosis factor-alpha inhibition therapy. Foot Ankle Int. 2004;25(5):331–5.
8. van Vugt T, Arts JJ, Geurts J. Antibiotic-loaded polymethylmethacrylate beads and spacers in treatment of orthopedic infections and the role of biofilm formation. Front Microbiol. 2019;10:1626. https://doi.org/10.3389/fmicb.2019.01626.
9. Anagnostakos K, Meyer C. Antibiotic elution from hip and knee acrylic bone cement spacers: a systematic review. Bio Med Res. 2017;
10. Bonnevialle P. Operative treatment of early infection after internal fixation of limb fractures (exclusive of severe open fractures). OTSR. 2017;103(1S):S67–73. https://doi.org/10.1016/j.otsr.2016.06.019.
11. Ferrao P, Myerson MS, Schuberth JM, McCourt MJ. Cement spacer as definitive management for postoperative ankle infection. Foot Ankle Int. 2012;33(3):173–8. https://doi.org/10.3113/FAI.2012.0173.
12. Donegan DJ, Scolaro J, Matuszewski PE, Mehta S. Staged bone grafting following placement of an antibiotic spacer block for the management of segmental long bone defects. Orthopedics. 2011;34(11):e730–5. https://doi.org/10.3928/01477447-20110922-16.
13. Kasha S, Rathore SS, Kumar H. Antibiotic cement spacer and induced membrane bone grafting in open fractures with bone loss: a case series. Indian J Orthop. 2019;53(2):237–45. https://doi.org/10.4103/ortho.IJOrtho_110_17.
14. Sekharappa V, James I, Amritanand R, Venkatesh K, David KS. Lumbar plexopathy following instrumented posterior lumbar interbody fusion: a complication with use of Hohmann's retractor. Eur Spine J. 2013;22(9):2039–46. https://doi.org/10.1007/s00586-013-2748-y.
15. Dydyk AM, Hameed S. Lumbosacral plexopathy. [Updated 2021 Apr 2]. In: StatPearls. Treasure Island, FL: StatPearls Publishing; 2021. Jan. Available from: https://www.ncbi.nlm.nih.gov/books/NBK556030/.

Part V

Tendinopathies

Case #38: Management of an Infected Achilles Tendon Rupture with Local Excision, V-Y Gastrocnemius Aponeurotic Lengthening and Flexor Hallucis Transfer

38

Case Presentation

This is a 50-year-old African American female who presented with a chronically draining wound and ulceration overlying her right Achilles tendon. She gave a history of prior surgery for a non-insertional rupture of the Achilles tendon approximately 1 year prior. This involved an open repair with utilization of an allomatrix graft, wrapped at the repair site [1]. A second surgery was performed 3 months later. This involved removal of the allomatrix graft wrap which had been deemed infected. An attempted secondary closure was performed. The wound again dehisced and she was sent for another opinion (Fig. 38.1).

Diagnosis and Assessment

Concerning her past medical history, she was not diabetic and was managed for hypertension and hyperlipidemia. Vascular exam noted full palpable pulses. Her neurological examination noted sensation to be completely intact. On her dermatologic exam, an open posterior wound directly over the Achilles tendon was present that measured 5 × 3 cm. The base was avascular and included the underlying Achilles tendon (Fig. 38.1). There was no drainage or other signs of gross infection. On her muscular exam, she had dysfunction of the gastroc-soleus muscle group via of the Achilles tendon and walked with a calcaneal gait. She required three-point crutch assistance during ambulation.

The magnetic resonance imaging (MRI) noted a large dorsal defect within the Achilles tendon which the radiologist interpreted as likely packing. There was no sign of an abscess. The Achilles tendon appeared "C" shaped about the ulceration (Fig. 38.2).

H. J. Visser, *Challenges in Foot and Ankle Reconstructive Surgery*,
https://doi.org/10.1007/978-3-031-07893-4_38

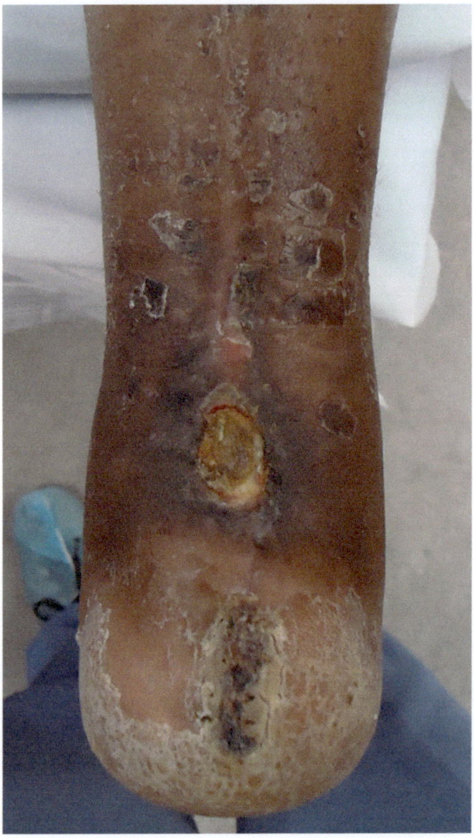

Fig. 38.1 5 × 3 cm ulceration, exposed Achilles tendon

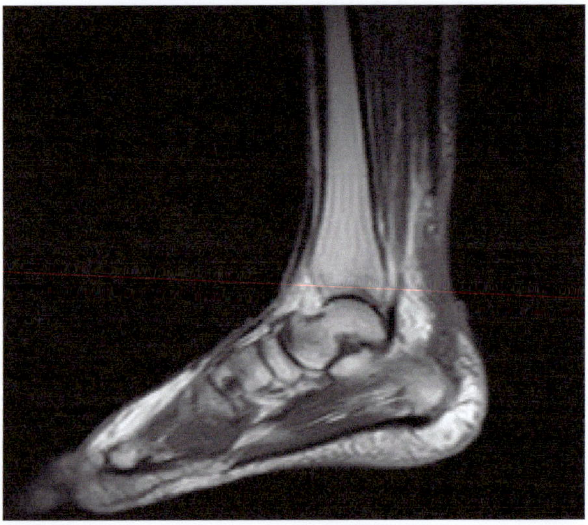

Fig. 38.2 Large defect within the Achilles tendon

The obvious issue was to assess the posterior wound/ulceration and manage the necrotic Achilles tendon. Also re-establishment of gastroc-soleus muscle function was critical.

Management

The initial incision was designed to excise the posterior ulceration. Also a long incision was made to allow undermining for closure at the end of the procedure (Fig. 38.3a, b). The skin was extremely indurated. The identified Achilles tendon underneath the wound/ulceration was found to be necrotic. The packing noted on the MRI proved to be residual allomatrix present from the primary procedure (Fig. 38.4a–c). At this point, the necrotic portion of the tendon was excised (Fig. 38.4d). The resected portion was measured (Fig. 38.4e). A long V-Y advancement of the gastrocnemius aponeurosis was utilized to allow restoration of healthy tendon at the insertion (Fig. 38.5a–c). Prior to Achilles tendon fixation, the flexor hallucis longus (FHL) tendon was recruited as a short harvest (Fig. 38.6). This was then secured with an interference screw at the superior portion of the calcaneus with the ankle positioned in maximal plantarflexion (Fig. 38.7). The advanced Achilles portion was secured to the posterior calcaneus with a 4.0 mm cancellous screw and a polyacetal washer [2]. The advanced aponeurosis was then secured to gastrocnemius aponeurosis proximally in retained full ankle plantarflexion (Fig. 38.8a, b).

The patient was kept non-weight bearing (NWB) with the ankle in 30° of plantarflexion for the first 6 weeks. Deep vein thrombosis (DVT) prophylaxis with lovenox was also performed [3]. At 6 weeks, the patient was placed in a boot with a 3 cm heel lift and began weight bearing (WB). At 9 weeks, the lift was removed and full WB in neutral position was performed. Physical (PT) was then performed over the next 2 months.

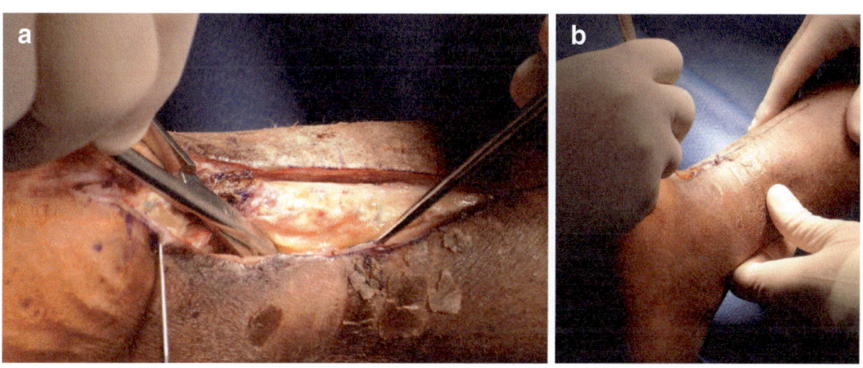

Fig. 38.3 (**a**, **b**) Large incision made to excise ulcer and expose underlying structures

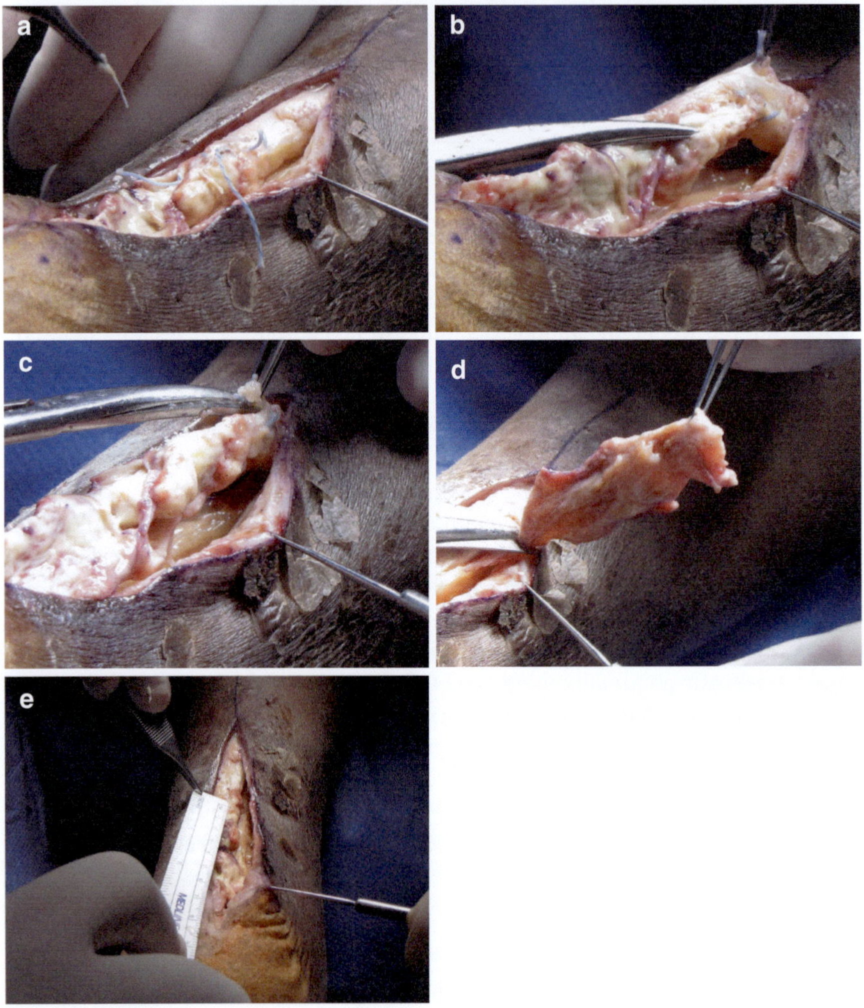

Fig. 38.4 (**a–c**) Necrotic Achilles tendon with infected allomatrix. (**d**) Resected necrotic Achilles tendon. (**e**) Measurement of resected area

Outcome

The patient did extremely well considering a very complicated situation. A wound dehiscence did occur which healed with local wound care. At 6 months, she walked with a mild limp. At 1 year, there were no noticeable gait disturbances. As can be seen, she was able to stand on her toes with full gastroc-soleus strength (Fig. 38.9a, b).

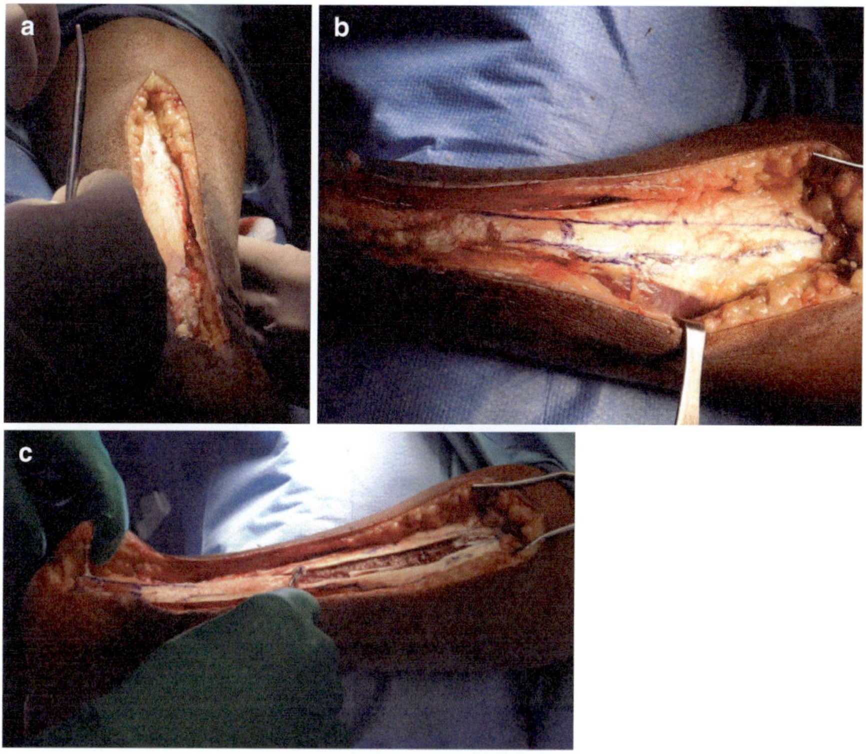

Fig. 38.5 (**a–c**) V-Y gastrocnemius aponeurotic advancement

Fig. 38.6 Short harvest FHL transfer

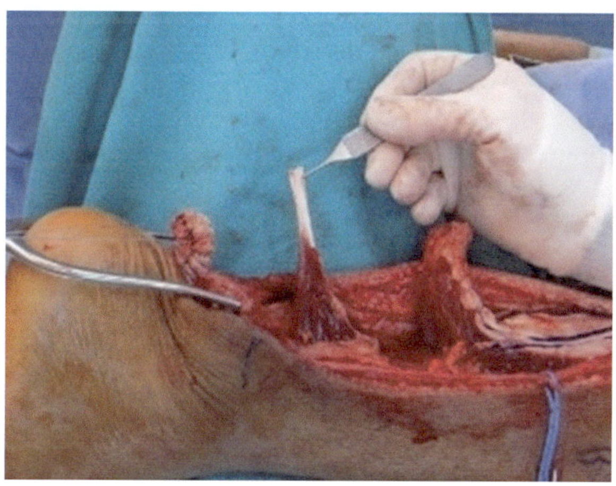

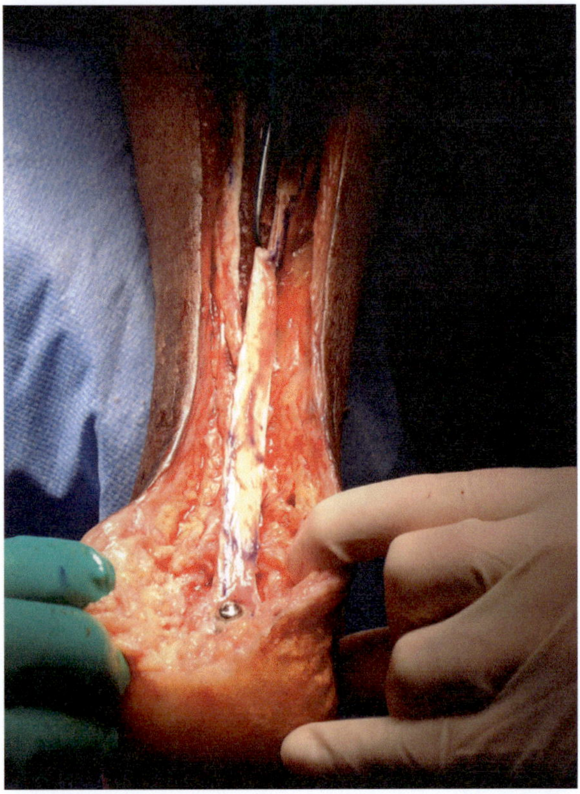

Fig. 38.7 Securing advanced aponeurosis and remaining Achilles tendon to calcaneus with 4.0 mm screw and polyacetyl washer

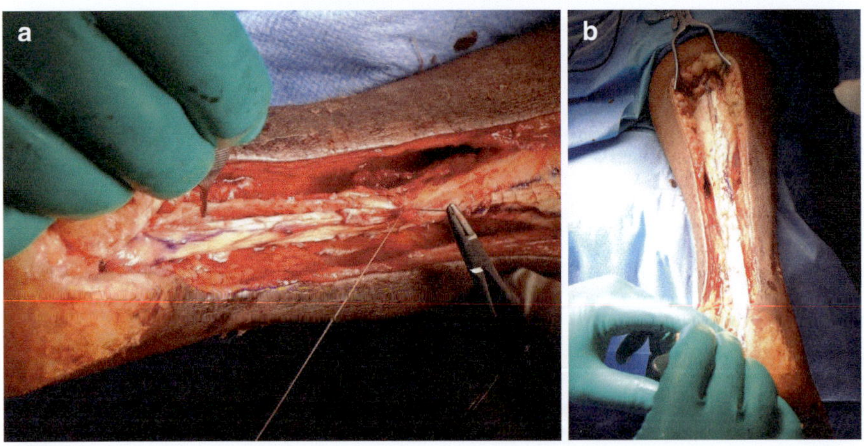

Fig. 38.8 (**a**, **b**) Suturing portion proximally with ankle in full plantarflexion

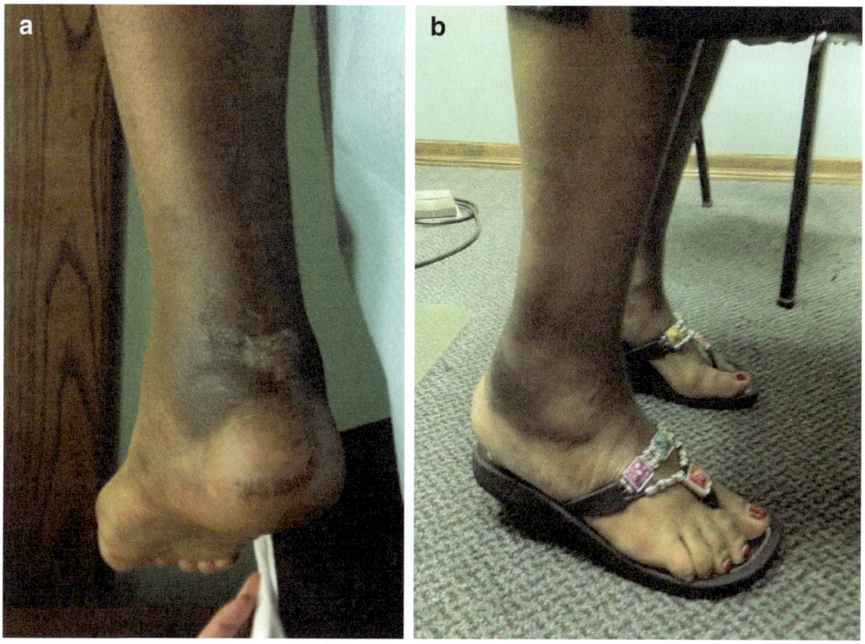

Fig. 38.9 (**a**, **b**) Full plantarflexion and heel lift

Clinical Pearls and Pitfalls

The use of allomatrix for augmented repair of an Achilles tendon at the ruptured site has been advocated in some circles [1–3]. The issue is that it also adds bulk to the repair site and can create tension at the wound repair site. If the wound as in this case dehisces, an avascular environment is created. This serves to leave exposed allomatrix grafts and tendons. Excision in this area of skin ulceration includes peritendon and subcutaneous dissection the length of the incision to allow closure.

Also another concern in this case was dysfunction of the Achilles complex (gastrocnemius soleus muscle). Restoration of graded muscle function depends on the condition of the muscle and re-establishing proper tension with restored tendon function [4, 5]. The degree of calf atrophy and findings of fatty infiltration of the muscle on the MRI indicate whether the restoration of strength may occur [6]. In this case, calf atrophy and a calcaneus gait with associated 25° of ankle dorsiflexion required attempts to provide reoccurring strength by proper tensioning and muscle transfer. Tensioning the FHL transfer was critical in this case and assists remaining muscle strength [7]. This along with attaining approximately one-third the strength with a V-Y tensioning to the gastroc-soleus allows much improved overall plantar flexion strength [8]. In this situation, the FHL is tensioned first with the ankle in maximal plantarflexion. The V-Y is sewn after the Achilles insertion is re-established. Again maximal plantar flexion is performed. As the repair must attempt to re-create normal gastroc-soleus function, this form of tensioning is required [9, 10]. "Over tensioning" will not occur.

References

1. Michael LS. Graft jacket augmentation of chronic Achilles tendon ruptures. Orthopedics. 2004;27(1):S151–3.
2. DeCarbo WT, Hyer CF. Interference screw fixation for flexor hallucis longus tendon transfer for chronic Achilles tendonopathy. J Foot Ankle Surg. 2008;47(1):69–72.
3. Kaboli P, Henderson MC, White RH. DVT prophylaxis and anticoagulation in the surgical patient. Med Clin North Am. 2003;87(1):77–110.
4. Chen C, Hunt KJ. Open reconstructive strategies for chronic Achilles tendon ruptures. Foot Ankle Clin. 2019;24(3):425–37. https://doi.org/10.1016/j.fcl.2019.04.002.
5. Lee DK. Achilles tendon repair with acellular tissue graft augmentation in neglected ruptures. J Foot Ankle Surg Surg. 2007;46(6):451–5. https://doi.org/10.1053/j.jfas.2007.05.007.
6. Lee DK. Achilles tendon repair with acellular tissue graft augmentation in neglected ruptures. J Foot Ankle Surg. 2007;46(6):451–5. https://doi.org/10.1053/j.jfas.2007.05.007.
7. Oksanen MM, Haapasalo HH, Elo PP, Laine HJ. Hypertrophy of the flexor hallucis longus muscle after tendon transfer in patients with chronic Achilles tendon rupture. Foot Ankle Surg. 2014;20(4):253–7. https://doi.org/10.1016/j.fas.2014.06.003.
8. Elias I, Besser M, Nazarian LN, Raikin SM. Reconstruction for missed or neglected Achilles tendon rupture with V-Y lengthening and flexor hallucis longus tendon transfer through one incision. Foot Ankle Int. 2007;28(12):1238–48. https://doi.org/10.3113/FAI.2007.1238.
9. Bäcker HC, Yenchak AJ, Trofa DP, Vosseller JT. Strength measurement after achilles tendon repair. Foot Ankle Spec. 2019;12(5):471–9. https://doi.org/10.1177/1938640018819779.
10. Maquirriain J. Achilles tendon rupture: avoiding tendon lengthening during surgical repair and rehabilitation. Yale J Biol Med. 2011;84(3):289–300.

39 Case #39: Management of an Infected Achilles Tendon Rupture with Secondary Allograft Associated with a Severe Allergic Dermatitis by Excision of Allograft and Transfer of the Flexor Hallucis Longus Tendon and Peroneus Brevis

Case Presentation

This is a 56-year-old Caucasian female who gives a history of a misstep and sustaining a rupture of her Achilles tendon. The patient had an open repair performed but was told that her rupture was "so bad" that an allograft was needed for the repair. The patient did reasonably well for the first 6 months but then began to develop reactive dermatitis. A wound/ulceration also occurred exposing the underlying allograft. The patient exhibited plantarflexion strength but could not rise up onto her toes. She was managed with mouth (PO) antibiotics, oral and topical steroids with no noted improvement.

Diagnosis and Assessment

On examination, the patient was healthy with only a history of hypertension. Her vascular and neurological examinations were normal with no signs of peripheral neuropathy. She had a large area of reactive dermatitis that was pruritic and erythematous. It was plaque-like extending from just above the calcaneus to the lower calf (Fig. 39.1). An ulceration measuring 3 × 3 cm with tendon exposed at its base was present (Fig. 39.2). The assessment was a reactive dermatitis created by the tendon allograft with a non-infected ulceration exhibiting exposed allograft tendon. There was mild dysfunction present.

H. J. Visser, *Challenges in Foot and Ankle Reconstructive Surgery*,
https://doi.org/10.1007/978-3-031-07893-4_39

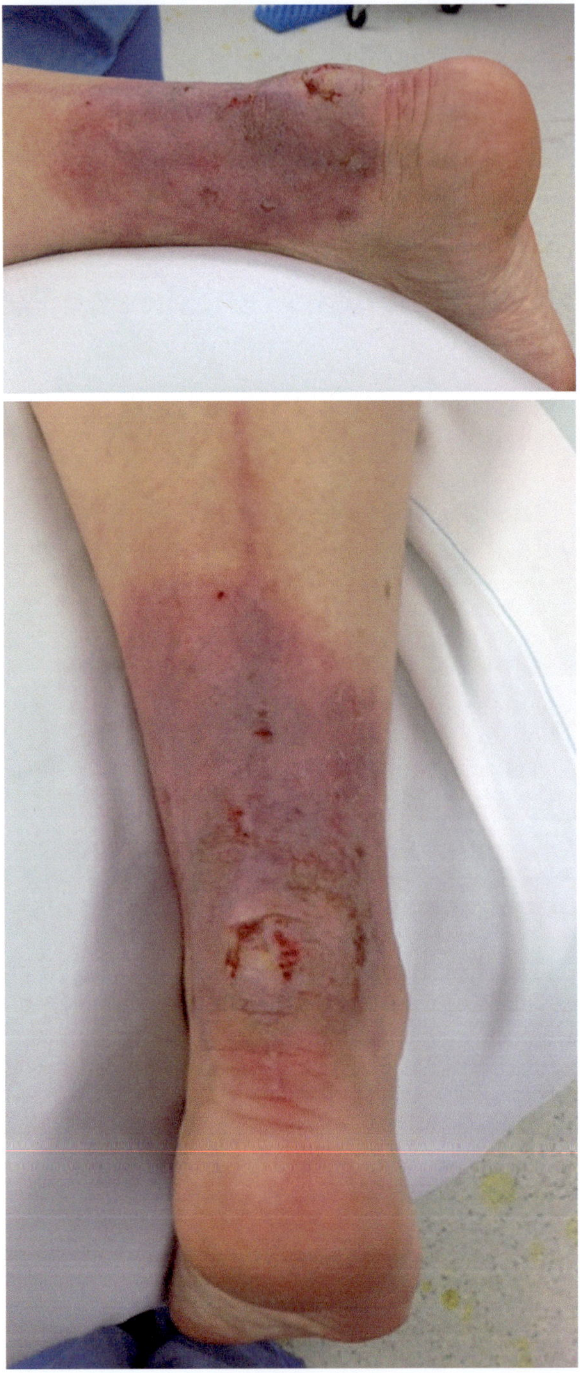

Figs. 39.1 and 39.2 Plaque-like reactive dermatitis with erythema extending from calcaneus to lower leg

Management

The approach was to remove the allograft as it served as the source of allergen. The sural nerve was identified and preserved (Fig. 39.3a, b). Since the entire Achilles tendon (allograft) was excised (Fig. 39.4), a dual transfer of the flexor hallucis longus (FHL) and the split anterior portion of the peroneus brevis was performed to establish posterior ankle strength (Figs. 39.5 and 39.6). Both tendons, the FHL medial and peroneus brevis lateral were routed through separate 4.5 mm drill holes in the calcaneus (Fig. 39.7a, b). They were tensioned in full plantarflexion (Fig. 39.8). Upon closure, the ulceration that was present centered over the transferred FHL muscle belly. The ulcer was debrided and a partial-thickness skin graft was applied.

The patient was kept on non-weight bearing (NWB) for 6 weeks in a posterior splint. She was then placed in a controlled ankle motion (CAM) boot with a 3 cm heel lift. At 9 weeks, the ankle was allowed to be neutral and active physical therapy (PT) was begun. Total immobilization was 12 weeks.

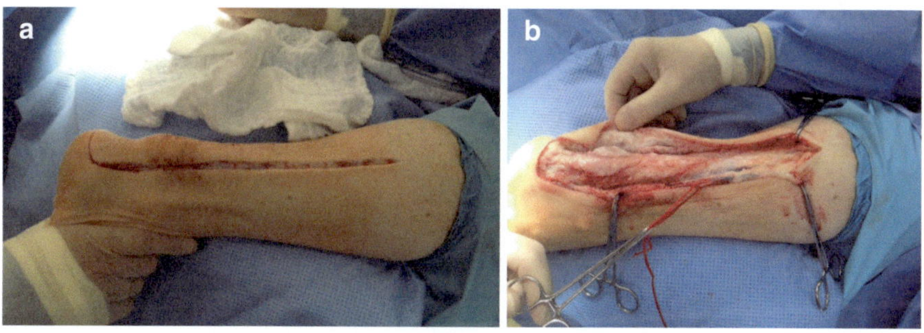

Fig. 39.3 (**a**) Incisional approach, (**b**) exposure of allograft

Fig. 39.4 Removal of allograft

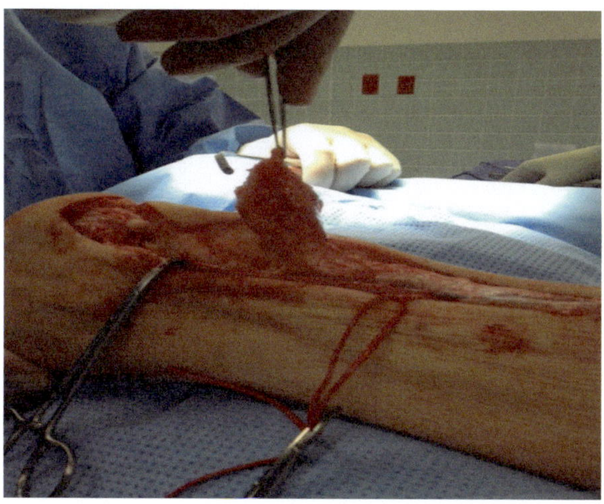

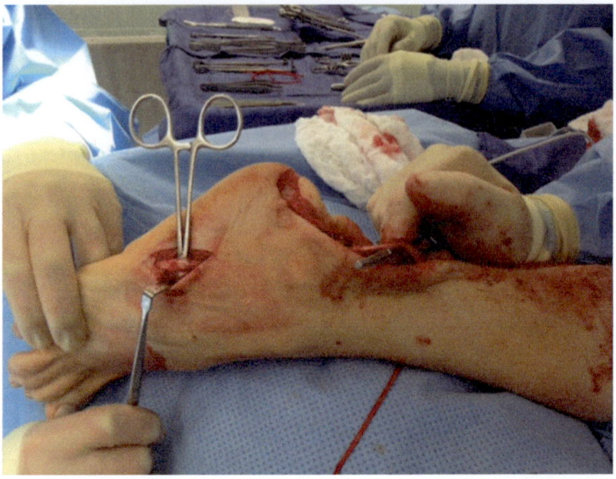

Fig. 39.5 Exposure of peroneus brevis

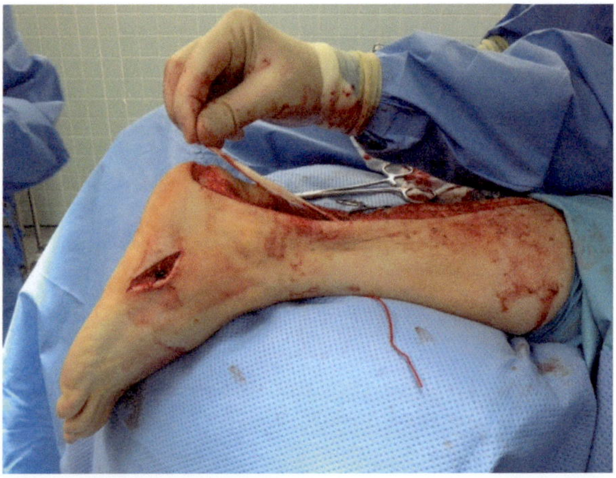

Fig. 39.6 FHL mobilized

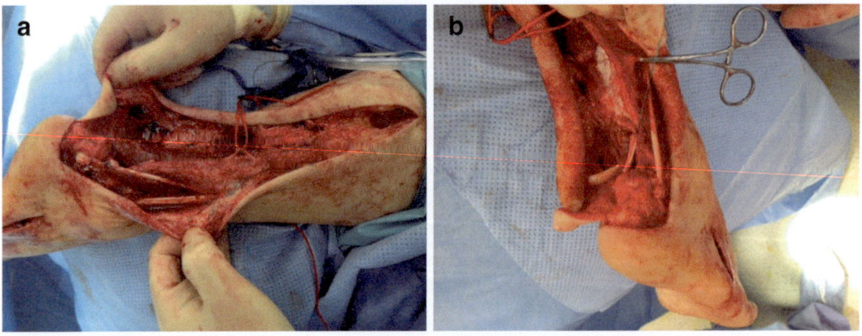

Fig. 39.7 (**a**) Tendon transfers through calcaneal bone tunnels. (**b**) Transfer of FHL with split peroneus brevis through calcaneal bone tunnels

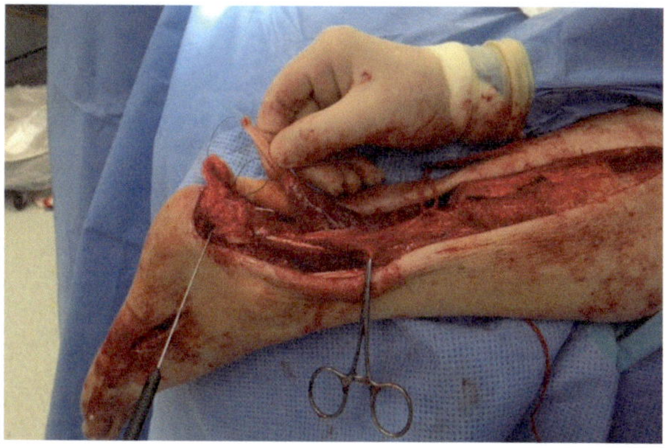

Fig. 39.8 Full plantarflexion tensions peroneus brevis and FHL

Outcome

The patient did very well with complete recovery of the dermatitis and functional ambulation. A wound dehiscence did occur involving the incision of 4 cm in length. It required wound care and one course of oral antibiotics. Overall complete recovery was noted at 9 months. The posterior ulceration healed and required 6 weeks. There were no issues with attaining a plantar grade foot despite maximal tendon tensioning.

Clinical Pearls and Pitfalls

This case represents another case of an allograft complication. Although allografts are quite useful and safe in most cases, complications can occur. The mystery in this case was why the allograft was needed in the first place. The patient was told that the full rupture was so bad that it needed to be excised and an allograft placed. The opposing ends of an Achilles rupture can appear as "degenerated mop ends of the tendon" but this only requires minimal debridement and direct anastomosis [1].

The main issue here was that a complete allograft was utilized to replace the rupture and Achilles tendon. The dermatitis would not resolve unless the allergen was eliminated. Note on the institution of application of the tourniquet the dermatitis "disappears."

When there is no available tendon to work with, a transfer of the FHL and peroneus brevis offers a good option for return of function [2, 3]. The FHL itself has been used for neglected Achilles tendon ruptures [4–6]. The addition of half of the peroneus brevis gives added power [7]. By routing the FHL medial and peroneus brevis lateral, adequate muscle strength can be attained [8]. Also full plantarflexion positioning is done in cases where smaller, weaker muscle groups are utilized. This also was a representation of a phasic transfer. In this case, I chose not to directly excise the posterior ulceration. A good option as in this case was to place the FHL muscle in direct proximity. This gave a good vascular bed for application of a split-thickness skin graft.

References

1. Yang X, Meng H, Quan Q, Peng J, Lu S, Wang A. Management of acute Achilles tendon ruptures: a review. Bone Joint Res. 2018;7(10):561–9. https://doi.org/10.1302/2046-3758.710.BJR-2018-0004.R2.
2. Sebastian H, Datta B, Maffulli N, et al. Mechanical properties of reconstructed Achilles tendon with transfer of peroneus brevis or flexor hallucis longus tendon. J Foot Ankle Surg. 2007;46(6):424–8.
3. Miskulin M, Miskulin A, Klobucar H, Kuvalja S. Neglected rupture of the Achilles tendon treated with peroneus brevis transfer: a functional assessment of 5 cases. J Foot Ankle Surg. 2005;44(1):49–56.
4. Wapner KL, Pavlock GS, Hecht PJ, Naselli F, Walther R. Repair of chronic Achilles tendon rupture with flexor hallucis longus tendon transfer. Foot Ankle. 1993;14(8):443–9. https://doi.org/10.1177/107110079301400803.
5. Kim JY, Lee I, Seo K, Jung W, Kim B. FHL tendon transfer in diabetics for treatment of non-healing plantar heel ulcers. Foot Ankle Int. 2010;31(6):480–5. https://doi.org/10.3113/FAI.2010.0480.
6. Ozer H, Ergisi Y, Harput G, Senol MS, Baltaci G. Short-term results of flexor hallucis longus transfer in delayed and neglected Achilles tendon repair. J Foot Ankle Surg. 2018;57(5):1042–7. https://doi.org/10.1053/j.jfas.2018.03.005.
7. Maffulli N, Oliva F, Costa V, Del Buono A. The management of chronic rupture of the Achilles tendon: minimally invasive peroneus brevis tendon transfer. Bone Joint J. 2015;97-B(3):353–7. https://doi.org/10.1302/0301-620X.97B3.33732.
8. Pintore E, Barra V, Pintore R, Maffulli N. Peroneus brevis tendon transfer in neglected tears of the Achilles tendon. J Trauma Acute Care Surg. 2001;50(1):71–8.

Case #40: Repair of an Attritional Rupture of the Tibialis Anterior Tendon

40

Case Presentation

This is a 55-year-old Caucasian male who was walking in a grocery store and felt a "sudden pop" in his right midfoot. He states that he had pain involving the midfoot area for about 3 months. He did not pursue medical care.

After the incident, the pain improved. He, however, felt "weak" and had trouble pulling his foot up. He stated that it now affected his gait. Mysteriously, his midfoot pain had resolved.

Diagnosis and Assessment

On examination, the patient's medical history was significant for cardiac disease. He had a 30 pack-year history of smoking. His neurovascular status was completely normal. A lab workup noted a hemoglobin A1C of 7.8. He was diagnosed as a non-insulin-dependent diabetic.

His muscular exam noted a palpable mass at the anterior ankle. Dorsiflexion strength was 3/5 and he was unable to recruit the tibialis anterior tendon. His contralateral foot and ankle demonstrated full strength and recruitment.

An MRI noted an insertional rupture of the tibialis anterior tendon with proximal retraction. Its retraction level was to the inferior band of the extensor retinaculum of the ankle joint (Fig. 40.1).

H. J. Visser, *Challenges in Foot and Ankle Reconstructive Surgery*,
https://doi.org/10.1007/978-3-031-07893-4_40

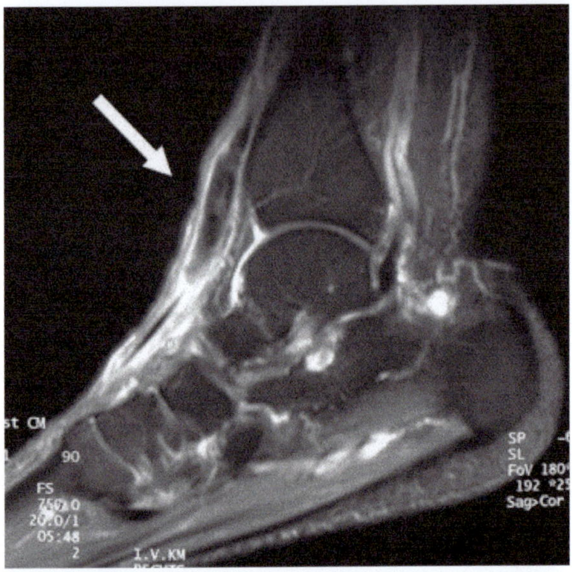

Fig. 40.1 Insertional rupture of tibialis anterior tendon with proximal retraction

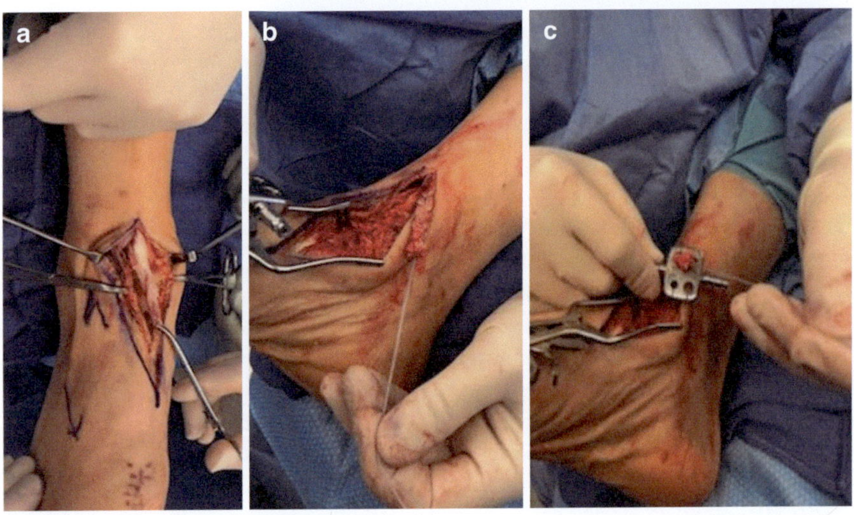

Fig. 40.2 (**a**) Insertional tibialis anterior rupture with proximal retraction. (**b**) Debridement to healthy tendon and insertion prepared with whip stitch. (**c**) Measuring tendon circumference for interference screw

Management

Surgically, the tibialis anterior was isolated with a direct incision along its course. The tendon was found completely ruptured at its insertion (Fig. 40.2a). It had retracted to just inferior to the superior band of the extensor retinaculum. Initial management was to debride the tendinopathic and ruptured portion to healthy tendon (Fig. 40.2b).

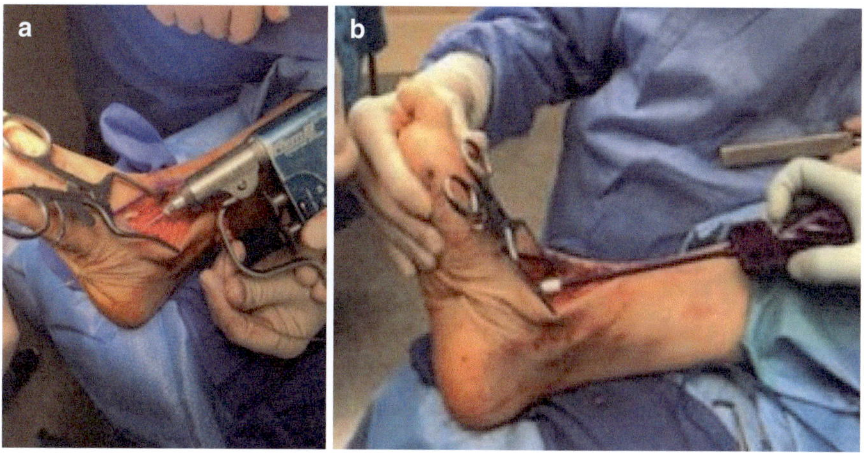

Fig. 40.3 (**a**) Guide pin for bone drill for 7.0 mm interference screw. (**b**) Placement of interference screw

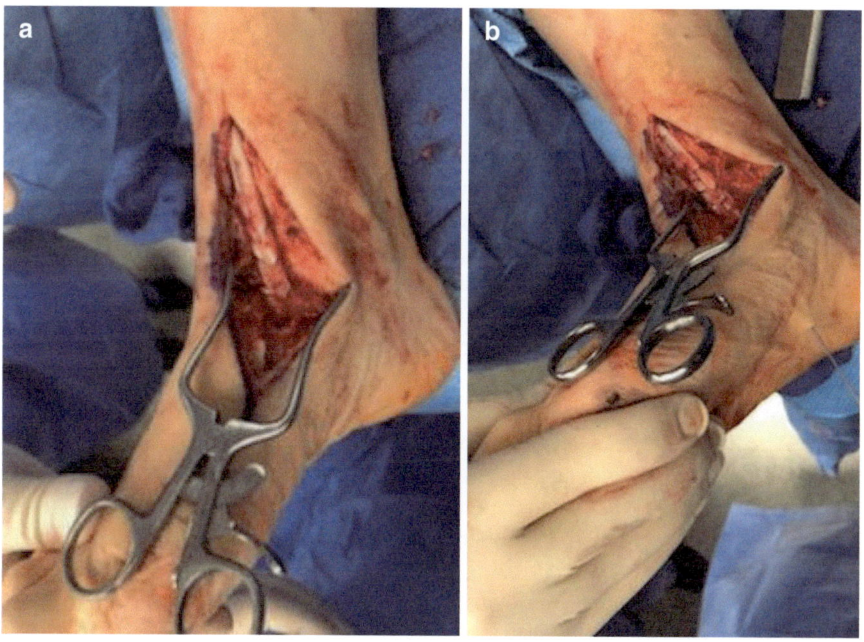

Fig. 40.4 (**a**, **b**) Tensioning tibialis anterior at neutral ankle joint position

A whip stitch was placed and the tendon measured for a proper sized interference screw (Fig. 40.2b, c). A 7 mm interference screw was used in this case (Fig. 40.3a, b). The tendon was tensioned with the ankle at neutral dorsiflexion. It was placed at the medial cuneiform site (Fig. 40.4a, b).

The patient was kept non-weight bearing for 4 weeks. He was then placed in a weight bearing boot for a further 4 weeks. Active range of motion began at 6 weeks.

Gait normalization and strengthening were then performed. He wore an ankle stabilizing orthosis (ASO) brace for support for 4 weeks when taken out of the controlled ankle motion (CAM) boot. He did have a small wound dehiscence. It healed with local wound care.

Outcome

The patient had physical therapy for 4 weeks. He then was fully ambulatory at 4 months postoperatively. He had no significant issues and his strength was 5/5 with no noticeable antalgia. There was no subsequent development of a hallux malleus deformity.

Clinical Pearls and Pitfalls

Insertional tibialis anterior tendon ruptures of a spontaneous nature are a well-known clinical entity [1]. Middle-aged and elderly individuals are the most commonly encountered. In this case, the patients smoking and undiagnosed diabetes may have contributed to this form of ischemic enthesopathy.

Patients with this condition often describe long-term pain that is confined to the midfoot. Once a rupture occurs, the pain resolves. This is due to the elimination of traction and strain at the insertion site.

In this case, with debridement, the remaining tendon could be advanced and properly tensioned at the medial cuneiform site. In cases where there is "inadequate" tendon available, a z-lengthening or a turn down technique can be used to gain native tendon length. The turn down technique involves splitting the tendon proximally in an anterior and posterior half. The anterior portion is then turned down leaving it attached at the distal cut tendon. This site must be reinforced with suture before the tendon is advanced and tensioned [2–5].

In cases of non-insertional rupture, degenerative tendons cannot undergo direct repair. An allograft or transfer of the extensor hallucis longus (EHL) can be chosen in these cases [6]. When using an allograft, it is first attached at its insertion (the medial cuneiform). The ankle is then brought to neutral dorsiflexion. The proximal portion of the allograft is then properly tensioned to the proximal portion of the native tibialis anterior tendon utilizing a Pulvertaft technique. If an EHL transfer is performed, it is secured to the base of the first metatarsal in full dorsiflexion tension. A hallux interphalangeal joint arthrodesis is also required [7, 8].

Success of the allograft depends on the integrity of the tibialis anterior muscle. This procedure seems to fare better concerning correction of the partial drop foot condition than the EHL transfer. However, if the tibialis anterior muscle is deemed to be insufficient by failure of response to intraoperative traction an EHL transfer is the best course of treatment [9].

Also consideration to lengthening the Achilles tendon must be addressed as it can serve as an antagonist to the transfer [10].

References

1. Harkin E, Pinzur M, Schiff A. Treatment of acute and chronic tibialis anterior tendon rupture and tendinopathy. Foot Ankle Clin. 2017;22(4):819–31. https://doi.org/10.1016/j.fcl.2017.07.009.
2. Kopriva JM, Cheesborough J, Frick SL. Tendon turndown to bridge a tibialis anterior gap and restore active dorsiflexion after degloving foot injury in a child: a case report. JBJS Case Connect. 2020;10(3):e19.00445. https://doi.org/10.2106/JBJS.CC.19.00445.
3. Otte S, Klinger H-M, Lorenz F, Haerer T. Operative treatment in case of a closed rupture of the anterior tibial tendon. Arch Orthop Trauma Surg. 2002;122(3):188–90. https://doi.org/10.1007/s004020100346.
4. Valisena S, Petri GJ, Ferrero A. Tancolli technique for delayed repair of tibialis anterior tendon rupture: a case report and literature review. Foot Ankle Spec. 2018;11(4):372–7. https://doi.org/10.1177/1938640017751539.
5. Trout BM, Hosey G, Wertheimer SJ. Rupture of the tibialis anterior tendon. J Foot Ankle Surg. 2000;39(1):54–8. https://doi.org/10.1016/s1067-2516(00)80065-4.
6. Huh J, Boyette DM, Parekh SG, Nunley JA. Allograft reconstruction of chronic tibialis anterior tendon ruptures. Foot Ankle Int. 2015;36(10):1180–9. https://doi.org/10.1177/1071100715589006.
7. Patel R, Fallat L. Surgical techniques for repair of atraumatic tibialis anterior tendon ruptures: a report of two cases. J Foot Ankle Surg. 2017;56(6):1343–9. https://doi.org/10.1053/j.jfas.2017.06.024.
8. Velan GJ, Hendel D. Degenerative tear of the tibialis anterior tendon after corticosteroid injection-augmentation with the extensor hallucis longus tendon, case report. Acta Orthop Scand. 1997;68(3):308–9. https://doi.org/10.3109/17453679708996711.
9. Ellington JK, McCormick J, Marion C, Cohen BE, Anderson RB, Davis WH, Jones CP. Surgical outcome following tibialis anterior tendon repair. Foot Ankle Int. 2010;31(5):412–7. https://doi.org/10.3113/fai.2010.0412.
10. Vosoughi AR, Heyes G, Molloy AP, Mason LW, Hoveidaei AH. Management of tibialis anterior tendon rupture. Foot Ankle Surg. 2020;26(5):487–93. https://doi.org/10.1016/j.fas.2019.06.003.

Part VI

The Cavus Foot and Ankle

Case #41: Management of Cavus Foot Deformity by a Two-Staged Approach—Stage 1: Correction of Rearfoot and Midfoot Deformities, Stage 2: Correction of Forefoot Deformities

41

Case Presentation

This is a 21-year-old male who presents with hammertoe deformities. He noticed they worsened and had developed considerable problems wearing shoes. He also noticed that his feet looked funny. He had symptoms also of spraining his ankles easily. His mother accompanied him and was very concerned about his pedal appearance. He was unable to participate in sports and noticed his feet worsening the past 2 years.

Diagnosis and Assessment

The patient exhibited significant bilateral cavus foot deformity and associated rigid hammertoe deformities (Fig. 41.1a–c). He was healthy and his mother said her father had really bad feet as well.

Initial exam noted excellent vascular perfusion. He did show signs of neurologic dysfunction. He was unable to fully perceive a Semmes-Weinstein monofilament of 5.09 to the midfoot level. He could not stand on one leg without falling (positive Romberg's test).

He had absent Achilles tendon reflexes but his patellar reflex was intact. Muscular exam noted 5/5 strength of all muscle groups, but there was weakness of the peroneus brevis (3/5) and of the tibialis anterior muscle (2/5). He did have weakness on eversion. He had further progression of first metatarsal plantarflexion when the ankle was fully dorsiflexed. No equinus was present. He had calf atrophy with preserved proximal thigh musculature. He exhibited the inverted champagne bottle deformity. He also demonstrated weakness of the pedal intrinsics.

H. J. Visser, *Challenges in Foot and Ankle Reconstructive Surgery*,
https://doi.org/10.1007/978-3-031-07893-4_41

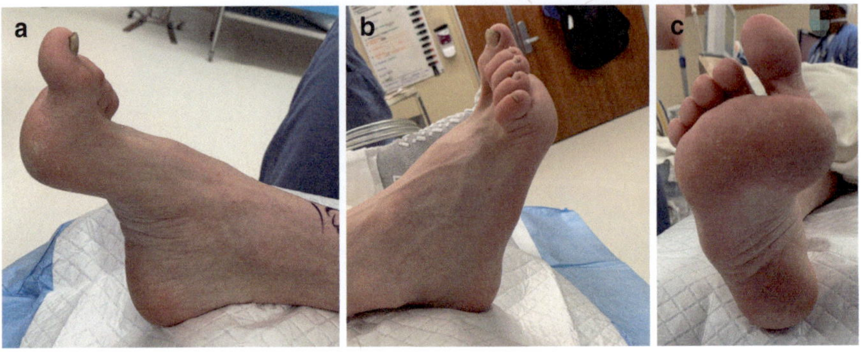

Fig. 41.1 (**a–c**) Significant cavus deformity

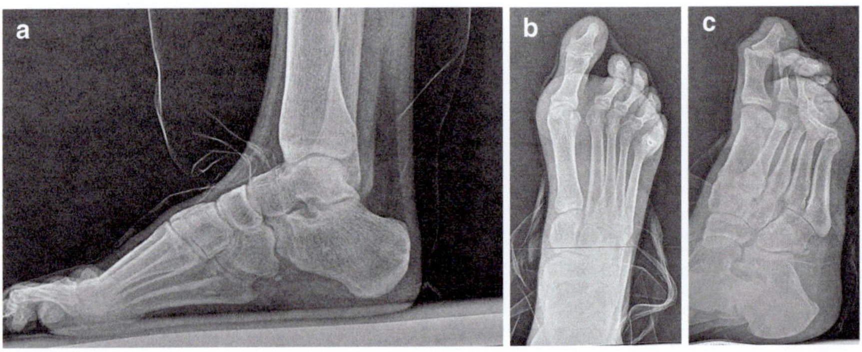

Fig. 41.2 (**a**) Radiographs demonstrating anterior form of cavus. (**b**) Gun barrel sign of proximal interphangeal joints of the digits. (**c**) Oblique view indicates severe subluxation at the MPJs

His biomechanical exam noted a plantarflexed first metatarsal and a fixed heel varus that did not reduce with the Coleman block test. He had semi-rigid plantarflexion of his forefoot that was centered at the Lisfranc joint. He had fixed hammertoe deformities. They were not reducible when performing a Kelikian push-up test.

X-rays noted an anterior cavus deformity. On the dorsoplantar view, convergence of the talus at the calcaneus was present. Gun barrel sign of the digits was also noted. On the lateral view, Meary's angle intersected at the first metatarsal cuneiform joint. This then signified an anterior form of cavus foot deformity (Fig. 41.2a–c).

An electromyography (EMG) and nerve conduction velocity (NCV) study was performed which was consistent with a sensory and motor peripheral neuropathy primary demyelinating.

Thus, a diagnosis of Charcot-Marie-Tooth (CMT) disease type I was made. The patient nor his mother were aware of this condition.

Management

The approach in this case was to first address the foot deformities in two stages. Stage 1 involved surgical correction of the rearfoot and midfoot deformity. The second stage addressed surgical correction of the forefoot deformity, primarily the hammertoes.

The first procedure involved a (Dwyer-type) calcaneal osteotomy (Fig. 41.3a, b). This was performed to address the fixed calcaneal and subtalar joint (STJ) varus deformity. The second procedure involved transfer of the peroneus brevis to the peroneus longus at the level of the cuboid groove (Fig. 41.4). This allowed strength to the weakened peroneus brevis. The third procedure involved a dorsiflexory wedge osteotomy of the first metatarsal. Fixation of the first metatarsal osteotomy utilized a tension band technique (Fig. 41.5). The fourth procedure involved a plantar fascial release (Figs. 41.6 and 41.7).

The second stage, then addressed the forefoot deformities of a plantarflexed forefoot and hammertoes. The first procedure which involved a Jones suspension and an interphalangeal hallux arthrodesis were performed to address the hallux malleus deformity. This further allowed positioning of the first metatarsal to the level of the heel. This eliminated the varus-creating force of the plantarflexed first metatarsal (Fig. 41.8a, b).

A second procedure, a Hibbs tenosuspension was performed through a long, third metatarsophalangeal joint (MPJ) centered incision. The extensor digitorum longus (EDL) tendons were transferred to the extensor digitorum brevis (EDB) at the level of the MPJ level distally. The proximal portion of the EDL tendons were then whip stitched and transferred to the lateral cuneiform with the foot at 90 ° to

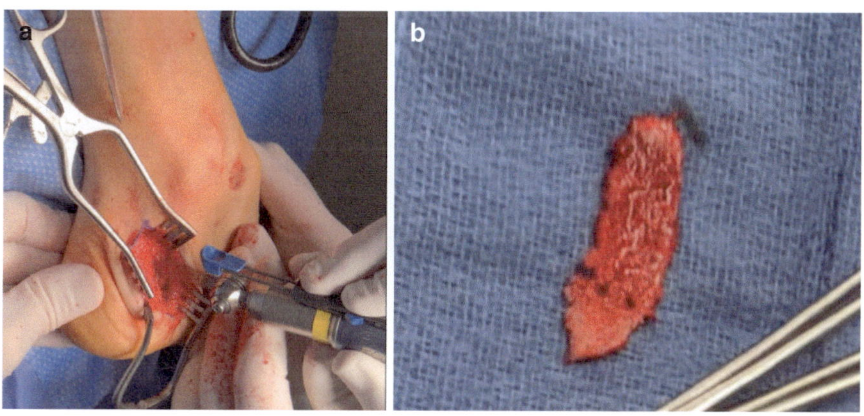

Fig. 41.3 (**a, b**) Dwyer calcaneal osteotomy

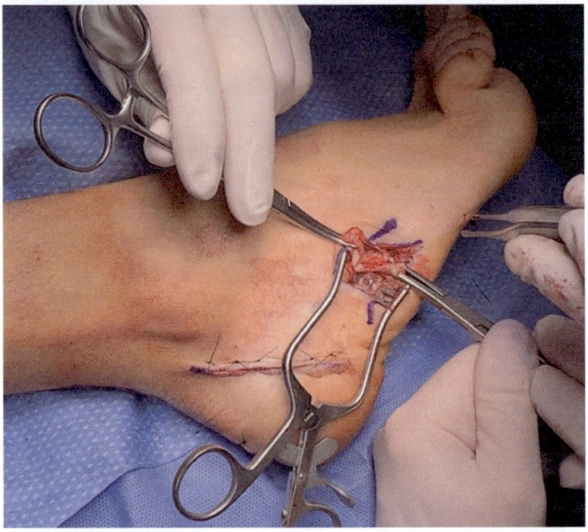

Fig. 41.4 Peroneus Brevis to longus transfer at level of cuboid groove

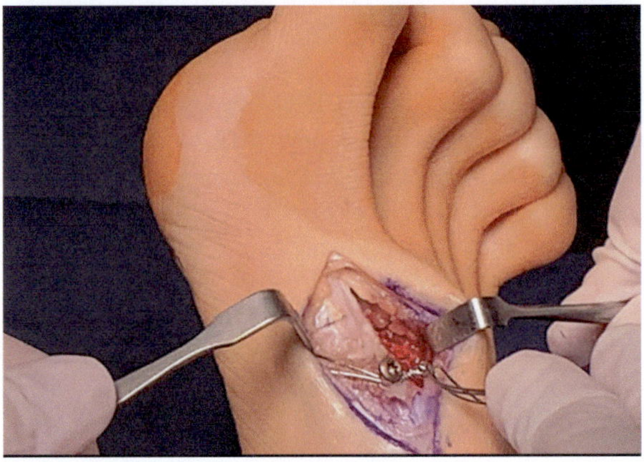

Fig. 41.5 Dorsiflexory first metatarsal osteotomy with tension band fixation

the ankle. Both procedures lent assistance to the weakened tibialis anterior. The hammertoes were repaired with a Taylor-type proximal interphalangeal joint (PIPJ) arthrodesis and 0.045" K-wires (Fig. 41.9a–e).

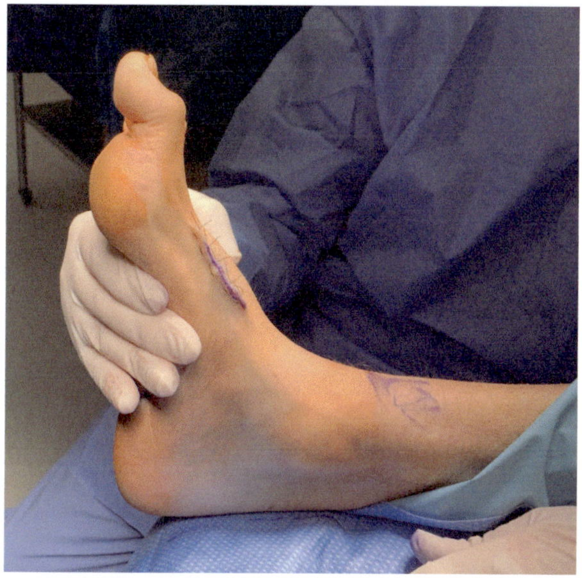

Fig. 41.6 Plantar fascia release

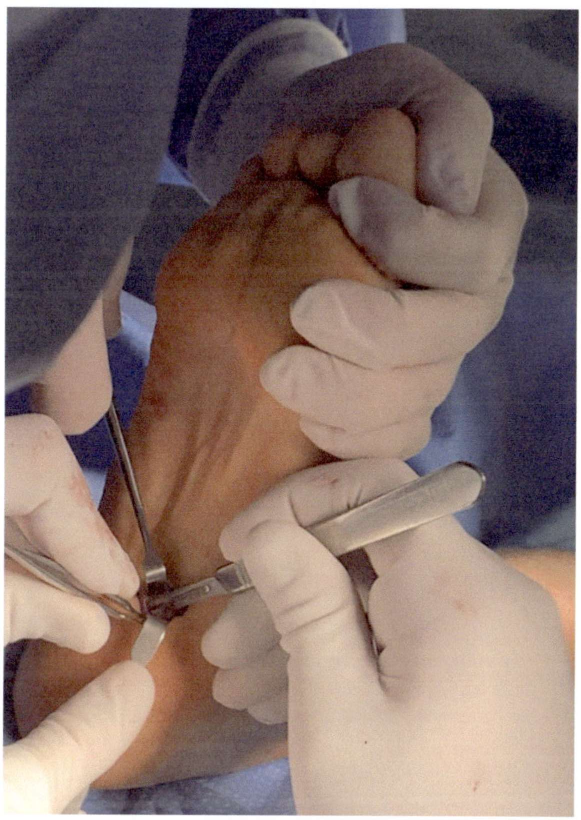

Fig. 41.7 Plantar fascia release

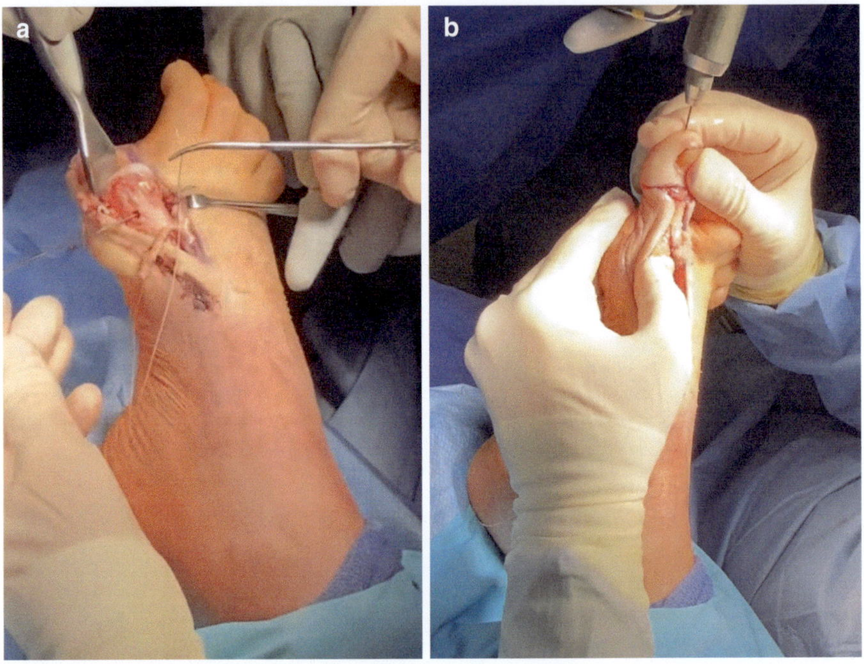

Fig. 41.8 (**a**) Jones tenosuspension. (**b**) Hallux interphalangeal joint arthrodesis

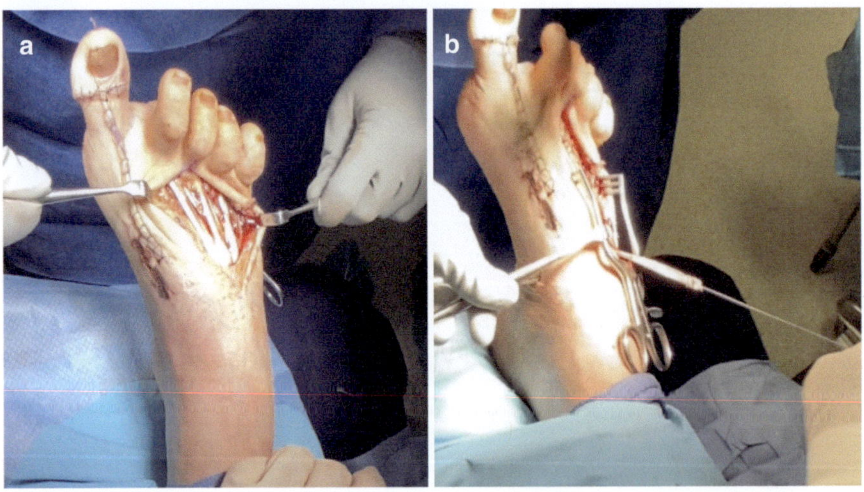

Fig. 41.9 (**a**) Anastomosis of EDB to EDL tendons distally. (**b**) Whip stitch of EDL tendons as bundles of tendons 2, 3, 4. (**c**) Guide pin for drill placed in lateral cuneiform. (**d**) Placement of interference screw at transfer site. (**e**) Forefoot correction with hammertoes repair

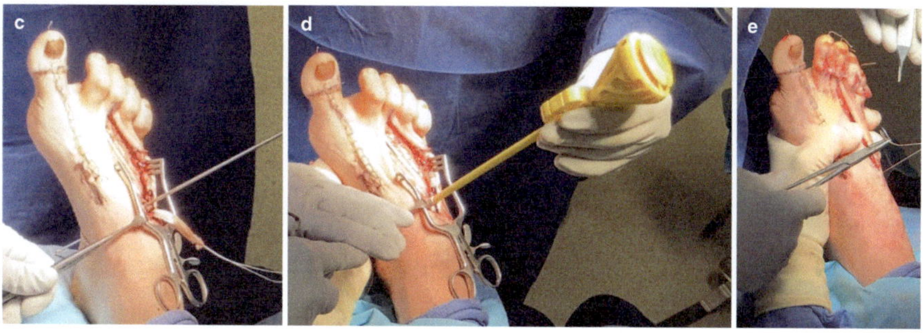

Fig. 41.9 (continued)

Outcome

The first stage was performed and then 4 weeks later the second stage. Weight bearing began at 4 weeks when the sutures and pins were removed. He began weight bearing immediately after the forefoot procedure. Physical therapy began at 8 weeks. He is in recovery at this time. Plans for the right foot are in 3–6 months.

Clinical Pearls and Pitfalls

This case represents a prototype of early CMT type I. This manifests as a demyelinating neuropathy usually in the teenage years. It exhibits an abnormal nerve conduction velocity (NCV). This differs from the type II where the axons are affected exhibiting normal NCV's but abnormal amplitudes [1–3].

The patient exhibited clinically significant hammertoe deformities and an unstable rearfoot. His heel varus was secondary to overpowering of the tibialis posterior and associated peroneus brevis weakness. It was also secondary to the plantarflexed first metatarsal. Creation of this deformity was also related to intrinsic weakness involving the abductor hallucis and flexor hallucis brevis (FHB) muscles, as well as weakness of the tibialis anterior [4, 5]. Also, his hallux malleus and hammertoes were secondary to intrinsic atrophy as well as tibialis anterior weakness. The result was the extensor substitution phenomenon [6]. A secondary equinus was not present due to the fact that there was still some strength to the tibialis anterior, 2/5, to serve as a restraint. When weakness of the tibialis anterior occurs, which is common in CMT, a distinct mechanical advantage of the peroneus longus occurs plantarflexing the first metatarsal [7]. The tibialis posterior unopposed by the weak peroneus brevis further accentuates the STJ into varus by closed kinetic chain supination and, thus, accentuates the longitudinal arch [8]. This causes posterior positioning of the fibula (noted on the lateral view) created by associated external leg rotation. The

Achilles tendon can then become contracted and must be evaluated as a deforming force. As the gastroc-soleus group is never affected in CMT the apex of Meary's angle will never be more proximal than the TN joint. The Hibbs tenosuspension takes the deforming force from the lesser digits and allows correction of intrinsic midfoot plantarflexion.

References

1. Dyck PJ. Lower motor and primary sensory neuron diseases with peroneal muscular atrophy. Arch Neurol. 1968;18(6):603. https://doi.org/10.1001/archneur.1968.00470360025002.
2. Davis CJ, Bradley WG, Madrid R. The peroneal muscular atrophy syndrome: clinical, genetic, electrophysiological and nerve biopsy studies. I. Clinical, genetic and electrophysiological findings and classification. J Genet Hum. 1978;26(4):311–49.
3. Harding AE, Thomas PK. The clinical features of hereditary motor and sensory neuropathy types I and II. Brain J Neurol. 1980;103(2):259–80. https://doi.org/10.1093/brain/103.2.259.
4. Tozza S, Aceto MG, Pisciotta C, Bruzzese D, Iodice R, Santoro L, Manganelli F. Postural instability in Charcot-Marie-tooth 1A disease. Gait Posture. 2016;49:353–7. https://doi.org/10.1016/j.gaitpost.2016.07.183.
5. Wicart P. Cavus foot, from neonates to adolescents. OTSR. 2012;98(7):813–28. https://doi.org/10.1016/j.otsr.2012.09.003.
6. de Retana PF, Poggio D. Charcot-Marie-tooth syndrome: orthopaedic considerations. Revista Española De Cirugía Ortopédica y Traumatología (English Edition). 2011;55(2):151–7. https://doi.org/10.1016/s1988-8856(11)70297-8.
7. Seaman TJ, Ball TA. Pes Cavus. In: StatPearls. Treasure Island, FL: StatPearls Publishing; 2021.
8. Joo SY, Choi BO, Kim DY, Jung SJ, Cho SY, Hwang SJ. Foot deformity in Charcot-Marie-tooth disease according to disease severity. Ann Rehabil Med. 2011;35(4):499–506. https://doi.org/10.5535/arm.2011.35.4.499.

Part VII

Complex Foot Deformity Correction with Hexapod External Fixator

42 Case #42: Two Stage Correction of Midfoot Charcot Deformity—Stage 1: Gradual Distraction and Correction of Deformity, Stage 2: Minimally Invasive Definitive Internal Fixation

Case Presentation

A 56-year-old long-term insulin-dependent diabetic who is also on a liver transplant list presents with a long-term midfoot Charcot osteoarthropathic deformity. The patient ambulates with a cane and protective shoe wear. He has a history on two prior occasions of a plantar cuboid ulceration that required contact casting for healing. The patient on weight bearing is very unstable due to the fact he demonstrates a lateral rocker bottom deformity. In this situation, the apex of the weight bearing deformity lies at the cuboid. Doppler and vascular evaluations noted a good peripheral perfusion with no signs of vascular compromise to the foot and limb. However, he demonstrates profound sensory, autonomic, and motor neuropathy. He was unable to perceive a 5.07 Semmes-Weinstein monofilament to the knee. He was cleared by his hepatologist for surgery.

Diagnosis and Assessment

As described the patient demonstrated a long-term history of midfoot Charcot osteoarthropathy secondary to long-standing type 1 insulin-dependent diabetes mellitus. He demonstrated profound symmetrical sensory, autonomic, and motor neuropathy of both extremities. His deformity at this juncture was classified as Eichenholz Stage 3 [1].

Radiographs on the DP view note essentially a Schon 1 type of deformity with breakdown and avascular changes at tarsometatarsal joints one through five [2]. There is residual midfoot abduction noted with an increased talocalcaneal angle

H. J. Visser, *Challenges in Foot and Ankle Reconstructive Surgery*,
https://doi.org/10.1007/978-3-031-07893-4_42

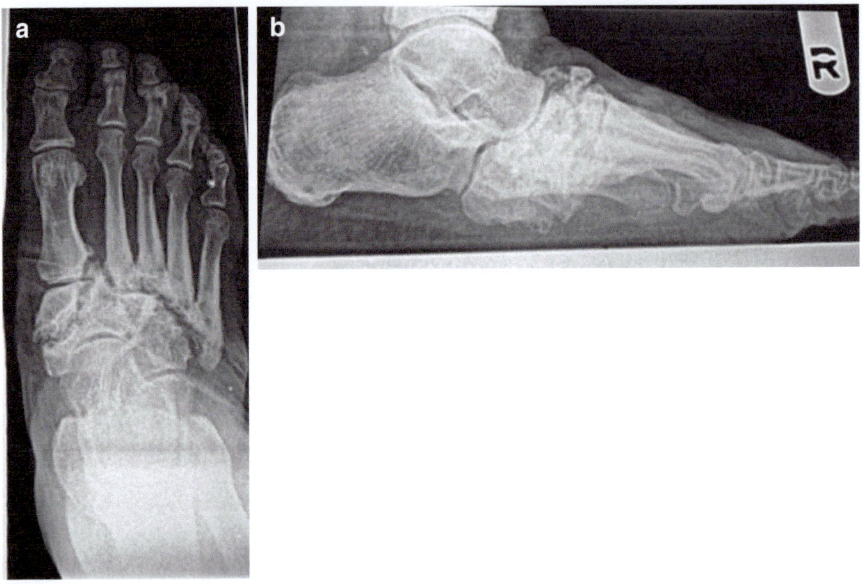

Fig. 42.1 (**a**) Schon 1 type of deformity with breakdown and avascular changes at tarsometatarsal joints one through five. (**b**) Rocker bottom deformity. Decreased calcaneal inclination and increased talar declination

(Fig. 42.1a). On the lateral view, he has loss of calcaneal inclination and increased talar declination. The talar first metatarsal angle is significantly decreased. Also noted is a rocker bottom deformity where the cuboid is the apex of weight bearing. Equinus is also a significant mitigating factor in the radiographic changes described (Fig. 42.1b).

Management

The patient underwent surgical reconstruction in two stages. The patient was done under a spinal anesthetic due to his hepatic compromise. The first stage involved performance of a percutaneous tendo Achilles lengthening [3, 4]. Then, a percutaneous midfoot osteotomy proximal to the tarsometatarsal joints one through five was performed. This involved the three cuneiforms and the cuboid. An incision was made medially and the dorsal and plantar soft tissues were released over the cuneiforms and cuboid with a large key elevator (Fig. 42.2a). A guide pin was then placed perpendicular to the medial tarsus across the cuneiforms and cuboid (Fig. 42.2b, c). An osteotome was introduced to create an osteotomy at the level following the guide pins (Fig. 42.2d).

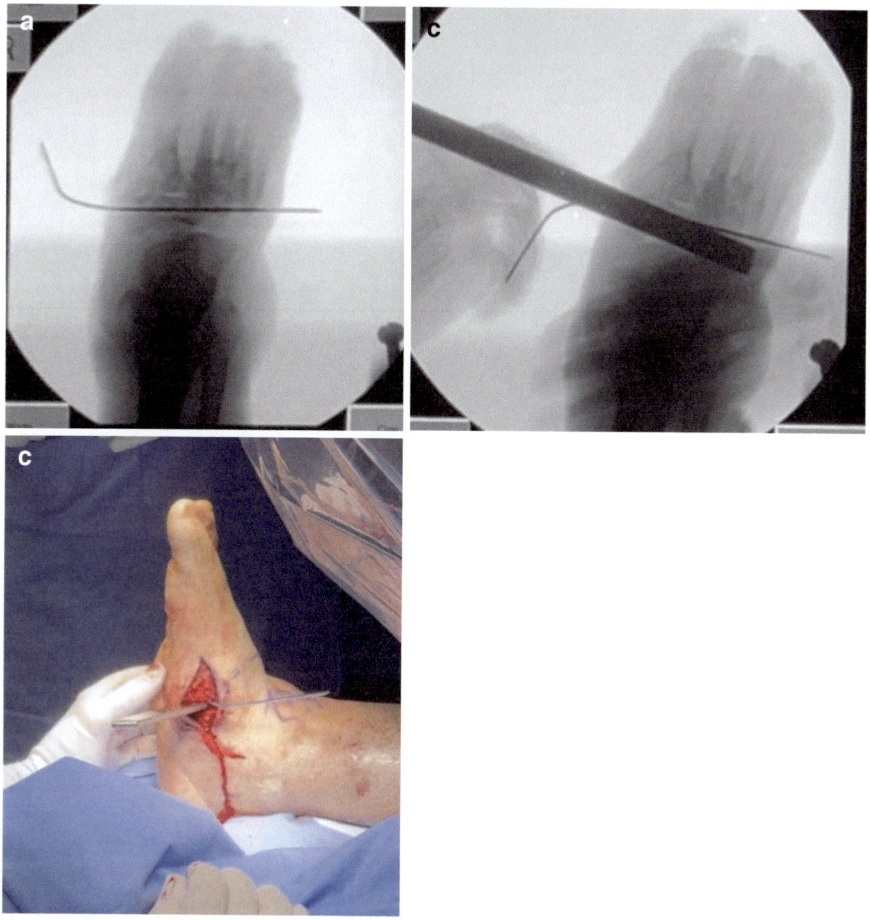

Fig. 42.2 (**a**) A guide pin was then placed perpendicular to the medial tarsus across the cuneiforms and cuboid. (**b**) Osteotome introduced to create an osteotomy at the level following the guide pin. (**c**) Recreation of the longitudinal arch

At this point, a hexapod butt external fixation frame was applied (Fig. 42.3a, b). Olive pins were utilized to engage the tibia, calcaneus, and metatarsals. Preoperative radiographs were analyzed by computer software. Corrections were then calculated per colored struts that connected the foot and tibial frame [3]. A guide sheet was provided to the patient and the patient instructed on which struts were turned at what particular time frame. The patient was discharged at 48 h after undergoing strut adjustment education and therapy. A knee scooter was utilized for non-weight bearing ambulation and thus the proximal wing was placed such that this could be carried out.

The distractions to correction were performed in 4 weeks. A radiograph of the lateral view (Fig. 42.4) noted restoration of talar and calcaneal inclination. The

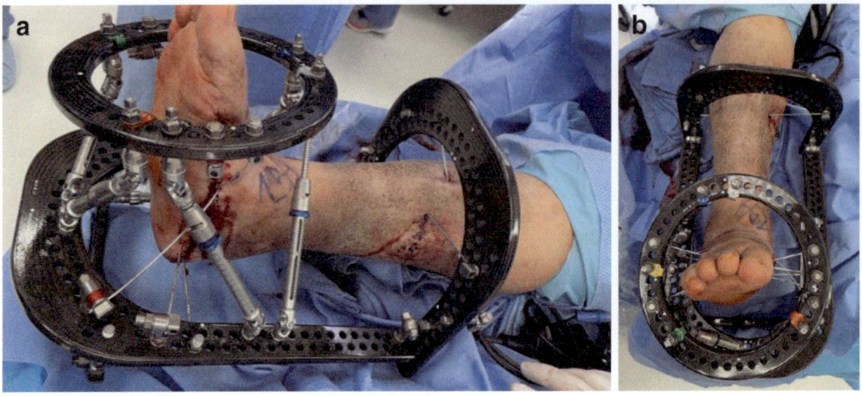

Fig. 42.3 (**a**, **b**) Hexapod butt frame external fixator

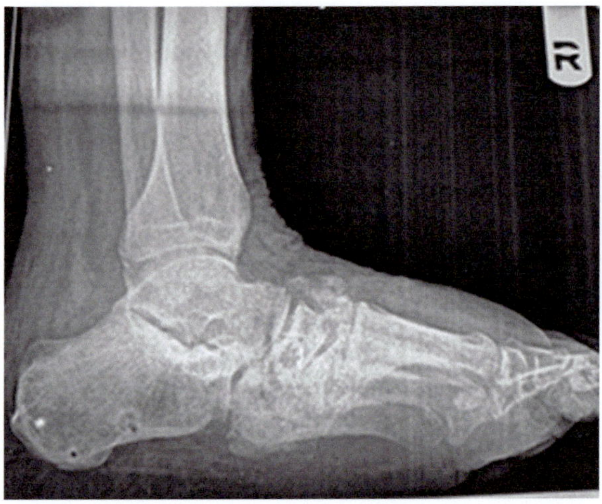

Fig. 42.4 Lateral radiograph demonstrates restoration of calcaneal inclination and talar declination angles and Meary's angle is normal

talar first metatarsal angle (Meary's Angle) was restored to normal alignment [4]. The frame was then removed and the patient given a 2-week holiday to restore skin integrity and allow pin tracts to heal. This was performed under monitored anesthesia care.

The second-staged procedure was then performed again under spinal anesthesia. A percutaneous MIS (minimal incision) approach was utilized to prepare the joints for arthrodesis. The subtalar joint and the midtarsal joint were exposed with a small lateral incision and the remaining hyaline articular cartilage was removed with high speed MIS burr (Fig. 42.5a). The talonavicular joint was also exposed through a minimal incision centered lateral to the tibial anterior tendon (Fig. 42.5a). The joint was also prepared in a similar manner. A 7.0 mm beaming screw was placed through the subtalar joint and the talonavicular joint (Fig. 42.6a). A 5.5 mm beaming screw was utilized for the tarsometatarsal 4 and calcaneal cuboid joint (Fig. 42.6a, b).

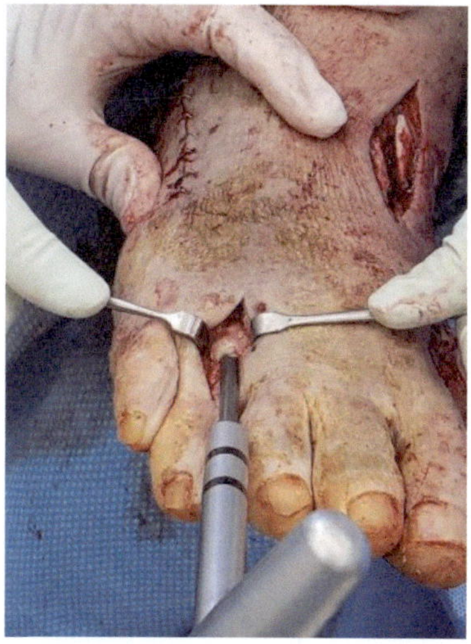

Fig. 42.5 Method of insertion of 5.5 mm beaming screw lateral column

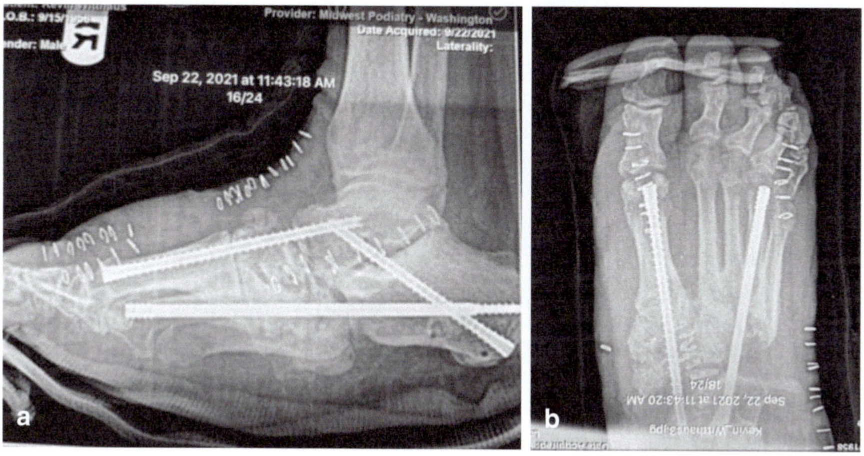

Fig. 42.6 (**a**, **b**) Beaming screws placed through the talonavicular, subtalar, fourth tarsometatarsal and calcaneocuboid joints

The postoperative radiographs show excellent restoration of the medial and lateral columns and the establishment of a plantigrade foot. Note calcaneal metatarsal weight bearing contact (Fig. 42.6a, b).

Outcome

The patient was then kept non-weight bearing for 12 weeks [4]. He was then placed in a CAM boot and allowed full weight bearing for 12 more weeks. An Arizona brace was constructed and worn for further 6 months. With excellent maintenance of deformity correction and stability, at 1 year he was then allowed to be placed in a functional orthotic device. However, for any increased excessive demand of walking or standing he was urged to use his Arizona brace. At this point, 1 year postoperatively he is fully functional and ambulating without cane assistance. A liver transplant was performed with good success some 8 months after the surgical procedure.

Clinical Pearls and Pitfalls

The advent of hexapod external fixation offers a new exciting approach to the condition of complex Charcot foot deformities [5]. Typical correction for lateral rocker bottom deformities at the midfoot level where the cuboid was the apex of weight bearing was a complicated condition to address. Exostectomy in general is ineffective in this general region. Primary approach often includes a midfoot closing wedge osteotomy through large incisions. This creates shortening and often causes ambulation problems with the more normal contralateral foot. The two-stage approach in this case allows gradual correction without bone loss [4]. In essence, creation of a near-normal biomechanically aligned foot can occur. With utilization of minimal incision technique, large open incisions are avoided for joint preparation for arthrodesis. This greatly limits the amount of soft tissue dissection and mobilization that is required with open one-stage arthrodesis techniques [4]. It is obvious patient selection is paramount. Despite hepatic compromise a gradual deformity correction was obtained. The patient must be compliant and aware of the longevity of recovery. One also must be able to tolerate functioning with an external fixator frame. This approach offers much less risk of deep infection with hardware and lessens chances of limb loss.

References

1. Eichenholtz SN. Charcot Joints, CC Thomas, Springfield, 1966.
2. Schon, Lew C. MD; Easley, Mark E. MD; Weinfeld, Steven B. MD. Charcot Neuroarthropathy of the Foot and Ankle. Clinical Orthopaedics and Related Research: April 1998 - Volume 349 - Issue - p 116–31
3. Cooper, Paul S. "Application of external fixators for management of Charcot deformities of the foot and ankle." *Foot and Ankle Clinics* 7.1;2002:207–54.
4. Lamm, Bradley M., II. David Gottlieb, and Dror Paley. "A two-stage percutaneous approach to Charcot diabetic foot reconstruction." *The Journal of foot and ankle surgery* 49 6;2010:517–22.
5. Wang, James C, Anthony W. Le, and Raymond K. Tsukuda. "A new technique for Charcot's foot reconstruction." *Journal of the American Podiatric Medical Association* 92.8;2002:429–36.

Case #43: Utilization of Hexapod Frame Following Failed Tibiocalcaneal Arthrodesis for the Treatment of Talar Body Avascular Necrosis

43

Case Presentation

A 54-year-old female non-diabetic patient who sustained a twisting injury several years prior while walking back to her car and fell into a hole. The patient was initially managed with CAM boot immobilization. The patient continued to have pain and at 6 weeks an MRI was performed which revealed a Hawkins 2 talar neck fracture of the left foot. No attempt of internal fixation was done. The patient continued to ambulate in CAM boot. Subsequently, 6–8 weeks later the talus began to demonstrate changes consistent with avascular necrosis. Note sclerotic talar body (Fig. 43.1a). MRI also notes decreased intensity on the T1 image consistent with advanced talar body avascular necrosis (Fig. 43.1b). Vascular and neurologic status were completely normal. The patient medically noted obesity, but however not other significant medical problems.

Diagnosis and Assessment

The lateral radiographs show (Fig. 43.1a) and T1 MRI (Fig. 43.1b), the condition of advanced AVN of the talus secondary to misdiagnosis of talar neck fracture. The patient was not ambulatory due to pain and collapse was beginning to occur. The lack of early non-weight bearing and no impending surgical stabilization led to this condition.

H. J. Visser, *Challenges in Foot and Ankle Reconstructive Surgery*,
https://doi.org/10.1007/978-3-031-07893-4_43

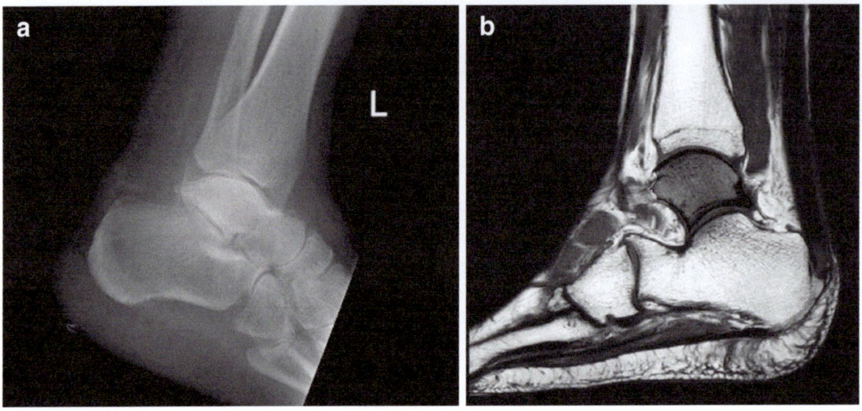

Fig. 43.1 (**a**) Radiograph demonstrates sclerotic talar body. (**b**) MRI T1 image consistent with advanced talar body avascular necrosis

Management

Due to the complete lack of viability of the talar body and signs of joint collapse, the talar body was excised [1]. A tricortical iliac autograft was utilized to restore the resected talar body. This was performed through a transfibular approach. A tibiotalar calcaneal arthrodesis was then performed. A 6.5 mm fully threaded cannulated screw was used for positioning. A 4.5 mm anatomic lateral locking plate was also applied. Note postoperative radiographs (Fig. 43.2a–c) where an anatomically aligned plantigrade left foot was attained.

Unfortunately, the patient began to note signs of infection at approximately 10–14 days. The wound was only mildly erythematous and copious amounts of serous drainage occurred. The wound probed to the lateral locking plate and cultures grew MRSA at this point in time. The plate and screws were removed as well as the autograft which was deemed also infected. A vancomycin-loaded PMMA spacer was then placed at the excision site [2]. A delta frame was applied to maintain stability to the spacer. Partial closure was performed over the spacer and the subcutaneous capsular portion of the wound was left open. A wound vac (NPWT) was then applied. The patient was then placed with a PICC line and 6 weeks of intravenous vancomycin was administered.

Outcome

Unfortunately, the patient did not show signs of complete wound healing. The lateral wound continued to drain a serous fluid that did not culture a bacteria. The wound did not show signs of inflammation but continued to produce a serous drainage which was noted in the wound vac containers. At this point, she was sent to plastic surgery. They performed a rotation flap to close the lateral wound. With this

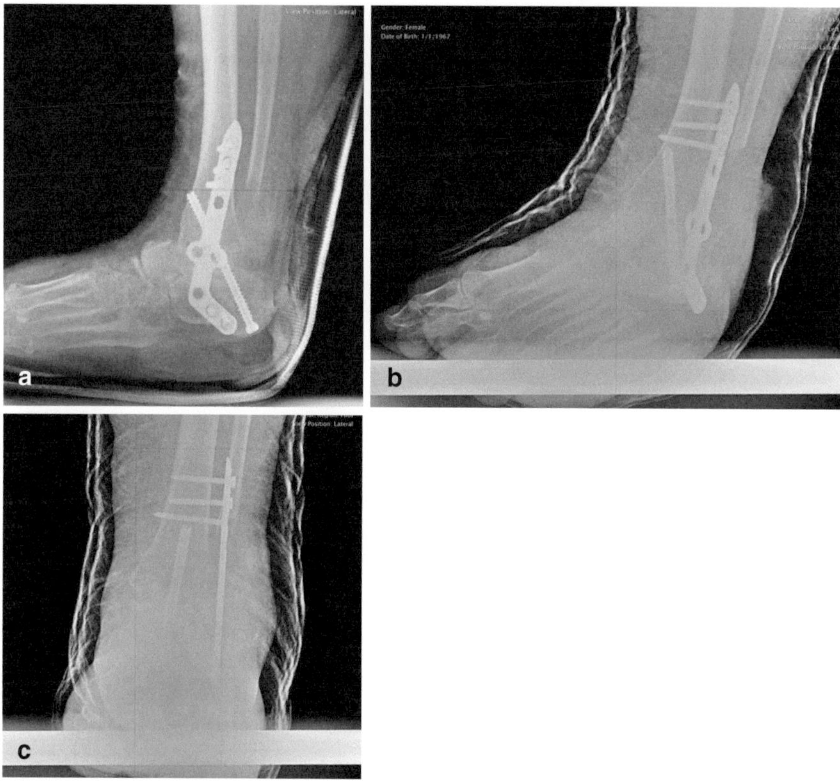

Fig. 43.2 (**a–c**) Anatomical plantigrade foot with tricortical iliac autograft performed through a transfibular approach

technique, they did not want fixation performed as they preferred the valgus unstable state to create relaxation for the lateral flap. This allowed lateral wound closure. However, this process took nearly 3 months for complete healing. Radiographs show the biomechanical alignment at this time. Note the sidecar deformity with no talar support (Fig. 43.3a, b). The AP (Fig. 43.3a) shows the bulk of the rotation flap.

At this point, the technology of computer-generated hexapod external fixation was utilized. A miter type frame was applied in this case to realign the ankle joint. This involved stretching the contracted soft tissue structures which involved the lateral ankle and the rotation flap (Fig. 43.4a–c). Olive pins were placed in the tibia, calcaneus, and metatarsals. It took 5 weeks to attain a corrected position. Note the aligned foot to ankle on the AP view and complete restoration of the tibia to calcaneus height. Note also, restoration of the joint space to allow restoration of the talar body (Fig. 43.5a, b). Contouring of the flap was also noted due to the distraction. The frame was again removed and the procedure was performed at the same time.

A posterior Gaille approach was made [3, 4]. The Achilles tendon was reflected superior ward. An acetabular reamer was utilized to create a space for the femoral head allograft (Fig. 43.6a). This removed the soft tissue occupying the distracted

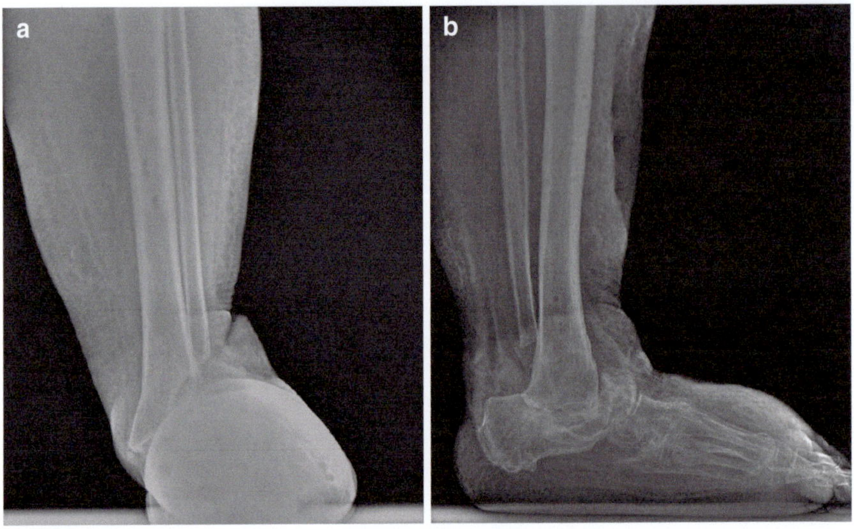

Fig. 43.3 (**a**, **b**) Side car deformity with no talar support

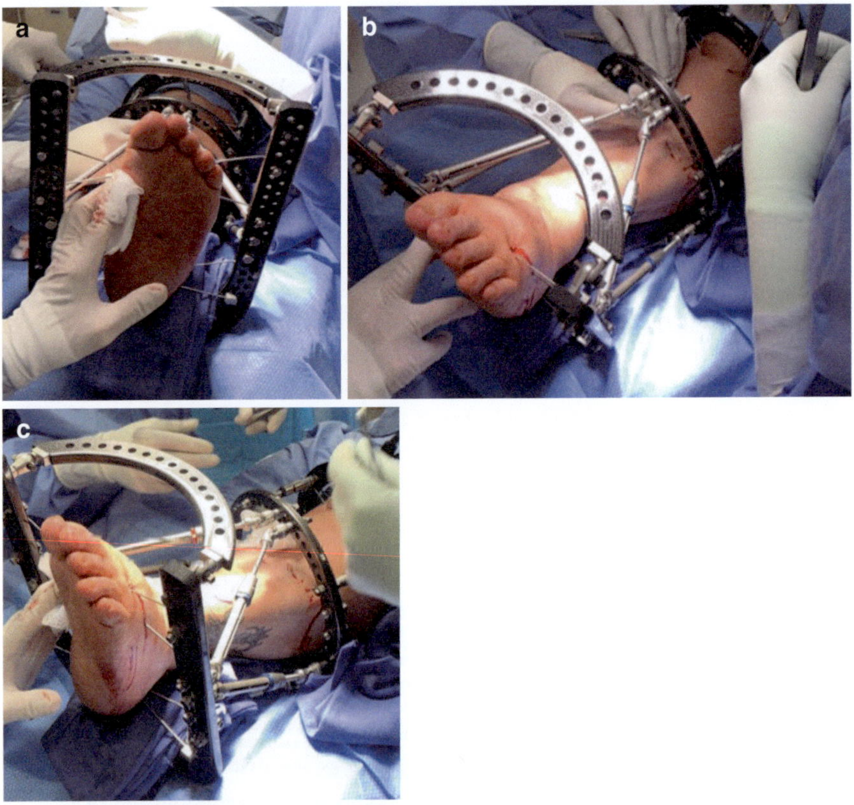

Fig. 43.4 (**a–c**) Application of hexapod for the purposes of re-aligning the ankle joint and stretching the soft tissues

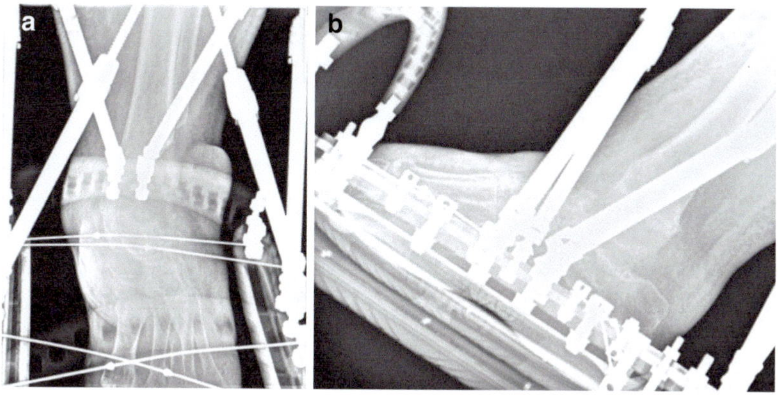

Fig. 43.5 (**a**, **b**) Restoration of joint space for planned definitive correction

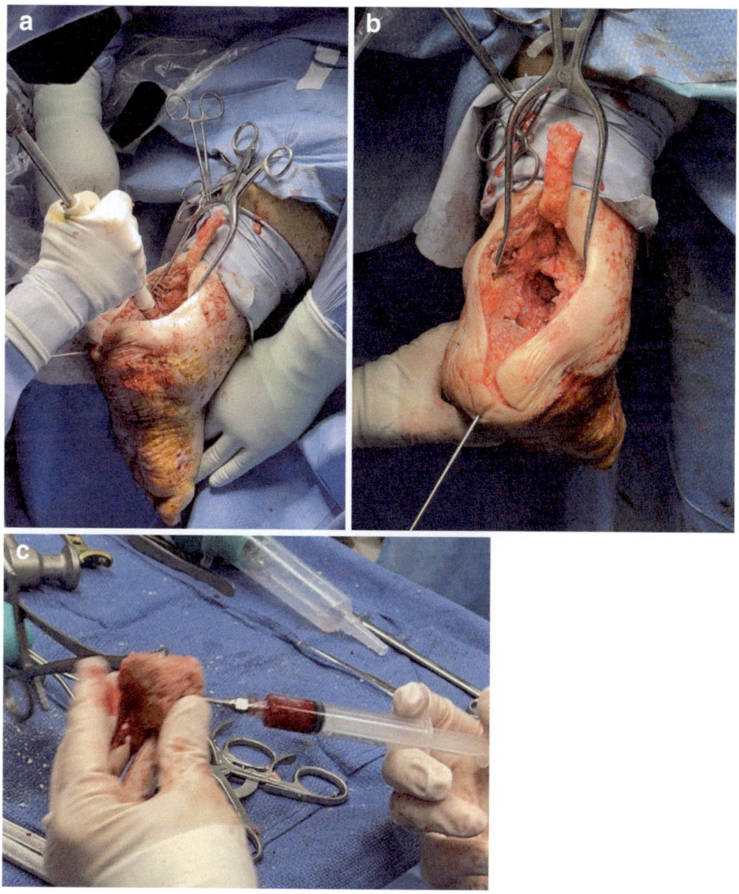

Fig. 43.6 (**a**, **b**) Joint space accessed through a Gaille approach. Acetabular reamer creating space for femoral head allograft. (**c**, **d**) Tibial, calcaneal and fresh frozen femoral head allograft surfaces injected with tibial bone marrow aspirate and Augment. (**e**) Securing of allograft with posterior anatomic locking plate

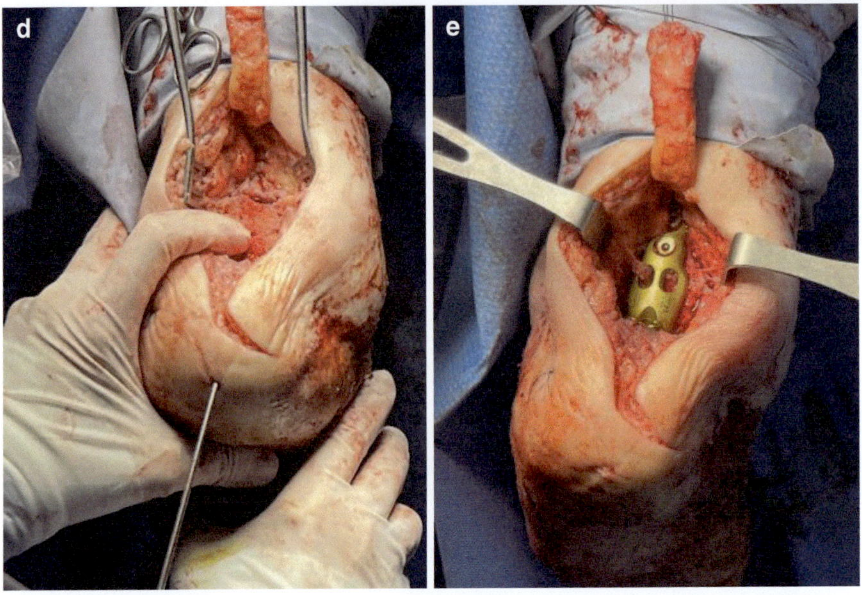

Fig. 43.6 (continued)

joint space (Fig. 43.6b). The fresh frozen femoral head allograft was injected with bone marrow aspirate from the tibia and placed in the created void [5]. Augment was also placed at the contact points between the allograft and tibiocalcaneal surfaces (Fig. 43.6c, d). A posterior anatomic locking plate and a 6.5 mm headless positioning screw were then applied to secure the graft (Fig. 43.6e). Note lateral radiograph exhibiting fixation and excellent restoration of height (Fig. 43.7a–d).

Again misfortune occurred at approximately 10 days postoperative, signs of wound dehiscence and necrosis began to occurs. The necrosis involved loss of epidermal-dermal tissue that extended well beyond the confines of the original incision (Fig. 43.8a). Also the positioning screw had become loose (Fig. 43.8b). The patient was then taken back to the surgical OR after having discontinued Eliquis for 48 h. Upon debridement of the skin edges, the Achilles tendon was found to be infected and affected by necrosis (Fig. 43.8c, d). The hardware was also deemed involved and the position screw and posterior locking plate and screws were removed (Fig. 43.8e). The graft was debrided was overall appeared unaffected. Deep bone cultures and bone biopsy were performed.

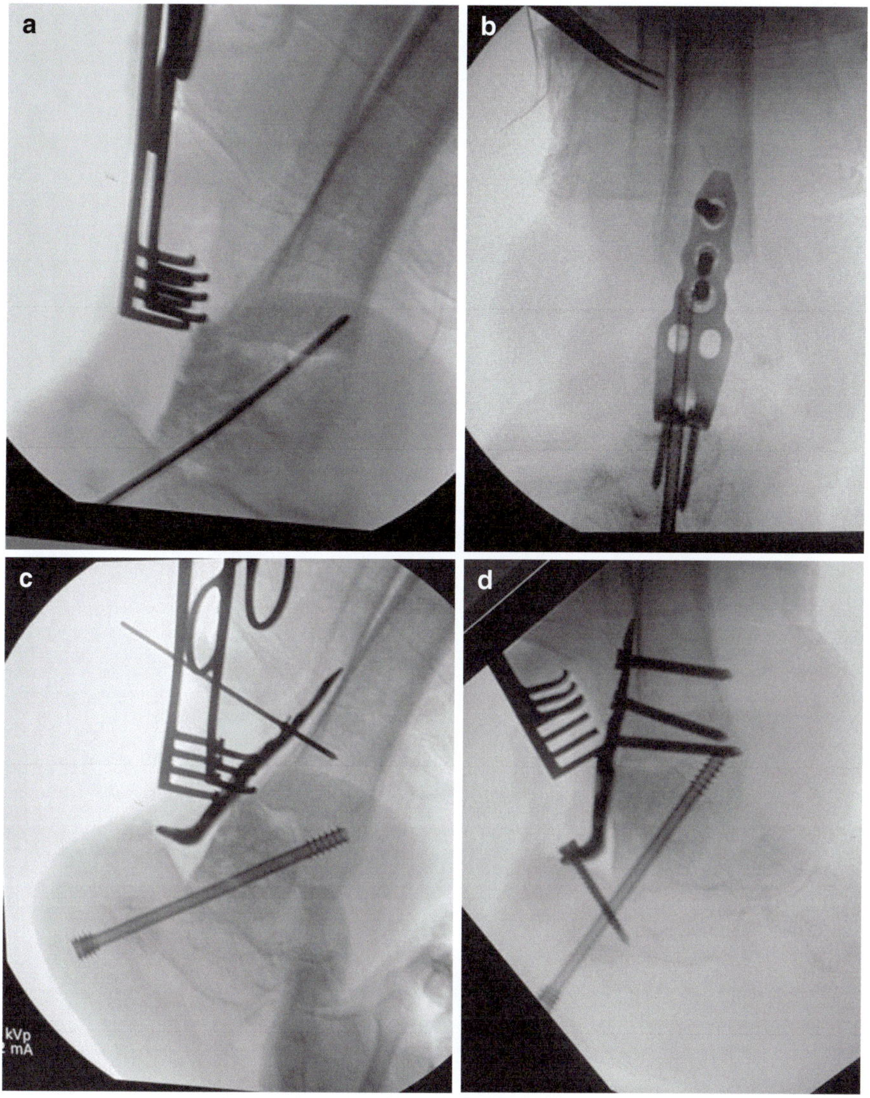

Fig. 43.7 (**a**–**d**) Stable fixation and restoration of height

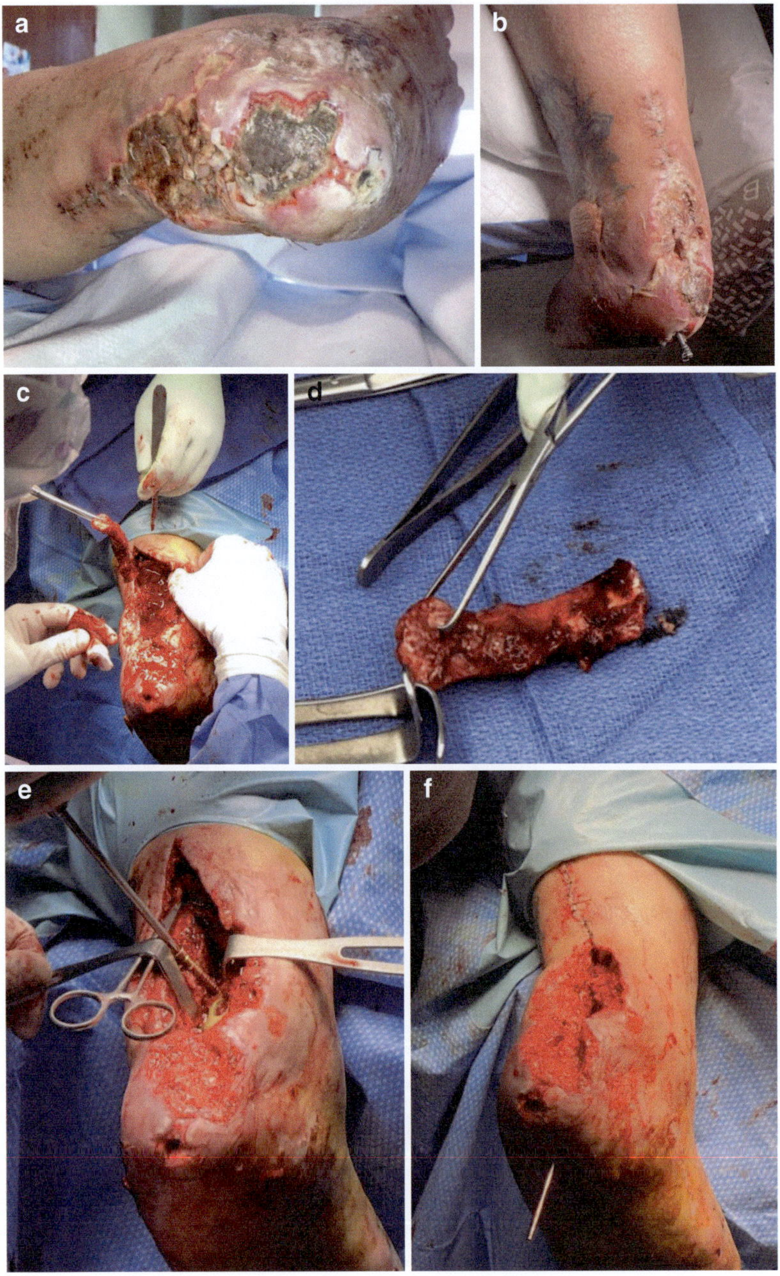

Fig. 43.8 (**a**) Post surgical epidermal-dermal necrosis. (**b**) Failure of positioning screw as seen protruding from wound. (**c–e**) Achilles tendon found to be infected, was resected. (**f**) All previously placed hardware was deemed involved and removed. Allograft left in place and secured in position with a pin

Clinical Pearls and Pitfalls

In this case, resolution of the infection became extremely difficult. Despite 6 weeks of intravenous antibiotics, the wound continued to drain a serous type of joint fluid. Cultures remained negative at this point, more than likely due to intravenous care. Thus, it was deemed “a wound problem” where granulation over the bone PMMA spacer did not occur despite NPWT. Referral to a plastic surgeon and a rotation flap ultimately solved the wound problem. The need for relaxation lateral for flap healing left the unstable ankle in a severe valgus, with the foot in a sidecar position (Fig. 43.4a, b). The ultimate problem now was to restore the tibial to floor height and create a space for the lost talar body. Options here included a bioengineered talus created by CT comparison to the opposite ankle. However with the long presence of infection, this did not appear to be a good choice. Thus, an allograft was chosen as insurance issues were also an issue. A posterior approach to the ankle was utilized to offer the best angiosome corridor. The procedure went extremely well. Soon after another postoperative infection occurred. This despite the wound being healed nearly 6 months. Obviously, the issue is a biomembrane (glycocalyx) that formed at the bone interface. Eukaryotic bacteria can live in a sessile state for years. Once an operative insult occurred, an explosion of bacteria extended into the reconstruction site. This led to further complications however as can be seen (Fig. 43.9a, b), the patient is well on her way to limb salvage.

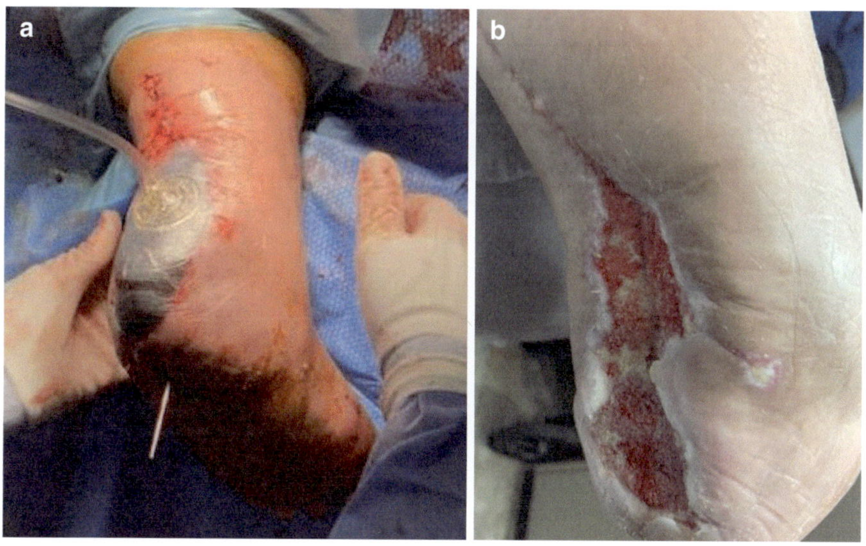

Fig. 43.9 (**a**, **b**) Negative pressure wound therapy

References

1. Gallie WE. Subastraglar arthrodesis in fractures of the os calcis. J Bone Joint Surg. 1943;25(4):731–6.
2. Wong TM, Lau TW, Li X, Fang C, Yeung K, Leung F. Masquelet technique for treatment of posttraumatic bone defects. Sci World J. 2014;2014
3. DeOrio JK, Leaseburg JT, Shapiro SA. Subtalar distraction arthrodesis through a posterior approach. Foot Ankle Int. 2008;29(12):1189–94.
4. Pollar JD, Schuberth JM. Posterior bone block distraction arthrodesis of the subtalar joint: a review of 22 cases. J Foot Ankle Surg. 2008;47(3):191–8.
5. Lee MS, Tallerico V. Distraction arthrodesis of the subtalar joint using allogeneic bone graft: a review of 15 cases. J Foot Ankle Surg. 2010;49(4):369–74.

Index

H. J. Visser, DPM, *Challenges in Foot and Ankle Reconstruction Surgery*, https://doi.org/10.1007/978-3-031-07893-4

K

L

M

N

O

P

R

MIX
Papier aus verantwortungsvollen Quellen
Paper from responsible sources
FSC® C105338

If you have any concerns about our products,
you can contact us on
ProductSafety@springernature.com

In case Publisher is established outside the EU,
the EU authorized representative is:
Springer Nature Customer Service Center GmbH
Europaplatz 3, 69115 Heidelberg, Germany

Printed by Libri Plureos GmbH
in Hamburg, Germany